D1130680

*Marcela Depiante*

# SPRINGER SERIES IN NEUROPSYCHOLOGY

Harry A. Whitaker, Series Editor

# Springer Series in Neuropsychology

Harry A. Whitaker, Series Editor

Jean-Luc Nespoulous    Pierre Villiard
Editors

# Morphology, Phonology, and Aphasia

Springer-Verlag
New York  Berlin  Heidelberg
London  Paris  Tokyo  Hong Kong

Jean-Luc Nespoulous
INSERM U.230
Service de Neurologie
31059 Toulouse Cedex
France

Pierre Villiard
Department of French
University of New Brunswick
Fredericton, New Brunswick E3B 5A3
Canada

Library of Congress Cataloging-in-Publication Data
Morphology, phonology, and aphasia/[edited by] Jean-Luc Nespoulous,
    Pierre Villiard.
        p.    cm. – (Springer series in neuropsychology)
        Based on papers from two symposia held in Krems, Austria, summer of
1988.
        Includes bibliographical references.
        ISBN 0-387-97183-1 (alk. paper)
        1. Aphasia–Congresses.   2. Psycholinguistics–Congresses.
    I. Nespoulous, Jean-Luc.   II. Villiard, Pierre.   III. Series.
        [DNLM: 1. Aphasia–congresses.   2. Linguistics–congresses.   WL
340.5 M871 1988]
        RC425.M599 1990        616.85′52–dc20        DNLM/DLC        89-26152

Printed on acid-free paper.

© 1990 by Springer-Verlag New York Inc.
All rights reserved. This work may not be translated or copied in whole or in part without
the written permission of the publisher (Springer-Verlag, 175 Fifth Avenue, New York, NY
10010, USA), except for brief excerpts in connection with reviews or scholarly analysis. Use
in connection with any form of information storage and retrieval, electronic adaptation, computer software, or by similar or dissimilar methodology now known or hereafter developed is
forbidden.
The use of general descriptive names, trade names, trademarks, etc. in this publication, even
if the former are not especially identified, is not to be taken as a sign that such names, as
understood by the Trade Marks and Merchandise Marks Act, may accordingly be used freely
by anyone.

Typeset by Best-set Typesetter Ltd., Quarry Bay, Hong Kong.
Printed and bound by Edwards Brothers, Ann Arbor, Michigan.
Printed in the United States of America.

9  8  7  6  5  4  3  2  1

ISBN 0-387-97183-1 Springer-Verlag New York Berlin Heidelberg
ISBN 3-540-97183-1 Springer-Verlag Berlin Heidelberg New York

# Contents

# Contributors

Josef Bayer   Max Planck Institute, Nijmegen, The Netherlands

Renée Béland   Laboratoire Théophile-Alajouanine, Université de Montréal, Montreal, Quebec, Canada

Daniel Bub   Montreal Neurological Institute, Montreal, Canada

Hugh W. Buckingham Jr.   Program in Linguistics and Department of Speech, Louisiana State University, Baton Rouge, Louisiana, USA

Brian Butterworth   Department of Psychology, University College of London, London, Great Britain

Alfonso Caramazza   Cognitive Science Center, The Johns Hopkins University, Baltimore, Maryland, USA

Ria de Bleser   Medizinische Fakultät, Abteilung Neurologie, Aachen, West Germany

Monique Dordain   INSERM, Hôpital Fontmaure, Clermont-Ferrand, France

Wolfgang U. Dressler   Institut für Sprachwissenschaft, Universität Wien, Vienna, Austria

Attie Duval-Gombert   Service de Neurologie, Hôpital Pontchaillou, Rennes, France

Tiziana Ferreri   Dipartimento di Psicologia Generale, Università di Padova, Padova, Italy

Hubert Guyard   Université Rennes 2 Haute Bretagne, UER du Langage, Rennes, France

GONIA JAREMA   Département de Linguistique et Philologie and Laboratoire Theóphile-Alajouanine, Montreal, Quebec, Canada

DANUTA KADZIELAWA   Faculty of Psychology, University of Warsaw, Warsaw, Poland

EVA KEHAYIA   Department of Linguistics, McGill University, and Laboratoire Théophile-Alajouanine, Montreal, Quebec, Canada

PÄIVI KOIVUSELKÄ-SALLINEN   Department of Phonetics and General Linguistics, University of Joensuu, Joensuu, Finland

MATTI LAINE   Department of Neurology, Turku University Central Hospital, Turku, Finland

MARIE-CLAUDE LE BOT   Université Rennes 2 Haute Bretagne, UER du Langage, Rennes, France

ANDRÉ ROCH LECOURS   Laboratoire Théophile-Alajouanine, Faculté de Médecine, Université de Montréal, Montreal, Quebec, Canada

GARY LIBBEN   Department of Linguistics, The University of Calgary, Calgary, Alberta, Canada

SONIA LUPIEN   Laboratoire Théophile-Alajouanine, Faculté de Médecine, Université de Montréal, Montreal, Quebec, Canada

EMANUELA MAGNO CALDOGNETTO   Centro di Fonetica CNR, Università di Padova, Padova, Italy

GABRIELE MICELI   Università Cattolica, Roma, Italy

JEAN-LUC NESPOULOUS   Laboratoire Jacques Lordat, Université de Toulouse-Le Mirail, and INSERM U.230, Toulouse, France; and Laboratoire Théophile-Alajouanine, Montreal, Quebec, Canada

JUSSI NIEMI   Department of Phonetics and General Linguistics, University of Joensuu, Joensuu, Finland

MARTA PANZERI   Dipartimento di Psicologia Generale, Università di Padova, Padova, Italy

MARJORIE PERLMAN-LORCH   Department of Speech Therapy, National Hospital for Nervous Diseases, and Applied Linguistics Department, Birkbeck College, University of London, London, Great Britain

CARLO SEMENZA    Dipartimento di Psicologia Generale, Università di Padova, Padova, Italy

HEINZ KARL STARK    Ludwig Boltzmann Institute for Cerebral Blood Flow Research, Vienna, Austria

JACQUELINE A. STARK    Brain Research Institute, Austrian Academy of Sciences, Vienna, Austria

LIVIA TONELLI    Facoltà di Lingue Moderne, Università di Trieste, Trieste, Italy

SYLVIANE VALDOIS    Laboratoire de Psychologie Expérimentale, U.A au CNRS 665, 38040 Grenoble, France; and Laboratoire Théophile-Alajouanine, Montreal, Quebec, Canada

PIERRE VILLIARD    University of New Brunswick, Fredericton, and Laboratoire Théophile-Alajouanine, Montréal, Canada

# Introduction

Starting with the pioneering work of Roman Jakobson and buttressed by the more recent birth and powerful surge of cognitive science, the interaction between linguistics, psycholinguistics, and aphasiology—sometimes labeled neuropsycholinguistics—has without any doubt gained its letters patent of nobility over the past two decades. Now, obviously, such a multidisciplinary "joint venture" has its own strict requirements, in the absence of which cognitive science would become nothing more than a "fashionable" topic of conversation for some pseudoscholars more attached to soft science fiction than to the hard—hopefully rigorous, verifiable, and replicable—facts of brain-mind-behavior relations.

Among such requirements, neuropsycholinguists have to place first the necessity to keep in constant touch with the most recent advances in *all* the various fields that are relevant to their broad domain of interest—easier said than done when one considers the unavoidable limitations to be found in a single scholar. Hence there is an obligation to (1) develop multidisciplinary research teams and (2) organize multidisciplinary meetings and conferences within which specialists readily share their respective expertise for the better understanding of aphasic patients' verbal behavior.

Such was the original idea that led us to organize two symposia—"Morphology and Aphasia" and "Phonology and Aphasia"—within the context of the international morphology and phonology meetings set up by Wolfgang Dressler and his colleagues (to whom we wish to express our warmest heartfelt thanks) in Krems, Austria, during the summer of 1988.

By bringing together "hard core" linguists and neuropsycholinguists, it was thus hoped that one would modestly but efficiently contribute to the mutual fertilization of general linguistics—in constant need, for many of its theoretical constructs, of external evidence that aphasiology is liable to provide—and aphasiology, which (again) must remain constantly informed of the current developments of linguistic theory, particularly in two fields, morphology and phonology, which have recently undergone substantial (r)evolution. The present volume is basically the outcome of those two symposia, in which participated some thirty scholars from all over the world.

JEAN-LUC NESPOULOUS and PIERRE VILLIARD

# 1
# Structure of the Lexicon: Functional Architecture and Lexical Representation

Alfonso Caramazza and Gabriele Miceli

One of the basic assumptions in cognitive neuropsychology is that we can characterize a cognitive process as a set of representations that are computed in the course of cognitive performance, i.e., in the course of object recognition, sentence understanding, and the like. A principal task of the cognitive neuropsychologist is to describe the series of representations ($R_2$) that are computed in the course of these cognitive activities. For any interesting cognitive process there are a series of representations that are assumed to intervene between the inputs and outputs of the process: $I(nput) \rightarrow R_1, R_2, \ldots R_i, \ldots \rightarrow O(utput)$.

This general assumption in cognitive science can be represented in the more familiar formalism of the information processing paradigm. In this formalism, a cognitive process consists of a set of subprocesses, or "stages," of processing. Given some input/output pair (e.g., producing a particular name for an object), there is a sequence of processes that are assumed to intervene between the input and output. The familiar way of schematically representing this assumption is through a flow chart of the process—the so-called box-and-arrow models. These models are intended to represent the sequence of processes that characterize a complex cognitive operation.

The model presented in Figure 1.1 represents a hypothesis about the structure of the lexical system. Two assumptions of this model are (1) lexical information is represented as independent sets of information—orthographic information is independent of phonological information—and these two, in turn, are independent of semantic information; and (2) the input lexicons are independent of the output lexicons. The reason for assuming separate input and output phonological processing lexicons stems from the fact that the processes engaged for recognizing an auditorily presented word use acoustic and phonetic information as input, whereas in the oral production of a word the information used as input for the phonological lexicon is not acoustic or phonetic but semantic in nature (a parallel argument applies to the case of the orthographic lexicons). We may entertain the alternative possibility that one need not distinguish between input

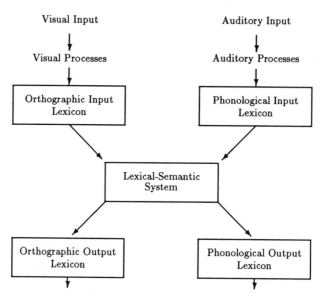

FIGURE 1.1. Organization of the lexical components that comprise the lexical system.

and output lexicons, but we would have to articulate this alternative in some detail: It is not sufficient to say that there is a single phonological lexicon; it must be shown how such a phonological lexicon could be accessed by both semantic and acoustic information in the case of production and perception, respectively. In the absence of adequate theoretical justification for the latter assumption, it seems appropriate to start with the assumption that there is a distinction between input and output lexicons and between phonological and orthographic lexicons.

Data from our laboratory (Caramazza and Hillis, in press; Hillis, Rapp, Romani, and Caramazza, in press) provide support for the proposed general architecture of the lexical system. Of course, there are many other observations in the literature that are relevant to this issue as well (see Caramazza, 1988, for review).

Subject K.E. (Caramazza and Hillis, in press; Hillis et al., in press) produced semantic errors in all single-word production tasks, independent of input and output modality, and in approximately the same proportion (Table 1.1). Furthermore, he made semantic errors in word comprehension as assessed through word/picture matching tasks.

The types of production error made by KE are exemplified in Table 1.2. For example, given "arm" as a stimulus, K.E. produced the following responses: "ear" when reading aloud, "finger" when oral naming, "leg" for written naming, and "hand" when writing to dictation. This example is intended only to illustrate that K.E. did not systematically give the same

TABLE 1.1. Distribution of semantic errors produced by K.E. in various tasks.

| Task | Total errors | | Semantic errors | |
|------|------|------|------|------|
| | No. | % | No. | % |
| Auditory comprehension | 61/144 | 42.4 | 61/144 | 42.4 |
| Reading comprehension | 53/144 | 36.8 | 52/144 | 36.1 |
| Verbal naming | 64/144 | 44.4 | 59/144 | 41.0 |
| Written naming | 67/144 | 46.5 | 50/144 | 34.7 |
| Oral reading | 60/144 | 41.7 | 52/144 | 36.1 |
| Writing to dictation | 60/144 | 41.7 | 40/144 | 27.8 |

TABLE 1.2. Examples of K.E.'s semantic errors across tasks for the same stimulus.

| Stimulus | Oral reading | Oral naming | Written naming | Dictation |
|----------|-------------|-------------|----------------|-----------|
| Arm | Ear | Finger | Leg | Hand |
| Elbow | Foot | Leg | Leg | Leg |
| Truck | Boat | Van | Bus | Truck |
| Apple | Peach | Peach | Pear | Apple |

response to the same word in different tasks. Of course, on various occasions he did make the same semantic error to a word in different tasks as exemplified in the case of the word "elbow," for which he gave the response "leg" in oral and written naming and in writing-to-dictation.

By contrast, subjects R.G.B. and H.W. (Caramazza and Hillis, in press) made semantic errors in tasks requiring oral output but did not make such errors in tasks requiring written output (Table 1.3). The types of incorrect response produced by these two subjects are reported in Table 1.4. For example, R.G.B. read "kangaroo" as "giraffe" and orally named it "raccoon," but his response to this stimulus in written naming, though spelled incorrectly (k–g–oo), clearly was the appropriate target response. Furthermore, both R.G.B. and H.W. could provide adequate definitions for words they could not name orally or read aloud. Asked to read "records," R.G.B. said "radio" and went on to define the word he was asked to read as: "You play them on a phonograph; it also means notes you take and keep" (Table. 1.5). This pattern of performance indicates that the two subjects knew the meanings of the target words but could not produce the appropriate phonological responses.

The performance observed in K.E. clearly differs from that observed in R.G.B. and H.W. Although all three subjects produced semantic errors in the spoken production of words, it is clear that the semantic errors produced by K.E. resulted from damage to a different component(s) of the lexical system than that responsible for the semantic errors produced by R.G.B. and H.W. In the case of K.E., it can be assumed that the locus of

TABLE 1.3. Performance across tasks on the same 47 items (given in proportion of total responses).

| Task | R.G.B. | | H.W. | |
|---|---|---|---|---|
| | Semantic errors (%) | Others (%) | Semantic errors (%) | Others (%) |
| Oral naming: pictures | 36 | 2 | 34 | 4 |
| Oral naming: tactile | 36 | 0 | 36 | 9 |
| Oral reading | 32 | 2 | 34 | 4 |
| Written naming | 0 | 6 | 0 | 2 |
| Dictation | 0 | 6 | 0 | 4 |
| Auditory word-picture matching | 0 | 0 | 0 | 0 |
| Printed word-picture matching | 0 | 0 | 0 | 0 |

TABLE 1.4. Examples of RGB's and HW's errors in oral versus written production tasks.

| Stimulus | Oral reading | Oral naming | Written naming |
|---|---|---|---|
| **R.G.B.** | | | |
| Sock | Stocking | Mitten | Sock |
| Cap | Hat | Stocking | Cap |
| Kangaroo | Giraffe | Racoon | Ka g oo |
| Donkey | Monkey | Monkey | Dokey |
| **H.W.** | | | |
| Lime | Lemon | Melon | Lime |
| Jar | Lunch | Bottle | Jar |
| Octopus | Clam | Squid | Octop |
| Shelf | Top | Book | Shef |

TABLE 1.5. R.G.B.'s and H.W.'s definitions of words following semanti errors.

| Stimulus | Oral reading response | Definition |
|---|---|---|
| **R.G.B.** | | |
| Records | Radio | You play 'em on a phonograph...can also mean notes you take and keep. |
| Tomato | Salad | You get 'em in the summer. Jackie used to grow 'em.... |
| Necklace | Necktie | You would wear...a woman would have around her neck...made out of metal...gold or silver. |
| Airport | Airplane | Where they're...airplanes are parked...where you go to get on a plane at. |
| **H.W.** | | |
| Scramble | Fry | Instead of in order, it's all mixed up. |
| Interest | Bank | You go to the bank and put it in and you get more money...not very much now. |
| Village | Live | Small city. |
| History | School | Find out things how they used to be. |

deficit is in the semantic system, as damage to this system is expected to affect all lexical comprehension and production tasks—the pattern of results observed for K.E.

For subjects R.G.B. and H.W., it can be hypothesized that brain damage has spared the semantic system but selectively disrupted the phonological output lexicon. The assumption that in these subjects the functional damage was restricted to the phonological output lexicon is supported by (1) the presence of semantic errors *only* in the oral production tasks and (2) the integrity of the semantic system as indicated by the subjects' ability to provide the correct definition of words they could not read or name. The hypothesis advanced here proposes that if a correct lexical item is not available for production in the phonological output lexicon a semantically related lexical entry may be produced in its stead (see Caramazza, 1988, for discussion). (These subjects also have damage at some level of the orthographic processing output system, resulting in the misspellings of correctly chosen target responses. However, this additional deficit is not of interest in the present context.)

The results we have briefly reviewed provide unambiguous evidence that a response scored as a "semantic" error may have different underlying causes. The contrasting patterns of performance observed in K.E. and in R.G.B. and H.W. may be used to distinguish between errors that arise from damage to the semantic component and those that arise from a deficit to the phonological output lexicon. Furthermore, the patterns of performance observed in these subjects provide convincing evidence in favor of the assumption that the orthographic output lexicon is independent of the phonological output lexicon.

The evidence reviewed to this point supports the multicomponent view of the lexical architecture presented in Figure 1.1, a cognitive architecture that includes separate input and output components and separate phonological and orthographic components, in both input and output. Some investigations have addressed more detailed tissues concerning the internal structure of the lexical components. For example, data from the Italian-speaking brain-damaged subject F.S. (Miceli and Caramazza, 1988) have been used to support hypotheses about the structure of the phonological output lexicon and in particular about the existence of morphological organization in the lexicon.

When repeating 1832 nouns, adjectives, verbs, and function words, F.S. made many errors for all classes of words (although he made more errors on verbs than on adjectives and more errors on adjectives than on nouns and function words), as shown in Table 1.6. Interestingly, these errors respected a specific constraint: Of a total of 893 incorrect responses to polymorphemic words, 637 (71%) could be construed as morphological errors, i.e., errors involving the suffixed part of the to-be-repeated word. The remaining incorrect responses (29%) consisted of phonological errors or unscorable responses. There was only one semantic error. The most

TABLE 1.6.  Performance by F.S.
in word repetition Tasks.

| Parts of speech | Errors | % |
| --- | --- | --- |
| Nouns | 121/409 | 29.6 |
| Adjectives | 290/589 | 49.2 |
| Verbs | 482/750 | 64.3 |
| Function words | 26/84 | 31.0 |
| *Total* | 919/1832 | 50.2 |

striking aspect of F.S.'s performance was that essentially all (615 of 637, 96.7%) of his morphological errors were inflectional. For example, asked to repeat a word such as "amavo" (I was loving), F.S. often produced in incorrectly inflected word such as "amasse" (that he loved) but essentially never produced a derivationally related word such as "amabile" (lovable).

These results, demonstrating a dissociation between inflectional and derivational processes, provide empirical support for the position that inflectional and deivational processes are distinct (Anderson, 1982; Lapointe, 1979; see Scalise, 1984, for review). Close analyses of F.S.'s performance allow us to address further issues about the morphological structure of the lexicon.

In Italian, most adjectives are marked for gender and number, and it was cear that F.S. did not make an equal number of errors on the various forms of the adjective. He was much more often correct when repeating adjectives in the masculine singular (m.sg.) than in the masculine plural (m.pl.) or in the feminine forms (f.sg. and f.pl.). This stimulus-error relation could reflect the effects of a morphological dimension on performance, but other possibilities had to be ruled out before such a conclusion could be reached. For example, it could be argued that F.S. repeated m.sg. forms better than other forms only because m.sg. for forms are more frequent in the language. To control for this possibility in a further experiment, F.S. was asked to repeat two sets of adjectives: For adjectives in the first set, the frequency of the m.sg. form was higher than the frequency of each of the non-m.sg. forms, whereas for adjectives in the second set the frequency of the m.sg. form was lower than the frequency of each of the non-m.sg. forms. The subject was asked to repeat both the m.sg. form and one non-m.sg. form of the adjectives included in each set (for adjectives in the second set the most frequency non-m.sg. form was chosen). The results were clear: The m.sg. form was repeated correctly most often, independent of its frequency of use in the language.

An analysis of all the adjective errors produced by F.S. (Table 1.7, top) revealed a striking pattern of performance that effectively ruled out the possibility that the subject's results could be accounted for by phonological factors. Table 1.7 (top) shows that F.S. was more often correct with the m.sg. form and that when he was unable to produce a response to other

TABLE 1.7. Confusion matrix for inflectional errors made by F.S. when repeating 4-ending and 2-ending adjectives.

| | Four-ending adjectives | | | | |
| | M.SG. | M.PL. | F.SG. | F.PL. | Total |
|---|---|---|---|---|---|
| m.sg. | **149 (94.9)** | 8 (5.1) | — | — | 157 |
| m.pl. | 40 (52.6) | **26 (34.2)** | 5 (6.6) | 5 (6.6) | 76 |
| f.sg. | 43 (48.9) | 1 (1.1) | **35 (39.8)** | 9 (10.2) | 88 |
| f.pl. | 34 (61.8) | 2 (3.6) | 5 (9.1) | **14 (25.5)** | 55 |
| Total | 266 (70.7) | 37 (9.8) | 45 (12.0) | 28 (7.4) | 376 |

| | Two-ending adjectives | |
| | SG. | PL. |
|---|---|---|
| sg. | 56 (81.2) | 13 (18.8) |
| pl. | 36 (65.5) | 19 (34.5) |

adjective forms (m.pl., f.sg., and f.pl.) he was not likely to produce one of the other adjectival forms at random. To the contrary, in these instances F.S. systematically produced the m.sg. form.

Could phonological principles account for this result? Could it be the case that F.S. was more often correct with m.sg. forms because, for example, it was easier for him to pronounce the word-final vowel /o/ in m.sg. adjectives than the other vowels (/a/,/i/,/e/) associated with the non-m.sg. form of adjectives? This possibility was ruled out by the analysis of F.S.'s performance on Italian adjectives that make a distinction only between singular and plural, such as the singular "forte" (strong) and the plural "forti." As may be seen in Table 1.7 (bottom), F.S. repeated the singular-form adjectives much better than the plural-form adjectives. (Note that the ending of the singular form of the latter adjectives is phonologically identical to the ending of the f.pl. form of the former, four-ending adjectives). Clearly, F.S.'s pattern of errors is best accounted for by a disruption of inflectional processes and supports the notion that one of the dimensions along which the lexicon is organized is morphology.

What these data suggest is that it is not possible to simply continue talking about phonological lexicon or orthographic lexicon; it is necessary to articulate stronger hypotheses about the structure of lexical components, i.e., to articulate hypotheses about the nature of the representations that are stored in the proposed lexical components. It is necessary to go beyond notions such as "logogen" (Morton, 1969) because these notions are much too general and unspecific—"logogen" simply stands for a response to a stimulus, but what the response actually is in representational and computational terms has never been articulated in any detail.

Other evidence from our laboratory favoring the hypothesis that lexical information is represented in morphologically decomposed form comes from the distribution of spelling errors in a dysgraphic subject, D.H. (Badecker, Hillis, and Caramazza, in press). A comparison of the distribution of D.H.'s errors in spelling suffixed words such as "ended" versus pseudosuffixed words such as "agent" revealed a theoretically significant contrast: D.H. made many fewer errors on the suffix part of suffixed words (-ed in ended) than on the pseudosuffix part of pseudosuffixed words (-nt in agent). This result could not be ascribed to differences in bigram frequencies of letter clusters in suffixed and pseudosuffixed words because the effect obtained even when bigram frequencies were strictly controlled. This pattern of results, together with the results reported earlier for F.S., strongly suggests that lexical entries are represented in morphologically decomposed form.

To this point, data from subjects K.E., R.G.B., and H.W. have been used to support some aspects of the general architecture of the lexicon, and data from F.S. and D.H. have helped us make the point that finer-grained hypotheses about the structure of the lexical system (in this case, morphological structure) must be proposed if we are to capture significant aspects of brain-damaged subjects' performance. In the next section, the results obtained from other cognitively impaired subjects are used to demonstrate that it is possible (and necessary) to further articulate our hypotheses about the structure of lexical representations. Because the relevant results in this section come from cases of acquired dysgraphia, a short presentation of the functional architecture of the spelling process that guides our research is in order.

There is ample evidence in the literature that the spelling system must be at least as complex as the functional architecture presented in Figure 1.2 (see Ellis, 1982, 1988, for review). This model assumes that different kinds of information and processes are involved in spelling familiar and unfamiliar words. Words are spelled by retrieving from memory lexical-orthographic representations: We know that /rId/ is spelled "read" or "reed," depending on which word we intend to produce. Considerations of this sort lead us to assume that we have word-specific orthographic knowledge; i.e., a particular meaning is associated with a particular lexical-orthographic representation. Furthermore, because unfamiliar words are not associated with any particular lexical-orthographic representation, the spelling of these words is assumed to involve the conversion of sublexical phonological units into graphemes. The latter claim is not noncontroversial but is not defended here as it does not bear on our present concerns (Campbell, 1983).

Another important aspect of the cognitive model of spelling depicted in Figure 1.2 concerns the hypothesis that buffer components (working memory components) must be included in the overall architecture of the spelling process. We assume that buffers must be postulated whenever a multiunit representation has to be processed sequentially over time or whenever several independent units must be processed simultaneously. In the case of spelling, it is assumed that, because the lexical representation of a word such as "read" consists of a series of graphemes, we must postulate

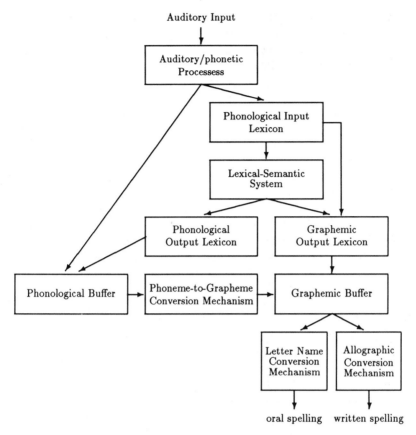

FIGURE 1.2. Functional organization of the spelling system.

a buffer where this information is temporarily held for the application of more peripheral spelling processes. This view receives considerable support from research showing that there are dysgraphic subjects whose spelling performance is explicated most plausibly by assuming that they have selective damage to the graphemic buffer (Caramazza, Miceli, Villa, and Romani, 1987; Hillis and Caramazza, 1989; Miceli, Silveri, and Caramazza, 1985; Posteraro, Zinelli, and Mazzucchi, 1988).

The pattern of performance of a dysgraphic subject with damage to the graphemic buffer is straightforwardly predicted from the functional architecture of the model presented in Figure 1.2. A functional lesion to this component of the spelling system should result in errors in all spelling tasks, independent of the input modality (e.g., writing-to-dictation or written naming) or the type of spelling mode (oral or written spelling); the spelling of familiar and unfamiliar words (the latter operationally represented by nonwords) should be affected equally because the representations computed for both familiar and unfamiliar words must be temporarily held in the buffer for more peripheral processes; stimulus length is a critical parameter in determining spelling performance—the longer the stimulus, the more errors that should be observed; and, most important, the quality of the errors should be identical for words and nonwords. Because the information available to the spelling system at the level of the graphemic buffer is orthographic (information concerning abstract letter identities or graphemes), only orthography-based errors should be observed. Thus errors should consist of letter substitutions, insertions, deletions, or transpositions, resulting mostly in the production of nonword responses and the violation of orthographic constraints (e.g., table → tbale). Semantically related errors such as table → chair should not be observed because at the level of the spelling process where we assume the damage to be located there are no possibilities for lexically based substitutions or confusions; nor should we observe phonologically plausible (or, more generally, phonology-based) errors (e.g., table → taybel) because, by hypothesis, phonological information is not available at the level of the graphemic buffer.

In a previous publication (Caramazza et al., 1987) we reported the performance of a dysgraphic subject, L.B., that closely conformed with the theoretical expectations of a functional lesion to the graphemic buffer in the proposed model of the spelling process. If our interpretation of this subject's performance as reflecting selective damage to the graphemic buffer is correct, his performance may be used to constrain hypotheses about the structure of orthographic representations.

According to the theory of spelling graphically summarized in Figure 1.2 (and fully supported by the pattern of errors observed in subjects such as L.B.), there is no semantic or phonological information in the graphemic buffer; the buffer contains only orthographic information, i.e., information about the graphemes (abstract letter identities) that constitute the spelling of a word. On this view, the performance of dysgraphic subjects with selective damage to the graphemic buffer provides a "window" to the structure of orthographic representations. Because the only information in the buffer consists of lexical-orthographic representations, the spelling errors produced by subjects with selective damage at this level of the spelling process should consist of *transformations* (or "deformations") of orthographic representations. The analysis of the patterns of transformations of orthographic structures in the spelling errors produced by dysgraphic subjects of this type may be used to constrain theoretical claims about the structure of lexical-orthographic representations. We have done just that (Caramazza and Miceli, 1989a, b) through the detailed analysis of the spelling performances of a dysgraphic subject, L.B., with selective damage to the graphemic buffer.

We have arugued that in the case of damage to the graphemic buffer the model schematized in Figure 1.2 allows us to predict that the errors made by subjects such as L.B. should *only* take the form of letter substitutions (e.g., ta*b*le → ta*n*le), insertions (e.g., table → t*n*able), deletions (e.g., table → ta*b*e), or transpositions (e.g., table → ta*lb*e). This model does not, however, allow us to make predictions that are more precise than those just presented. In other words, the state of our theorizing is such that we are essentially unable to provide answers to questions concerning the distributional properties of spelling errors beyond the gross claim that they should be insertions, deletions, transpositions, or substitutions of letters.

Consider in this context the case of substitution errors. Let us suppose that L.B. makes a substitution error to the word "tavolo" (table). The error may take one of four forms. L.B. may substitute (1) a consonant for a consonant, as in ta*v*olo → ta*s*olo; (2) a vowel for a vowel, as in tav*o*lo → tav*a*lo; (3) a consonant for a vowel, as in tav*o*lo → tav*s*lo; or (4) a vowel for a consonant, as in ta*v*olo → ta*e*olo. Clearly, so far as the model in Figure 1.2 is concerned, there is no reason for not expecting that these four types of error should occur with equal probability. In other words, our expectations concerning the types of error we should observe depend on the assumptions we have made concerning the kind of information represented in the buffer. If the assumption is made that orthographic information in the buffer represents only an ordered set of graphemes, and if the deficit in this subject involves loss of information stored in the buffer, any grapheme may be substituted for any other grapheme—the four types of substitution errors described above should then occur with equal probability (at least, we have no grounds for assuming otherwise). This expectation was not confirmed in our analysis of the spelling performance of L.B.

The substitution errors produced by L.B. were essentially all (640 of 643, 99.5%) vowels for vowels or consonants for consonants. So the simple claim that the only information at the level of the graphemic buffer consists of an ordered set of graphemes is not supported by our results. Instead, we must assume that the information contained at the orthographic level of representation includes a distinction between consonants and vowels—a much stronger assumption about the structure of orthographic representations than we had previously made. A crucial implication of this assumption is that we must distinguish between two types of information in orthographic representations: information specifying the ordered set of graphemes that comprise a lexical item and information about the consonant-vowel (C-V) status of individual graphemes. The proposed distinction may be captured through the assumption that graphemic and consonant-vowel information constitute *separate but linked levels* of representation (or "tiers," as they are called in the phonological theory that has inspired the proposed hypothesis). The assumption is that orthographic representations are multidimensional: One dimension specifies graphemic structure (graphemic level), and the other specifies C-V structure. (However, as noted below, a two-dimensional structure is insufficient to capture the relevant information in orthographic representations.) Thus, for example, the orthographic representation for the word "tavolo" would be

$$[T]\ [A]\ [V]\ [O]\ [L]\ [O] \quad \text{Grapheme tier}$$
$$|\quad|\quad|\quad|\quad|\quad| \quad \text{Association lines}$$
$$C\quad V\quad C\quad V\quad C\quad V \quad \text{C-V tier} \qquad\qquad (1)$$

where the top tier consisting of the bracketed letters represents the graphemes (or abstract letter identities) that comprise the word, and the bottom tier represents the C-V structure associated with the word, through a one-to-one mapping of grapheme to C-V unit.

This hypothesis about the structure of orthographic representations provides the basis for a motivated explanation of the observed pattern of substitution errors in L.B. If we assume that damage of the buffer results in the loss (or inefficient use) of orthographic information, when information about a specific grapheme is inadequate for further processing there would be C-V information that could be used to determine whether a consonant or a vowel should be produced at that point in the word. An example of how this hypothesis would work is as follows.

$$[T]\ [A]\ [-]\ [O]\ [L]\ [O] \rightarrow \text{TASOLO}$$
$$|\quad|\quad|\quad|\quad|\quad|$$
$$C\quad V\quad C\quad V\quad C\quad V \qquad\qquad (2)$$

If information about the grapheme [V] in the word tavolo is missing, C-V information indicating that a consonant should occupy the insufficiently specified grapheme would lead to the production of a consonant in its place (in our example, an [S], resulting in the incorrect response "tasolo").

The hypothesis about the structure of orthographic representations entertained here also allows us to provide a motivated explanation for another nonobvious experimental result obtained with L.B. The experimental result in question concerns the contrast in L.B.'s spelling performance for words with geminate (double) consonants, e.g., as in the word stella (star), versus nongeminate words, e.g., stanco (tired). His performance was much better for geminate than for nongeminate words of equal length. Thus he correctly spelled 78% of the six-letter geminate words (e.g., stella) but only 57% of the six-letter nongeminate words (e.g., stanco). L.B.'s spelling performance with six-letter geminate words was comparable to his performance with five-letter nongeminate words, e.g., stile (style)—78% versus 77% correct, respectively. This pattern of results does not find a principled explanation within a theory of spelling that assumes that orthographic representations specify only an ordered set of graphemes. By contrast, the hypothesis that C-V and grapheme information represent autonomous but associated levels of orthographic structure allows a motivated explanation of the reported results, provided we further assume that geminate consonants are represented only *once* at the graphemic level but are associated with two positions at the C-V level, as shown here.

$$[S] \; [T] \; [E] \quad [L] \quad [A]$$

$$
\begin{array}{ccccc}
| & | & | & \diagup\diagdown & | \\
C & C & V & C \quad C & V
\end{array} \qquad (3)
$$

The spelling performance of L.B. was strongly affected by word length. His performance was worse for long than for short words, a result consistent with the hypothesis of selective damage to the graphemic buffer. However, depending on the assumptions we make about the nature of orthographic representations placed in the buffer, there are different expectations concerning spelling performance for words with geminate and nongeminate consonants. Specifically, on the assumption that spelling performance is a function of the number of grapheme units in the buffer, our expectations are that (1) if both consonants of a geminate cluster are represented at the grapheme level, spelling performance should be poorer for six-letter geminate (e.g., stella) and nongeminate (e.g., stanco) words than for five-letter nongeminate words (e.g., stile), whereas (2) if only one consonant of the geminate cluster is represented at the grapheme level spelling performance should be poorer for six-letter nongeminate words than for six-letter geminate and five-letter nongeminate words. At issue is whether six-letter words with double consonants are represented as strings of five or six graphemes. The expectations of the two hypotheses are summarized below.

$H_1$: Each letter is represented by a grapheme:
$$\text{STANCO} = \text{STELLA} < \text{STILE}$$

$H_2$: Double letters are represented by one grapheme:
$$\text{STANCO} < \text{STELLA} = \text{STILE}$$

As already noted, the experimental results strongly favor the view that L.B.'s performance for six-letter words with geminate consonants is comparable to his performance with five- and not six-letter nongeminate words ($H_2$). The conclusion that geminate clusters are represented by a single consonant grapheme ($H_2$) leads us to assume that orthographic representations contain *other* information that allows the single consonant grapheme to be spelled as two letters in output. Note, however, that this kind of information is not specified at the grapheme level. In fact, the hypothesis we have proposed for the structure of orthographic representations distinguishes between levels at which grapheme and other relevant orthographic information is represented. In the case of gemination, the hypothesis is that consonant doubling is indicated in the C-V tier where two consonant units (or slots) are associated with a single grapheme (see (3) above).

The results we have reported for words with geminate consonants, together with the previously reported observation of consonant-for-consonant and vowel-for-vowel substitutions, argue strongly for the existence of separate C-V level and grapheme level representations. The assumption of separate C-V level and graphemic level representations accounts for data on spelling performance far better than the assumption of a single level of representation, consisting of only a sequence of graphemes. However, even this richer assumption is not sufficient to account for various other aspects of L.B.'s spelling performance. These other observations require us to make still stronger assumptions about the structure of orthographic representations.

In Italian, there are words with a "simple" C-V structure (i.e., words that contain *n* sequences of one consonant and one vowel, e.g., "tavolo") and words that have an "complex" C-V structure, i.e., words that contain vocalic or consonantal clusters, e.g., "fiasco" (flask), "tempio" (temple), "strano" (strange), "nostro" (our), "onesto" (honest), and "albero" (tree), in addition to words with geminate consonants. On the assumption that the representations used in spelling contain information only about grapheme units and C-V structure, the performance obtained with words containing the same number of letters (with the exception of words with geminate letters, see above) should be the same, independent of whether they have a simple or a complex C-V structure. This case is not what we found. L.B.'s performance with simple six-letter words was far superior to his performance with complex six-letter words: Words such as "tavolo" were written correctly substantially more often than words such as "onesto" or "fiasco" [1300 of 1777 (73%) versus 579 of 1024 (57%) correct]. Once again, if we were to assume that orthographic representations consist only of an ordered set of graphemes, this result would not be expected, nor would it be expected even if, in addition, we were to assume a C-V level of representation.

The analysis of the type of errors made by L.B. when spelling words with simple and complex C-V structure provides important clues to the organization of orthographic representations. The distribution of error types differed markedly as a function of whether the to-be-spelled word had a simple or a complex C-V structure, as may readily be seen in Table 1.8.

TABLE 1.8. Effect of orthographic structure on writing performance: incidence of various error types in incorrect responses to CVCVCV and to non-CVCVCV stimuli.

| Performance | Orthographic structure | |
|---|---|---|
| | CVCVCV | Non-CVCVCV |
| Substitutions | 386 (70.6)[a] | 122 (28.6) |
| Insertions | 4 (0.7) | 32 (7.5) |
| Deletions | 2 (0.4) | 141 (33.0) |
| Exchanges (nonadjacent letters) | 155 (28.3) | 96 (22.5) |
| Transpositions | 0 (0.0) | 36 (8.4) |
| *Total* (No. of simple errors) | 547 (100) | 427 (100) |

[a] Numbers in parentheses are percentages.

L.B. did not produce letter deletion or insertion errors for simple C-V words, nor did he produce adjacent-letter exchange errors (e.g., errors such as tavolo → taovlo) for these words. However, he did produce insertion, deletion, and adjacent-letter exchange errors for complex C-V words. Thus essentially all of L.B.'s spelling errors for simple C-V structure words were either substitutions (e.g., tavolo → tapolo) or exchanges of *nonad*-jacent letters, e.g., sirena (siren) → sinera or sirane, but not sierna. Why should there be such a difference in the distribution of spelling errors for the two types of word?

Let us consider first, briefly, the case of exchange errors. One reason for the absence of adjacent-letter exchange errors is that these errors do not occur because they would involve a consonant/vowel exchange. This reason cannot be the whole explanation, however, because when spelling words with complex C-V structure L.B. produced adjacent-letter errors that involved consonant-vowel exchanges, e.g., premio (prize) → permio. A more likely reason for the asymmetrical distribution of exchange errors appeals to the possibility of orthosyllabic structure constraints on the production of errors. That is, the reason for the absence of adjacent-letter exchange errors for simple C-V structure words is that such errors would result in the violation of the orthosyllabic structure of the target words. For example, the incorrect spelling of "sirena" as "sierna" not only involves the exchange of the positions of a consonant and a vowel (i.e., CVCVCV → CV*V*CCV) but also a change in the orthosyllabic structure of the word sirena—a change from three (si-re-na) to two (sier-na) syllables. In other words, if lexical-orthographic representations specified not only grapheme and C-V information but also orthosyllabic structure, the latter information could serve to constrain the types of error produced by the subject when grapheme or C-V information is underspecified as a consequence of brain damage. This point may more readily be appreciated by considering the distribution of deletion errors.

The deletion of a single consonant or vowel in words with simple C-V structure almost always results in a change in the orthosyllabic structure of the word (e.g., si-re-na → sir-na, sie-na). It need not be the case for words with complex C-V structure, e.g., destra (right) → detra, desra, desta; compie (completes) → compi, compe. Consequently, if orthographic representations contain orthosyllabic structure, we would expect deletion errors only (or mostly) to occur for complex C-V words. In fact, among a body of several hundred errors, L.B. made only two omission errors on simple C-V words, both involving deletion of the entire first syllable, as in "cugino" (cousin) → "gino," but he made 141 single-letter deletion errors on complex C-V words. Most single-letter deletions (128/141, 90.8%) were consonant deletions in consonant clusters, as in "destra" (right) → "desta" (he awakes). These errors did *not* lead to a change in the orthosyllabic structure of the target response. Similarly, of the 13 single-letter deletions (9.2%) involving vowels, 12 (8.5% of the total number of deletions) consisted in the deletion of one of two vowels in vowel digraphs, as in "compie" → "compe." As in the case of the consonant deletion errors, these vowel deletion errors also respect the orthosyllabic structure of the target response. Of the 141 single deletion errors for complex C-V words, only one vowel deletion error resulted in a violation of syllabic structure (0.7% of the total number of deletions). These results provide strong evidence for the hypothesis that orthosyllabic structure constitutes an autonomous level of orthographic representation.

The hypothesis we have formulated for the structure of orthographic representations provides a motivated account of the distribution of L.B.'s spelling errors. Consider, for example, the expected performance when spelling a word such as "stanco" (tired). Suppose that the only information available to the subject was that: (1) the word has two syllables ($\sigma$); (2) the first two graphemes in the response are consonants, and the last two graphemes are a consonant and a vowel, respectively; and (3) the first grapheme is [S] and the last grapheme is [O] (this information is represented in [4], below). Information on C-V structure would force the production of consonants in the second and in the penultimate position, even though information about specific graphemes is unavailable. Information on syllabic structure would induce the production of a vowel between the initial CC cluster and the final CV sequence. (If there is a syllable, there has to be a vowel.) These constraints would lead to the production of a CCVCV sequence, resulting in a consonant deletion and substitutions (e.g., stanco → stoto). Alternatively, a -VC- or a -CV- sequence may be produced to fill the empty slots, resulting in more complex errors, which would, nonetheless, respect the orthosyllabic structure of the target response (e.g., stanco → stpodo, stopdo), in the sense that the sequence of Cs and Vs satisfy graphotactic constraints in terms of the number of such elements that can occur in sequence. The outcome of these "repairs" would be substitution errors or letter exchanges, with or without letter substitutions, that respect orthosyllabic structure. These error types are

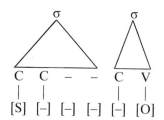

|   |   |   |   |   |   |   |           |     |
|---|---|---|---|---|---|---|-----------|-----|
| s | C |   | V |   | C | o | (deletion) |     |
| s | C | C | V |   | C | o | (exchange) |     |
| s | C |   | V | C | C | o | (exchange) | (4) |

precisely those that were observed in L.B.'s performance. In other words, if we assume a richly articulated orthographic representation that specifies information on orthosyllabic structure, C-V structure, and abstract letter identities, we are able to account for the vast majority of the letter substitutions and deletions made by the subject.

One last remark is in order. We have used terms and concepts that were developed in an area different from that which has been our concern here. Indeed, the concepts of orthosyllabic level, C-V level, and graphemic level were proposed by analogy to developments in phonological theory (van der Hulst and Smith, 1982). However, we must emphasize that the multi-dimensional structures proposed for orthographic representations are orthographic and not phonological in nature (see Cummings, 1988, for discussion; for experimental evidence on the structure of orthographic representations in reading, see Prinzmetal, Treiman, and Rho, 1986, and the references cited therein). What is exciting about our results is that similar general principles of lexical representation may be needed to account for phonological *and* orthographic processing. In other words, our results may be taken as evidence in favor of a general hypothesis about the form of lexical representations.

## Conclusions

We have reviewed some results, mostly from our laboratory, that speak to the general issue of lexical processing. We have shown that there is compelling evidence for the hypothesis that lexical information is represented in independent, modality-specific input and output lexicons. More importantly, however, we have gone on to show that it is possible to articulate more detailed hypotheses about the structure of the information represented in the proposed lexical components. Indeed, unless we articulate detailed claims about the structure of lexical mechanisms, as we have done herein, it is not possible to capture systematic regularities in the pattern of errors produced by brain-damaged subjects. The last point was amply demonstrated by our analysis of the spelling performance of a dysgraphic subject, which showed that we must make highly specific assumptions about orthographic representations in order to account for the observed patterns of spelling errors. To the extent to which specific hypotheses about the structure of lexical representations and about the organization of lexical components allow us to explicate the observed patterns of impaired performance, we may conclude that those hypotheses constitute valid aspects of a theory of lexical processing. In this context, we suggest that the research reviewed here provides strong support for the proposed hypotheses about the organization of the lexical system and the structure of lexical representations.

*Acknowledgments.* The work reported here was supported in part by NIH grants NS22202 and NS23836 and by a grant from the Seaver Institute to the first author. This support is gratefully acknowledged.

# References

Anderson, S.R. (1982). Where's morphology? *Linguistic Inquiry, 13,* 571–612.

Badecker, W., Hillis, A., & Caramazza, A. (in press). Lexical morphology and its role in the writing process: evidence from a case of acquired dysgraphia. *Cognition.*

Campbell, R. (1983). Writing nonwords to dictation. *Brain and Language, 19,* 153–178.

Caramazza, A. (1988). Some aspects of language processing revealed through the analysis of acquired aphasia: the lexical system. *Annual Review of Neuroscience, 11,* 395–521.

Caramazza, A., & Hillis, A. (in press). Modularity: a perspective from the analysis of acquired dyslexia and dysgraphia. In R. Malatesha Joshi (ed.), *Written Language Disorders.* Dordrecht: Kluwer Academic Publishers.

Caramazza, A., & Miceli, G. (1989a). Orthographic structure, the graphemic buffer and the spelling process. In C. von Euler, I. Lundberg, and G. Lennerstrand (eds.), *Brain and Reading.* Wenner-Gren International Symposium Series. Volume 54. New York: Macmillan.

Caramazza, A., & Miceli, G., (1989b). The structure of orthographic representation in spelling. *Reports of the Cognitive Neuropsychology Laboratory.* Baltimore: The Johns Hopkins University.

Caramazza, A., Miceli, G., Villa, G., & Romani, C. (1987). The role of the graphemic buffer in spelling; evidence from a case of acquired dysgraphia. *Cognition, 26,* 59–85.

Cummings, D.W. (1988). *American English Spelling.* Baltimore: The Johns Hopkins University Press.

Ellis, A.W. (1982). Spelling and writing (and reading and speaking). In A.W. Ellis (ed.), *Normality and Pathology in Cognitive Functions.* London: Academic Press.

Ellis, A.W. (1988). Normal writing processes and peripheral acquired dysgraphias. *Language and Cognitive Processes, 3,* 99–127.

Hillis, A., & Caramazza, A. (1989). The graphemic buffer and mechanisms of unilateral spatial neglect. *Brain and Language, 36,* 208–235.

Hillis, A., Rapp, B., Romani, C., & Caramazza, A. (in press). Selective impairment of semantics in lexical processing. *Cognitive Neuropsychology.*

Lapointe, S.G. (1979). A Theory of Grammatical Agreement. Unpublished doctoral dissertation, University of Massachusetts, Amherst.

Miceli, G., & Caramazza, A. (1988). Dissociation of inflectional and derivational morphology. *Brain and Language, 35,* 24–65.

Miceli, G., Silveri, M.C., & Caramazza, A. (1985). Cognitive analysis of a case of pure dysgraphia. *Brain and Language, 25,* 187–212.

Morton, J. (1969). The interaction of information in word recognition.

*Psychological Review 76*, 165–178.

Posteraro, L., Zinelli, P., and Mazzucchi, A. 1988. Selective impairment of the graphemic buffer in acquired dysgraphia: a case study. *Brain and Language, 35*, 274–286.

Prinzmetal, W., Treiman, R., & Rho, S.H. (1986). How to see a reading unit. *Journal of Memory and Language, 25*, 461–475.

Scalise, S. (1984). *Generative Morphology*. Dordrecht: Foris.

Van der Hulst, H. & Smith, N. (1982). *The Structure of Phonological Representations* (Part 1). Dordrecht: Foris.

# 2
# Morphological Representations and Morphological Deficits in Aphasia

GARY LIBBEN

A major goal in the study of language disorders by linguists is to develop an understanding of the functional architecture of language competence. Specifically, it is hoped that the study of language breakdown in aphasia will shed light on certain questions: In what form is linguistic knowledge represented in the brain? What role do linguistic representations play in the process of language comprehension and production?

A crucial assumption in this approach to linguistic aphasiology is that there is a significant relation between the units of linguistic theory and units appropriate to the functional characterization of language in the brain. In this chapter it is argued that it is profitable to characterize language competence in terms of theoretically motivated modules (i.e., phonology, morphology, syntax, semantics) and that theoretically motivated characterizations of language modules contribute significantly to the explanation of language disturbance in aphasia. However, it is also argued that this contribution requires neither the postulation of linguistic representations in the brain nor the postulation of a modular brain with respect to language.

The position is presented in the context of the investigation of morphological competence and its breakdown in aphasia. The chapter presents a case study of a patient, J.Z., who exhibited an interestingly specific production deficit. It is argued that, although this deficit was, in terms of a linguistic characterization, specifically morphological, the deficit was not related to any representation of morphological competence in the brain but, rather, resulted from an interaction between the demands of English morphology and the essentially nonmodular computational resources of the patient.

## Morphological Competence

In the generative morphology literature (Di Sciullo and Williams, 1987; Lieber, 1981; Selkirk, 1982; Williams, 1981a,b) it has been assumed that words have internal structure such as that displayed in Figure 2.1. In the

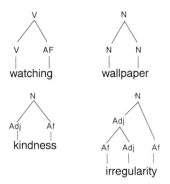

FIGURE 2.1. The representation of inflected and derived words in generative morphology.

psycholinguistic literature the question has been asked: What is the relation between these (and similar) characterizations of word structure and the representation and processing of words in the brain? In other words, do these structures have psychological reality?

It has been suggested by Murrel and Morton (1974), Taft and Forster (1975), and Taft (1979) that in the process of word recognition complex words are not accessed by their full forms but, rather, are decomposed and recognized in terms of their constituent morphemes. This position claims that the representations in Figure 2.1 are psychologically real to the extent that they have as their basic unit the morpheme and represent a word as an arrangement of morphemes. The findings of the above studies are to be contrasted, however, to findings which suggest that complex words are accessed and represented by their full forms in the mental lexicon. In a series of studies that investigated the recognition of pseudo-affixed and truly affixed words, Mandelis and Tharp (1977) and Henderson, Wallis, and Knight (1984) found no evidence for a morphologically organized mental lexicon.

A possible explanation for the lack of empirical consensus in this area might be that the early questions were too broad—that there is no statement possible about the psychological reality of morphological structure in general, and there are significant differences that correspond to the morphologically different types of structures in Figure 2.1. It can be seen that the word "watching" represents an example of inflection, the word "kindness" an example of derivation, and the word "wallpaper" an example of compounding. Finally the word "irregularity" represents a case of derivation in which affixation changes the phonological properties of the stem and the affix. Given these types of linguistic difference between complex words, a reasonable formulation of the question of psychological reality might be: Do the differences between types of morphological structures correspond to differences in the representation and processing of complex words in the brain.? In other words, are these distinctions psychologically real? There has been some experimental support for the claim that they *are* real. Bradley (1980), using a frequency mapping paradigm, found a processing difference between affixed words in which affixation does not affect the stem ("#" boundary affixes) and affixed words in which affixation does affect phonological properties of the stem ("+" boundary affixes). Stanners, Neiser, Hernon, and Hall (1979), using a priming paradigm, found a distinction between derived forms and inflected forms. They concluded that only the base forms of regularly inflected verbs are represented in the mental lexicon. Inflectional suffixes are stripped from the stem in the process of word recognition. Derivational affixes, on the other hand, are not stripped from their stems because derived words are represented in the mental lexicon by their full forms.

What is the status of such findings? Assuming, for example, that the above claims are correct, does it mean that derived forms are listed in the mental lexicon because they are derived forms? If Bradley's (1980) conclusions are correct and there is a psychologically real distinction between "+" boundary and "#" boundary affixes, does it mean that boundary type is represented in the mind?

In this chapter it is argued that the answer to both these questions is "no." With respect to the boundary distinction in particular, Bradley's findings indicated only that there is a correlation between the binary distinction in linguistic theory and computational processes of the mind such that one form takes longer to compute than the other. Her findings did not provide evidence for a type reductionistic (Fodor, 1975) view that the boundary distinction itself is represented in the mind.

These issues and arguments related to linguistic representations in the mind are also relevant to the interpretation of language loss in aphasia. Indeed the attention received by the putative syndrome of agrammatism in both the aphasiological and linguistic literature (Bradley, Garrett, and Zurif, 1980; Caplan, 1983; Caplan and Hildebrandt, 1988; Grodzinsky, 1984; Kean, 1977) is attributable to the fact that the syndrome's existence points to a significant relation between the units of linguistic theory and units appropriate to the characterization of language in the brain.

In the case study below, evidence is provided that supports a correlation between the units of linguistic theory and mental representations. The patient has exhibited a loss of morphological competence, but the data do not demonstrate that he has lost morphology (or that he was ever in possession of morphology). Rather, it appears that he has lost the ability to *do* morphology.

## Case Study (J.Z.)

J.Z. is a left-handed college-educated man who in 1986 at the age of 48 suffered a cerebrovascular accident due to an embolic infarction of the right middle cerebral artery. He was initially diagnosed as a Broca patient who showed severe expressive difficulties characterized by agrammatic speech and anomia. He did show a less severe but nevertheless significant deficit in comprehension. His comprehension difficulties were sensitive to message length, syntactic complexity, and semantic anomaly.

Now, 2 years after onset, J.Z. has recovered such that he is attending and passing undergraduate university courses. His speech is still slightly less fluent than before, and he reports difficulty attending to complex lecture material. In sum, he shows little language disability save for the communicatively irrelevant but linguistically significant one described below.

## Word Production

J.Z. showed difficulty in the production of words that could be characterized as having a complex form in the mental lexicon. J.Z.'s difficulty manifested itself only in production, but it appeared to be central to the extent that the degree of impairment was invariant across all production modalities. The words he could not repeat he also could not write to dictation and could not correctly produce spontaneously.

The complex word repetition impairment of J.Z. is outlined in Table 2.1. It can be seen that he showed difficulty with derived forms in which affixation results in a phonological change in the stem or affix.. He produced errors in the repetition (and writing) of "irregularity," "illegible," "irrefutable," and "illegality." In contrast, J.Z. showed no difficulty with equally long words in which affixation did not involve phonological adjustment. He produced error-free repetition of "unhappiness," "materialism," and "ungratefulness."

The typical word repetition errors he made are provided in Table 2.1. An interesting characteristic of his errors is that he showed a tendency to produce the canonical (or linguistically underlying) forms of the constituent morphemes of a complex word. His repetition of "irregularity," for example, was often "inregularity." A theoretical characterization (Chomsky and Halle, 1968)[1] of the word "irregularity" would claim that it is underlyingly the form /in + regular + ity/, and that in surface form the final phoneme /n/ of the prefix has completely assimilated to the first phoneme /r/ of the root. This production of an underlying prefix form could also be seen in J.Z.'s repetition of "irreparable." Here, however, he also showed a tendency to produce the underlying form of the root. Specifically, his production maintained phonological stress on the syllable "pair," such as it would be in the unaffixed form "repair." He did not shift stress to the syllable "re" as a result of the affixation of "-able."

---

[1] For discussion of alternative and more recent formulations of underlying forms see Caisse and Shaw (1985).

TABLE 2.1. J.Z.'s oral repetition of words.

| Target | Successful repetition rate | | Typical errors |
|--------|------|-----|----------------|
|        | No.  | %   |                |
| Happy | 10/10 | 100 | N/A[a] |
| Happiness | 10/10 | 100 | N/A |
| Unhappiness | 10/10 | 100 | N/A |
| Regular | 10/10 | 100 | N/A |
| Regulárity | 8/10 | 80 | Regularity |
| Irregular | 17/20 | 85 | Inregular |
| Irregularity | 8/20 | 40 | Inregularity |
| Legal | 9/10 | 90 | /Liygər/ |
| Legality | 16/20 | 80 | Inlegal |
| Illegal | 11/15 | 73 | Inlegal |
| Illegality | 8/15 | 53 | Inlegality |
| Legible | 10/10 | 100 | N/A |
| Illegible | 7/10 | 70 | Unlegible |
| Repair | 10/10 | 100 | N/A |
| Irreparable | 3/10 | 30 | Irrepair; inrepairable |

[a] Not available.

The word repetition performance of J.Z. suggested that his production of complex words was affected by the underlying form of constituent morphemes. This finding may be taken as evidence for the correspondence between morphological theory and morphological representations in the mind. Can J.Z.'s impairment, however, be characterized as the loss of linguistic knowledge? Could he, for example, have lost the knowledge that the prefix "in-" assimilates to the first phoneme of the root in words such as "irregular," "illegal," and "irrefutable"?

It seems impossible that J.Z.'s difficulty results from knowledge loss. An important characteristic of the pattern of errors presented in Table 2.1 is that repetition difficulties seem to map onto discrete types of morphological representations, but the performance cost associated with these representations appears to be additive. As has been discussed above, J.Z. showed difficulty with the attachment of "in-" and with stress shifting as a result of affixation. He also seemed to allow blocked affixation, producing a form such as "unlegible" which would normally be disallowed in English because of the existence of the form "illegible." Note, however, that although J.Z.'s production was systematically related to these morphological types, it was highly variable. For some words J.Z. produced the assimilated form of the prefix "in-" perfectly well, whereas for other words his ability to produce the correct form was greatly impaired. An examination of this variability leads to the view that J.Z.'s performance is negatively correlated with the number of the above-mentioned morphological processes in a particular word. Thus he could produce the word "regular" perfectly. He showed a success rate of 80% with the word "regularity," a success rate of 85% with the word "regular," but a success rate of only 40% with the word "irregularity." A similar pattern was seen with all other forms in Table 2.1 with the exception of the affixed forms of "happy," which do not involve assimilation or stress shift.

This pattern of performance does not seem consistent with a characterization of the deficit as a loss of specific linguistic representations (i.e., a knowledge loss). A more adequate explanation of J.Z.'s behavior is that he has suffered a decrease in lexical processing resources such that he can no longer produce computationally complex words. Computational complexity of particular lexical items, in this case, is a measure of the computations required in word production.

Does this finding suggest that words such as "irregularity" are not represented in the mental lexicon and that J.Z. was actually composing them on-line in the process of word production? There has not been support for such a view in the psycholinguistic research on normal subjects. The possibility remains, however, that J.Z.'s performance did not reveal the functional architecture of the normal lexicon but that he developed a particular adaptive strategy to his language deficit, and that it is this adaptive strategy that was revealed by his pattern of errors. This explanation too seems unlikely because the putative adaptive strategy would have to involve a development of fundamentally different representations in the mental lexicon and a fundamentally different mechanism of lexical access. It is expected that such global reorganization would produce widespread observable deviations from normal language functioning. J.Z. showed minimal language impairment save for the specific morphological structures discussed above and the idiomatic phrases discussed below.

## Idiomatic Phrase Production

The pattern of J.Z.'s idiomatic phrase repetition is presented in Table 2.2. He was completely unable to correctly repeat the phrase "no ifs, ands, or buts." He also showed difficulty with the other idiomatic expressions in Table 2.2. Note, however, that although J.Z. was not able to produce "no ifs, ands, or buts" correctly over 64 trials, he had complete comprehension of the meaning. When asked to paraphrase the expression he responded: "it's like when a mother says to a child to do something and he has to do it—no discussion."

J.Z. also showed difficulty with other idiomatic expressions but virtually no difficulty in the repetition of non-idiomatic phrases. By definition, idiomatic phrases are those phrases whose meaning cannot be determined by normal lexical and syntactic analysis but must be learned. If J.Z.'s inability to repeat "no ifs, ands, or buts" is related to his difficulty repeating "irre-

TABLE 2.2. J.Z.'s oral repetition of phrases.

| Target | Successful repetition rate | | Typical errors |
|---|---|---|---|
| | No. | % | |
| No ifs, ands, or buts | 0/64 | 0 | But no ifs. No ifs and no buts |
| A horse of a different color | 7/10 | 70 | A different horse |
| No doubt about it | 8/10 | 80 | Not doubt it |
| He kicked the bucket | 13/15 | 85 | He kicked it |
| The ins and outs of life | 6/15 | 40 | In and out of life |

gularity," we may safely abandon the hypothesis that J.Z.'s errors are a result of his on-line composition of complex morphological forms. If he were composing "no ifs, ands, or buts" from its constituent morphemes, he would not show perfect comprehension of the noncompositional meaning of the phrase.

The view that a single deficit accounts for J.Z.'s word and idiomatic phrase production is consistent with the view that the mental lexicon is the repository of all language units that must be learned and subsequently "listed" in memory. Under this view, "irregularity," "kick the bucket," and "no ifs, ands, or buts" are all listemes. They have in common the fact that they are listed in memory—nothing more (Di Sciullo and Williams, 1987). It remains for us to demonstrate, however, the computational relatedness of the phrases and words with which J.Z. has particular difficulty.

## Morphological Representations and the Mental Lexicon

It is argued here that J.Z.'s repetition difficulties are best understood in terms of the interaction between properties of English morphology and his diminished computational resources. It is also claimed that J.Z.'s impairment supports a particular view of the organization of the mental lexicon.

This view considers the mental lexicon, at a level of abstraction appropriate to the characterization of functional architecture, to be a store of entries. Entries can be either simple or complex. The simple entries are individual morphemes (roots and affixes). Each simple entry minimally contains the morpheme's underlying phonological form, its lexical category, and the categories to which it can attach. We may represent this information in the following manner: In (1), below, the phonological form of the word "happy" is given in phonemic slashes. Its lexical category [Adj] is represented immediately to the right in square brackets. The representation of the entry "regular" in (2) is of the same format. Entry (3), which presents the suffix "-ness," however, is of a slightly different format. The suffix is also assumed to have a lexical category (in this case N), but it additionally contains a specification of the lexical categories to which the suffix may attach (in this case Adj). The specification is represented as the lexical category {Adj} in brace brackets on the appropriate side (in this case, left) of the representation. The entry for the suffix "-ity" in (4) is of an identical format.

An example of the format of prefix entries is presented in (5). The difference between this representation and the representation of a suffix is that the square bracket is empty because prefixes do not determine lexical category in English and that the specification of the category to which the prefix can attach is on the right.

$$\text{-/hæpiy/[Adj]-} \tag{1}$$
$$\text{-/rɛgyulər/[Adj]-} \tag{2}$$
$$\text{-\{Adj\}/nəs/[N]-} \tag{3}$$
$$\text{-\{Adj\}/Itiy/[N]-} \tag{4}$$
$$\text{-/ʌn/[ ]    \{Adj,} \tag{5}$$
$$\text{V\}-}$$

Complex entries in the mental lexicon are of the same general format as simple entries. It is assumed, however, that a complex entry is one that contains a set of pointers (or associations) to its constituent morpheme entries. Each constituent morpheme contributes the contents of its lexical entry to the representation of the complex word. A complex word is therefore compositional to the extent that its entry contains the unaltered sum of the information contained in the constituent morpheme entries. In the area of lexical semantics, for example, a complex entry is perfectly semantically compositional if nothing but the understanding of the constituent forms is required to understand the complex word. In the area of phonological representation, which is the focus of this chapter, a complex word is perfectly compositional if the complex form contains all and only the phonological representations of the constituent forms. An example of this type of complex word is "unhappiness." Its representation is presented in (6).

$$\text{-/ʌn/[ ] \{Adj, V\}--/hæpiy/[Adj]--\{N\}/nəs/[N]-} \tag{6}$$

Recall that this word is precisely the type of complex word J.Z. showed no difficulty producing. The complex words that he did have difficulty producing are those whose phonological forms are not transparently related to the phonological forms of their constituent morphemes. An example of this type is the word "irregularity." The representation of this form is given in (8), below. Note that the underlying form of the word is provided by the constituents. Because we are assuming that a complex word such as "irregularity" has an individual entry in the mental lexicon and that it is understandable as "the state of not being regular," we require that its lexical entry contain both the correct complex (surface) form and its relation to its constituents (underlying form). The underlying form of "irregularity" is given in (7). In (8) the difference between underlying phonological form and surface phonological form is represented in "adjustment brackets" which have the general form: $(X \rightarrow Y)$. The form $(X \rightarrow \emptyset)$ indicates deletion, an the form $(\emptyset \rightarrow X)$ indicates insertion.

$$-/\text{In}/[\ ]\ \{Adj\}--/\text{rɛgyulər}/[Adj]--\{Adj\}/\text{Itiy}/[N]- \tag{7}$$

$$-/\text{I}\ (n>\emptyset)/[\ ]\ \{Adj\}--/\text{rɛgyul}\ (ə>æ)\ r/[Adj]--\{Adj\}/\text{Itiy}/[N]- \tag{8}$$

The representation in (8) contains more information than the transparent phonological form in (7), which J.Z. produces as a repetition error. The form in (8) is thus computationally complex owing to the additional representations needed to fulfill the requirement stated above, i.e., that a complex entry specify the correct surface form and its relation to its constituent morphemes. Thus J.Z.'s repetition impairment may be explained without reference to the loss of morphological knowledge. It is claimed here that J.Z. simply had difficulty producing lexical items that contain adjustment brackets. If so, we have provided a unitary explanation of his sensitivity to the otherwise dissimilar phonological processes of stress adjustment and assimilation.

At the level of abstraction of this formalism, it remains unclear exactly how the adjustment brackets contribute to the computational complexity of a lexical entry or why their contribution is so great. For the present, however, it may suffice to state that they increase the information load in a representation. This first approximation seems to accord with J.Z.'s general sensitivity to unusually long lexical entries, i.e., the idiomatic phrases, and may also account for his difficulty with "no ifs, ands, or buts."

As is claimed above, it is assumed that the mental lexicon is a store of listemes. Complex listemes are lexical chains. Most lexical chains are words, although some may be phrases or sentences. Under this view the idiomatic phrase "kick the bucket" would have the lexical representation in (9).

$$-/\text{kIk}/[V]--/\text{ðə}/[Det]--/\text{bʌkIt}/[N]- \tag{9}$$

Now the phrase "no ifs, ands, or buts" appears to be a special case. The first thing we note is that it is long, containing eight morphemes. If we assume, as we have been, that the functional architecture of the mental lexicon is such that each constituent morpheme of the entry must contribute the information in its lexical entry to the entry of the complex form, a number of adjustment brackets are required. The entry for the suffix "-s" has as part of its entry the specification that it must attach to nouns. The lexical entries for "if," "and," and "but" do not provide the lexical category "N." The categories therefore have to be converted by adjustment brackets in the entry for the complex form. The lexical entry for the phrase is presented in (10).

$$-/\text{now}/[Spec]--/\text{If}/[(Comp>N)]--\{N\}/s/[N]--/\text{ænd}/[(Conj>N)]-$$
$$-\{N\}/s/[N]--/\text{or}/[Conj]--/\text{bʌt}/[(Conj>N)]--\{N\}/s/[N]- \tag{10}$$

The representation in (10) is clearly complicated. The computation required for its production appears to exceed J.Z.'s on-line computational resources. The fact that (10) is complicated and is therefore difficult, falls out from the general principles of the organization of the mental lexicon outlined above. If it is the correct lexical representation of "no ifs, and ands, or buts," we may take J.Z.'s performance as offering support for the psychological reality of lexical categories. The categories must be represented in the mind if it costs him computational resources to change them as we have shown in (10).

## Where is Morphology?

The account presented here offers a single explanation for the pattern of J.Z.'s word repetition and idiomatic phrase repetition. It also offers an explanation of the apparent variability of his performance by operationalizing the notion of additive processing cost. The account takes a paradoxical position, however, with respect to the role of theoretical linguistics in the characterization of language in the brain. On the one hand, we appear to have support for the mental representations of lexical categories; and on the other, we have claimed that a computational view of the mental lexicon is more appropriate than a morphological view. This paradox may be due to the fact that theoretical morphology and syntax are designed to capture the generative properties of language but by definition, the mental lexicon contains those language structures that are not generated but, rather, are listed in memory. The complex words in the mental lexicon may be morphologically well formed, but morphology is not there. The listed phrases such as "a horse of a different color" may be syntactically well formed, but syntax is not represented in the mental lexicon. It may be that morphological knowledge can be lost in aphasia, but the patient who has lost this knowledge would be likely to present intact word comprehension and production. It would be expected that the knowledge deficit would manifest exclusively in the patient's ability to create and comprehend new (but morphologically legal) English words.

*Acknowledgments.* This research was supported in part by a Social Sciences and Humanities Research Council of Canada General Research grant 871423 to the author.

## Summary

The case of an aphasic patient who shows a morphological deficit in language production is presented. Although the patient's morphological deficit was related to specific affix types, his performance depended on the overall complexity of the word formation process. He showed no general difficulty producing multisyllabic words, and his sensitivity to morphological structure was evident only in production. It is argued that the pattern of impairment in this patient is not due to damage to the representation of morphology in the brain but, rather, reflects the interaction between linguistic properties of English morphology and computational properties of the brain.

## References

Bradley, D.C. (1980). Lexical representation of derivational relation. In M. Aronoff and M. Kean (eds.), *Juncture*. Saratoga, CA: Amma Libri & Co.

Bradley, D.C., Garrett, M.F., & Zurif, E.B. (1980). Syntactic deficits in Broca's aphasia. In D. Caplan (Ed.), *Biological Studies of Mental Processes*. Cambridge Mass: MIT Press.

Caiss, E.M., & Shaw, P. (1985). On the theory of lexical phonology. *Phonology Yearbook, 2*, 1–30.

Caplan, D. (1983). A note on the "word order problem" in agrammatism. *Brain and Language, 20*, 155–165.

Caplan, D. & Hildebrandt, N. (1988). *Disorders of Syntactic Comprehension*. Cambridge, MA:MIT Press.

Chomsky, N., & Halle, M. (1968). *The Sound Pattern of English*. New York: Harper & Row.

Di Sciullo, A.M., & Williams, E. (1987). *On the Definition of Word*. Cambridge, MA: MIT Press.

Fodor, J.A. (1975). *The Language of Thought*. New York: Crowell.

Grodzinsky, Y. (1984). The syntactic characterization of agrammatism. *Cognition, 5*, 9–46.

Henderson, L., Wallis, J., & Knight, D. (1984). Morphemic structure and lexical access. In H. Bouma & D. Bouwhuls (eds.), *Attention and Performance X*. Hillsdale, NJ: Lawrence Erlbaum.

Kean, M.L. (1977). The linguistic interpretation of aphasic syndromes: agrammatism in Broca's aphasia, an example. *Cognition, 5*, 9–46.

Lieber, R. (1981). On the Organization of the Lexicon. Unpublished doctoral dissertation, MIT, Cambridge, MA.

Mandelis, L., & Tharp, D.A. (1977). The processing of affixed words. *Memory and Cognition 5*, 690–695.

Murrell, G.A., & Morton, J. (1974). Word recognition and morphemic structure. *Journal of Experimental Psychology, 102*, 963–968.

Selkirk, E.O. (1982). *The Syntax of Words. Linguistic Inquiry Monograph I.* Cambridge, MA:MIT Press.

Stanners, R.F., Neiser, J.J., Hernon, W.P., & Hall, R. (1979). Memory representation for morphologically related words. *Journal of Verbal Learning and Verbal Behavior, 18*, 399–412.

Taft, M. (1979). Recognition of affixed words and the word frequency effect. *Memory and Cognition, 7*, 263–272.

Taft, M., & Forster, K.I. (1975). Lexical storage and retrieval of prefixed words.

*Journal of Verbal Learning and Verbal Behavior, 14,* 638–647.

Williams, E. (1981a). Argument structure and morphology. *Linguistic Review, 1,* 81–114.

Williams, E. (1981b). On the notions "lexically related" and "head of a word". *Linguistic Inquiry, 12,* 245–274.

# 3
# Morphological Reading Errors in a German Case of Deep Dyslexia

RIA DE BLESER AND JOSEF BAYER

The case presented in this chapter is used to compare agrammatisms in speech and reading. The criteria for the diagnosis of deep dyslexia are also explored and the examination procedure for establishing the location of the functional disorder is described. The main interest of the case, however, lies in the analysis of the morphological reading errors and in the determination of their linguistic and psycholinguistic status. These areas are covered in depth.

## Agrammatisms in Speech and Reading

The patient, H.J., a seamstress from a small town around Aachen, had had a cesarean section at the birth of her son when she was 22 years old. During delivery she suffered from a lung and brain embolism, which led to a relatively large perisylvian left hemisphere lesion with right hemiparesis and aphasia. In June 1978, which was 3 years after onset, she came to the RWTH hospital in Aachen for examination because of aphasia. The patient was diagnosed as a Broca's aphasic with agrammatic speech production, and she was subsequently given intensive speech therapy. During this 7-year therapy period the main improvement was in her spontaneous speech. At the time of the examination for dyslexia in 1985, agrammatic symptoms in her spontaneous speech were hardly noticeable.

Agrammatism is traditionally characterized by the lack of function words and inflected forms in speech production. The patient H.J. occasionally fit this characterization, but she also produced incorrect inflected forms. Her spontaneous speech was characterized mainly by the rare presence of complex sentence structures, which, for example, led to the frequent use of direct speech where indirect speech would have been more appropriate. In addition, she had noticeable word-finding difficulties. The following is a typical example of the patient's spontaneous speech.

*Frage*: Will Ihr Sohn abends nicht ins Bett?
*Reaktion*: Nee, freiwillig, nee ich bin nicht müde, aber jetzt habe ich gesagt, du

32

mußt im Bett, du mußt morgen Schule, Wochenende darf er dann länger aufbleiben, aber so, das geht ja nicht, die halbe Nacht.

*Question*: Doesn't your son want to go to bed at night?

*Reaction*: No, volontarily, no, I am not tired, but now I said, you have to go to bed [case error], you have to go school tomorrow, weekend he can stay up longer, but this way, it doesn't work, half the night.

*Frage*: Wer kam auf die Idee, einen Hund zu kaufen?

*Reaktion*: Also erst Tino [der Sohn]. Ich hab gesagt, hier vorm Herzen da hab ich gesagt, wenn alles vorbei ist, dann kaufen wir einen Hund, ja, und dann, Operation gut überstanden und da fing er, wann krieg ich ihn denn, ja und da konnt' ich auch nicht so, nee, sag ich, zuerst müsse wir warten, ja und dann, mein Mann sagte auch ich möchte gern nen Hund.

*Question*: Whose idea was it to buy a dog?

*Reaction*: Oh, first [the name of the son]. I said, here before my heart [means: heart attack], there I said, when everything is over, then we'll buy a dog, yes, and then, operation succeeded, then he started, when will I get it then, yes and there I couldn't very well either, no, I said, first we have to wait, yes and then, my husband also said, I would like to have a dog.

The mildly agrammatic features of this conversation sample stand in strong contrast to the pronounced agrammatisms produced in reading.

"Mir    wird    schlecht": Mir ... schlecht
Me  becomes    bad      Me ...    bad    (I'm getting ill)

"Er  schrie  er  sei  blind": Er  schreien  er  blind
He  shouted he were blind   He    shout   he blind

"Wir liebten diese Rose": Lieben .. Rose
We  loved  this  rose    Love      rose

" Du  mußt ihm den Stuhl verkaufen": Du  .. Stuhl verkaufen
You  must him the chair      sell     You    chair    sell

The reason for this discrepancy, as we will show, is the peculiar reading disorder of the patient.

During H.J.'s aphasia therapy, semantic paralexias were occasionally noted, e.g., *Kaiser* (*emperor*) for *König* (*king*) or *Vogel* (*bird*) for *Adler* (*eagle*). This finding motivated a further examination for deep dyslexia.

## Assessment of Deep Dyslexia

Apart from typical semantic paralexias, the following symptoms are also characteristic for deep dyslexia (Patterson, 1981).

1. Deep dyslexics are unable to read nonwords.

2. "Semantic" features, such as degree of abstractness, play an important role when reading words; concrete nouns are read correctly more often than abstract ones.
3. The word category of the stimuli influences the reading performance. Content words are generally read correctly more often than function words, and there is a severity hierarchy within the group of content words; nouns are read correctly more frequently than adjectives and adjectives more frequently than verbs.
4. The frequency with which morphological errors occur depends on the structure of the stimulus word: Simple morphemes without inflectional or derivational affixes provoke relatively few morphological errors, whereas they may constitute up to 50% of the reactions for words with affixes (Patterson, 1980).

For the assessment of deep dyslexia, the patient was requested to read 80 nouns, e.g., *Kunst* (*art*), and 20 noun-like nonwords with German phonotactics, e.g., *Funst* (*ort*). The nouns were subdivided into 40 concrete nouns, e.g., *Beil* (*axe*), and 40 abstract words, e.g., *Norm* (*norm*). In addition, 60 minimal pairs of content words and function words were presented, e.g., *Sieb* (*sieve*) versus *Sie* (*she*). The percentage of correct responses is listed below:

| | | | |
|---|---|---|---|
| Words (n = 80) | .635 | Nonwords (n = 20) | 0 |
| Concrete Nouns (n = 40) | .875 | Abstract Nouns (n = 40) | .375 |
| Content Words (n = 60) | .87 | Function Words[1] (n = 60) | .47 |

The percentage of semantic paralexias to the total amount of errors was remarkably high, even for deep dyslexics.

| | | | |
|---|---|---|---|
| Words (n = 80) | .53 | Nonwords (n = 20) | 0 |
| Concrete Nouns (n = 40) | 1.00 | Abstract Nouns (n = 40) | .44 |
| Content Words (n = 60) | .68 | Function Words (n = 60) | .47 |

According to the cardinal symptoms given by Patterson (1981), this patient clearly suffered from deep dyslexia.

We then examined the influence of word category, which is said to constitute a severity hierarchy in patients with deep dyslexia (nouns > adjectives > verbs > function words, wherein ">" is defined as "more correct responses than"). The patient was requested to read underived and uninflected word forms. The percentage of correct reactions to the various word categories was as follows.

---

[1] The category "semantic paralexias to function words" includes substitutions of one function word by another, e.g., *mir* (me$_{dative}$) for *mein* (my$_{possessive}$), *du* (*you*$_{nominative}$) for *dir* (*you* $_{dative}$).

Nouns (n = 55)              .74
Adjectives (n = 72)         .50
Infinitive Verbs (n = 91) .47
Function Words (n = 80).36
    Prepositions (n = 28) .57
    Conjunctions (n = 12) .33
    Pronouns (n = 24)      .29
    Modal Verbs (n = 16) .13

The proportion of semantic paralexias to the total incorrect responses was again high, but the percentage varied across the various types of content words.

Nouns              .79
Adjectives         .44
Infinitive Verbs .33

Following are some examples of semantic reactions.

| *Stimulus* | *Reaction* |
|---|---|
| Nouns | |
| Beil (axe) | Hammer (hammer) |
| Grund (ground) | Boden (floor) |
| Eisen (iron) | Stahl (steel) |
| Fürst (sovereign) | Prinz (prince) |
| Menge (mass) | Gruppe (group) |
| Herd (stove) | Ofen (oven) |
| Dunst (vapor) | Qualm (smoke) |
| Adjectives | |
| tapfer (courageous) | mutig (courageous) |
| düster (dark) | dunkel (dark) |
| trübe (overcast) | das wetter, bewölkt (the weather, cloudy) |
| ledig (single) | nicht verheiratet (not married) |
| sanft (soft) | zärtlich (tender) |
| gering (few) | wenige (few) |
| Verbs | |
| retten (save) | helfen (help) |
| kosten (cost) | zahlen (pay) |
| läuten (ring) | klingeln (ring) |
| rennen (race) | laufen (run) |
| saufen (drink a lot) | trinken (drink) |
| stechen (stick) | Messer irgendwas, schneiden (knife something, cut) |
| sinken (sink) | kentern (sink) |

The word category effect was nevertheless not as pronounced as might have been expected according to the predictions in the English literature.

There was no big difference between adjectives and verbs, whereas there was a lot of variance within the category of function words. For example, prepositions were read better than the infinitive of verbs, and modal verbs were much more severely affected than main verbs.

One factor that may help to explain these different results for function words could be referential content, which is much stronger in prepositions than, for instance, in conjunctions. The word category effect could thus be related to the concreteness effect. It is important to note that the disorder cannot be explained by a general impairment of phonological access, but that it is restricted to processing written material. H.J. could easily repeat every function word spoken to her.

The results for verbs and adjectives may be related to the fact that in German few adjectives are underived. We therefore had to include low frequency words in our corpus of underived adjectives. It is well known that frequency plays a role in the reading of deep dyslexics.

Strikingly, only a small portion of the responses to our word category corpus could be considered morphological errors (nouns: 1% morphological versus 18% semantic; adjectives: 3% morphological versus 22% semantic; verbs: 15% morphological versus 18% semantic). In this corpus, only underived and uninflected word forms were presented. Therefore the relatively small number of morphological errors corresponds to the observation made by Patterson (1980) that morphological errors are most frequent in morphologically complex words. The higher amount of morphological errors in the responses to infinitival verbs may be related to the fact that the infinitive is already a morphologically complex form itself. This subject is discussed in greater detail later in the chapter.

## Assessment of the Functional Locus of the Disorder

First, a paradigm of lexical decision was used, whereby the patient is requested to decide if a written or spoken letter or sound chain is a word. The stimulus material consisted of chains of four syllables, constructed in the following manner.

1. EK: existing compounds consisting of two content morphemes and a (variable) number of grammatical morphemes, e.g., *Kugelschreiber* (ballpoint), *Schlagersänger* (hit singer).
2. PA: nonwords constructed by substituting the initial phonemes of the composite parts of the compound words, e.g., *Wugelkreiber*.
3. PE: nonwords constructed by substituting the final phoneme of the composite parts of the compound words, e.g., *Schlagessängel*.
4. SPK: nonexisting compounds in which the composite parts were phonemically correct and semantically meaningful, but the compounded product makes no sense, e.g., *Kugelsänger*.

5. NS: nonsense words constructed after a phonemically illegitimate CVCV pattern, e.g., *Kupäwagü*.

Each category contained 15 items and was offered twice. Altogether 150 items were presented to the patient in randomized order, with the request to judge their correctness. The lexical decision task was performed in auditory and written presentation.

In the auditory modality, H.J.'s results were entirely normal. When given PA, PE, and NS nonwords in written presentation, H.J. made no incorrect decisions either. For real compounds, she made 3 incorrect decisions of 30 by visual presentation. Interestingly, she rejected all semantic pseudocompounds (SPK) upon visual presentation. In some cases, she commented, "not those two together," or else she would try to construct some compositional semantics but she would finally reject the composition.

Sammlerhochzeit (collector wedding): When many get married, maybe, but no.

Geschenkskrümel (present crumb): Too few presents, but no.

Nadelfeuer (needle fire): When there are too many, but no.

Pflanzenwohnung (plants dwelling): Could exist, but never heard of it.

These results indicate that H.J. could provide a rather specific semantic interpretation for an input chain upon auditory as well as graphemic presentation. Therefore her deep dyslexia does not seem to arise on the input side, between the graphemic stimulus and the semantic system, or in the semantic system itself, as the patient could even make judgments of semantic anomaly for compounds. The disturbance is more likely situated between the semantic representation and the phonological word form because, like semantics, the phonological word form itself is also undisturbed, as shown by the fact that H.J. can repeat all of the SPK pseudowords without problems, although typical reading reactions were the following.

| Sammlerhochzeit (collector wedding) | Sammeln-hochzeit (collect-wedding) |
| Kugelsänger (ball singer) | Bleistift irgendwas, Sänger (pencil something, singer. (Note the semantic similarity between *Kugel–Schreiber*, or (ballpoint) and *Bleistift*, (pencil). |
| Kleiderbesteck (clothes cutlery) | Kleider-Porzellan (clothes-porcelain) |
| Pflanzenwohnung (plants appartment) | Wohnung-Blumen nicht (appartment, flowers not) |
| Bienentabak (bees tobacco) | Bienen und Zigarren-innen (bees and cigars . . . in them) |

The patient was further tested for reading comprehension of the classes of words she could hardly read aloud, i.e., modal verbs and pronouns. It was done using a sentence/picture matching paradigm. For the modal verbs, there was a choice of only two pictures. Modal verbs are difficult to depict; and if one were to include several distractors, there would be more than one plausible target candidate. Our set included items such as (1) a boy with his leg in a cast and hung in a traction sling (target: der Junge *kann* nicht laufen—the boy is unable to walk), and (2) a boy who has a sour face while being pushed to move by his father (target: Der Junge *will* nicht laufen—the boy is unwilling to walk). Even with this restricted set, the target picture can be chosen only by comparing the two pictures and picking the one that most plausibly fits the sentence. Among the 22 sentences to be matched, the patient made five errors.

The task for reading comprehension of pronouns was more easy to develop. A group of 22 simple semantically reversible SVO sentences were constructed with a pronoun as subject and another pronoun as object, e.g., *Sie* sucht *ihn*—she searches him. There were two distractor pictures, one with a distractor for the subject (*Er* sucht *ihn*—He searches him) and one with a distractor for the object (*Sie* sucht *sie*—She searches her). On this task, the patient made 4 errors among 22 which is significantly above chance.

Thus the patient's poor performance regarding reading aloud modal verbs and pronouns does not stand in proportion to her rather mild disorder in grasping their meaning from graphemic presentation.

Additional data show that the route H.J. utilizes for reading proceeds as follows.

1. Segmentation of the letter chain is performed with the help of the semantic-lexical system.
2. The graphemic segments so identified are matched with an appropriate (concrete and referentially transparent) meaning.
3. The semantic content so identified is matched with a corresponding entry in the phonological lexicon.

H.J. did not segment graphemic chains by identifying the syllabic or morphemic structure as such, but only through interaction with the semantic lexical system. When reading neologisms, H.J. chose any part of the letter chain that could function as a word. For instance, when reading the stimuli of the lexical decision task described previously, she produced the following reactions.

| Gasenläher: | Gas | (gas) |
| Säkelradel: | Rad | (bicycle) |
| Hogelpäfig: | Gel | (wet gel) |
| Mutafazö: | Mut | (courage) |
| Kauchiräpo: | Po-kau | (the behind-chew) |
| Rasiemwasset: | Was | (what) |

Probleslösunt:   Pro        (pro)
Binaifodü:       Bin        (am)

The last three responses, where the patient picked up a function word, are comparatively rare. Usually these choices are ignored during segmentation.

Real words are segmented by H.J. under semantic guidance. When morphologically ambiguous words are offered in which both a function word and a content word can be identified (e.g., *Beil-Eid* versus *bei-Leid*, *axe-oath* versus *with-suffering* = condolences), the composite semantics is decisive for segmentation. This situation is no different from what normal people do. "Gardenpath" words such as the following were used to examine this effect.

Her-z-eigen                    *Herz. . zeigen, her. zeigen*
  her/herz, zeigen/eigen      heart show      to show = show up
  (to/heart, show/own)

Bei-l-eid                      *Mitleid*
  bei/beil, leid/eid             with suffering = pity
  (with/axe, suffering/oath)

Only in the case of low frequency words or abstract words could semantics not provide the necessary information for correct segmentation.

Ab-t-rudeln                    *abt*  (as in church) *. .ruder*
  ab/abt, trudeln/rudeln         *abbot*                        oar
  (off/abbot, move/packs)

Zu-g-riff                      *Zug. . ∅*
  zu/zug, griff/riff             train
  (to/train, grip/reef)

As the direct phonological-lexical route is missing, H.J. proceeded with the identified graphemic segments to the cognitive system and combined them with their referential semantics. It was then often linked to the wrong phonological form, resulting in semantic paralexias. Segments without clear referential semantics cannot be realized phonologically, which explains the following.

1. *Differences between proper names and common nouns.* H.J. could read only 6 of 70 proper nouns; the remaining 64 produced no response. When asked to identify the sex, she made only 8 errors. Twenty of the names had been chosen because they were exceptions to the German rule that names ending on consonants are masculine, and names ending on vowels are feminine. Examples of the irregular pairs are *Otto* (male ending on a vowel), *Gertrud* (female ending in a consonant). Another 20 names

showed no differences in form between male and female, e.g., *Martin*, *Karin*. The remaining 30 names were regular, e.g., *Josef*, *Claudia*.

For the simple common nouns in this test material, 20% of the responses were semantic paralexias, which was about 50% of the total error rate, zero reactions included. Most reactions were related to the stimulus item by coordination/synonomy. The second most frequent type of semantic paralexia were paraphrases.

2. *Differences between derivational affixes.* H.J. paraphrased the diminutive endings *-chen* and *-lein* with "klein" (small). Both endings were sometimes realized phonologically as *-chen* after such circumscription: in 8 of 15 cases of the *-chen* diminutives and in 6 of 15 of the *-lein* diminutives.

Briefchen (small letter)     Brief.kleines.chen (letter small.diminutive
                                     affix)
Männlein (small men)         kleiner Mann.Männchen (small man.man+
                                     diminutive affix)
Türchen (small door)         Tür.kleine.Türchen (door.small.door+
                                     diminutive affix)

The prefix *un-* was also paraphrased semantically with the free morpheme *nicht* (not). H.J. resorted to this strategy not only to describe the transparent derivations but often also in pseudoderivations.

unmutig (displeased)         nicht mutig (not couragous)
unbillig (unfair)            nicht billig (not cheap)
unwegsam (impracticable)     nicht Weg irgendwas (not way something)

The phonological form *un-* was not produced once in 45 cases, *nicht* in 15 of 30 derivations and in 7 of 15 pseudoderivations.

The suffix *-bar* (-able) was treated differently again. Although it can be paraphrased semantically, it cannot be done so with a single word. A paraphrase occurred only once in 30 cases: *kann man mischen* (one can mix it) for *mischbar* (mixable). However, *-bar* was often realized phonologically (in 13 of 30 cases). Because *-bar* also has a homophonous noun, which H.J. could read (e.g., *Bühnenbar* was read as *Theater..bar*), the interpretation of *-bar* as a suffix was unlikely at least in some of the reactions.

machbar (doable)             bar aber..keine Ahnung (bar but..no idea)
trinkbar (drinkable)         trinken..bar (drink..bar)
ergreifbar (graspable)       greifen..wieder bar (grasp..again bar)

The suffixes *ig*, *-isch*, and *-lich* can hardly be paraphrased semantically. These suffixes have the syntactic category of adjective and are used to derive adjectives from nouns. They were rarely realized phonologically (of 30 items each, 4 for *-ig*, 0 for *-isch*, and 5 for *-lich*). Reactions were mainly restricted to the nominal root.

| | |
|---|---|
| staubig (dusty) | Staub (dust) |
| heimisch (homy) | Heim (home) |
| mündlich (orally) | Mund (mouth) |

So far, the differential treatment of the above suffixes seems to be compatible with an alternative explanation to the "semantic content" hypothesis. The diminutive and negation affixes are category-preserving, whereas the adjectival suffixes -ig, -isch, and -lich have a syntactic function converting nouns into adjectives. The patient might have a particular inability to read syntactic affixes. To test this assumption, we presented words with other negation affixes, 10 with the adjectival -los (-less), and 10 with the verbal prefix ent- (de-), e.g., herz-los (heart-less), ent-gift-en (de-poison: to take the poison out).

The patient correctly read 3 of 10 -los items and 3 of 10 ent- items. The remaining reactions provoked semantic paraphrases, as in the case of the nonsyntactic un-:

| | |
|---|---|
| zahn-los (tooth-less) | Zahn. . .ohne Zähne (tooth. .without teeth) |
| brot-los (bread-less) | Brot. . .frei.ohne Brot (Bread. .free.without bread) |
| ärmel-los (sleeveless) | Arm. .frei (arm. .free) |
| herz-los (heart-less) | Herz. .arm (heart. .poor) |
| ent-haupten (be-head) | . .Tod (gestures "Head off") (death) |
| ent-fett-en (de-grease) | nicht fettig (not greasy) |
| ent-gift-en (de-poison) | Gift. .nicht giftig jetzt, aber früher war das giftig (poison. .not poisonous now, but before it was poisonous) |

These examples indicate that semantically paraphrasable affixes were processed by the patient irrespective of their syntactic status.

## Morphological Reading Errors

The morphological structure of words is richer in German than in English. This fact motivated us to take a closer look at the interaction between the internal structure of the morphological lexicon and the direct, semantic-lexical route for reading.

The starting point of our own examination and of the current debate in the literature was a descriptive study by Patterson (1980) on the "derivational" errors two English-speaking deep dyslexics had produced. The term "derivational error" used by the author included both inflectional and linguistically speaking derivational morphological relations between stimulus and response. In her study of the two patients with deep dyslexia, P.W. and D.E., who like our patient were also of the output kind, Patterson concluded that the derivational paralexias collected from the reading

TABLE 3.1.  Reading of affixed words–affix responses of two English deep dyslexics.

| Response \ Target | -ing | -er | -ly | -y | -ed | -est | -tion | Other | Delete | Total No. |
|---|---|---|---|---|---|---|---|---|---|---|
| -ing | .58 | .07 | — | .02 | .04 | — | .02 | .02 | .25 | 53 |
| -er | .13 | .57 | .10 | — | — | — | — | — | .20 | 30 |
| -ly | .09 | .05 | .48 | — | — | — | — | — | .38 | 21 |
| -y | .07 | — | — | .80 | — | — | — | — | .13 | 15 |
| -ed | .09 | — | — | .05 | .05 | — | .09 | .09 | .64 | 22 |
| -est | — | .45 | — | — | — | .09 | — | — | .45 | 11 |
| -tion | — | — | — | — | — | — | .22 | .56 | .22 | 9 |
| *Total* | 40 | 27 | 13 | 14 | 3 | 1 | 5 | 8 | 50 | 161 |

© From Patterson (1980). With permission from Routledge & Kegan Paul Ltd.

data revealed a systematic pattern. Seven productive suffixes were available for analysis, and all of them were frequently deleted. There were, however, differences in the correct production of the various suffixes; for example, the suffixes -*ing*, -*er*, -*ly*, and -*y* were often read correctly, whereas -*ed* and -*st* were never produced correctly. Also, the suffixes -*ing* and -*er* were frequently used as substitutes for other suffixes (Table 3.1).

The author herself did not offer any theoretical explanation for the observation of these patterns. An attempt at a theoretical explanation for the Patterson data was later made by Futter and Bub (1986). These authors used the framework of lexicalist morphology/phonology (Kiparsky, 1982). In the next section we will evaluate their proposal.

## Morphological Errors and Linquistic Models

### MORPHOLOGICAL ERRORS AND LEXICAL MORPHOLOGY

Lexical morphology adopts three layers in the lexicon that have different functions in word building.

Level 1 contains derivational and inflectional word formation with root-changing affixes (e.g., *decide*/*decision*).
Level 2 contains phonologically neutral affixation processes for derivation and compounding (e.g., *man*/*manly*).
Level 3 contains regular inflectional processes.

On the basis of such a model, Futter and Bub (1986) assumed that morphological paralexias would reveal the following characteristics.

I.  Simplifications, i.e., suffix deletions, would occur most frequently, whereby the suffixes of level 1 would be omitted more often than those of level 2, and the latter, again, more often than those of level 3.

II. In cases of suffix substitution, affixes of levels 2 and 3 would be used for those of level 1 and not the reverse (e.g., *decision* → *deciding*).

On the whole, there would exist a hierarchy of disturbance in which the n − 1 level would always be more prone to disturbance than level n, i.e., level 1 > level 2 > level 3 (> = more disturbance prone).

Both assumptions can be examined in German by means of inflected verbs, which may follow a regular or irregular paradigm.

| Condition | Regular | Irregular I | Irregular II |
|---|---|---|---|
| Infinitive | spülen | bringen | fahren |
| | (rinse) | (bring) | (drive) |
| Present, 3rd person singular | spült | bringt | fährt |
| | (rinses) | (brings) | (drives) |
| Past simple | spülte | brachte | fuhr |
| | (rinsed) | (brought) | (drove) |
| Past participle | gespült | gebracht | gefahren |
| | (rinsed) | (brought) | (driven) |
| Imperative | spül | bring | fahr |
| | (rinse) | (bring) | (drive) |

According to I., the imperative form of the verb would be expected to be the most frequent default form, as it is the only existing form with possible homophony to the stem; e.g., *gehen* (to go)/*geh* (go).

According to II., one would expect a difference between regular and irregular inflection forms. Futter and Bub did not assume a general lexical disturbance in cases of deep dyslexia, i.e., no regularizations of irregular forms should occur as, for example, *lief* → *läufte* (ran → *runned*). They, rather, assumed that when a patient reads a word all morphologically related words are activated as well. Contrary to normal readers, however, the patient is unable to filter out the inadequate forms. When deciding which form to choose from the variety of candidates, he picks out the more regular form. Accordingly, quantitatively more errors would have to be expected when irregular forms are read, and irregular forms should occur less often as reactions as well.

H.J. read a total of 316 verb forms (infinitive, present, imperfect, and perfect participle—79 of each). For the infinitive, there were 16% morphological errors and for the other forms, 49%, 43%, and 46% were morphologically incorrect, respectively. None of these morphological errors consisted in the production of an imperative or a verbal root. The responses were restricted exclusively to infinitives, present tenses, morphologically related nouns, participles, and the past tense form. The frequency of occurrence of these forms is given as a percentage in Table 3.2. The number of items includes correct and morphologically related re-

TABLE 3.2. H.J.'s responses when reading 4 different verb forms.

| Target \ Response | Inf. | Pres. | Imperf. | Partic. | Noun |
|---|---|---|---|---|---|
| Inf. (n = 50) | .74 | .10 | .00 | .02 | .14 |
| Pres. (n = 49) | .59 | .21 | .00 | .12 | .08 |
| Imperf. (n = 40) | .50 | .18 | .15 | .02 | .15 |
| Partic. (n = 49) | .55 | .12 | .00 | .25 | .08 |

(n = number of items which did not attract semantic or visual errors or zero-responses; correct responses are boxed.)

actions to a specific verb form. Those errors showing semantic or visual similarity and zero reactions are not considered here.

The system in H.J.'s reading is obvious. The patient reads approximately 20% of the target forms correctly, whereas in over 50% of the reactions the infinitive is used as a default form. This explains why in the case of infinitive forms "apparently correct" responses are so frequent.

The analysis of the patient's responses to regular and irregular imperfect tense forms provided the results shown in Table 3.3. None of the 30 regular imperfective forms was read correctly. In 11 of 30 cases the infinitive was substituted; in 2 of 30 cases a present tense was substituted; and in 5 of 30 cases the substituted form was a morphologically related noun. The remaining reactions were either visually (n = 1) or semantically (n = 6) related words or zero reactions (n = 5). Of the 49 irregular imperfect forms, 6 were read correctly, 9 were realized as an infinitive, 5 as present tense, 1 as a participle, and 1 as a noun. Of the remaining responses, 10 were visually related, 3 were semantically related, and there were 14 zero reactions.

These results contrast sharply with the expectations set up by Futter and Bub. If an imperfective form was read at all, it was an irregular, phonologically marked form, not a regular one.

Additional evidence concerning a difference between reactions to inflectional forms of level 1 and those of level 3 can be obtained by comparing the plural forms of nouns to the comparative and superlative forms of adjectives.

TABLE 3.3. H.J.'s reading of regular and irregular imperfective forms.

| Target \ Response | Imperf. | Inf. | Pres. | Partic. | Noun | θ | Other |
|---|---|---|---|---|---|---|---|
| Imperf. reg. (n = 30) | 0 | .36 | .07 | .00 | .17 | .17 | .23 |
| Imperf. irreg. (n = 49) | .12 | .18 | .10 | .02 | .02 | .29 | .27 |

With the exception of the -s plural, German plural forms are largely unpredictable and must thus be localized in level 1 of the lexicon.[2] In contrast, the comparative and superlative form of adjectives may count as regular inflection and would thus be located in level 3 of the lexicon.

The patient was offered 10 singular forms and 30 plural forms to read. The plural forms were composed as follows: ⁻ə (*Stock/Stöcke*), ⁻∅ (*Vater/ Väter*), and ⁻ər (*Glas/Gläser*). Of the 10 singular forms, 9 were read correctly; and in one case there was a semantic paralexia in the singular. In contrast, only 5 of the 30 plurals were read correctly (*Züge, Hüte, Bücher, Häuser, Gärten*); and in four additional cases, the first reaction was a singular noun that was then changed to a plural, whereas in two cases a paraphrase with *viele* (many) intervened. In 20 of 30 cases, only the singular form was provided; and in one case there was a zero reaction.

This performance was restricted exclusively to phonological output by graphemic input, however. When the patient was requested to orally pluralize singular forms (the 30 stimuli were the same as those in the graphemic plural reading task), 27 of 30 correct plural forms were produced; in only 3 cases did a stimulus remain unchanged. The patient thus shows only minimal impairment in her ability to produce plural forms. Therefore the morphological errors produced during reading are not caused by disturbances of the morphophonological representation itself but by the ability to adequately process graphemic stimuli. Once more, it could be shown that this disorder must be on the output side of the semantic system by asking the patient to match word cards with a singular versus a plural noun (18 items each) to pictures with one or several objects. In this task, H.J. only made 1 of 36 possible errors, which means that she grasped well the plural versus the singular meaning of the graphemic input that she could not transform phonologically.

Regular inflection (level 3) applies in the case of comparative and superlative forms of adjectives. Patterson (1980) had reported that her two English patients almost never produced the superlative affix -est and that the comparative ending -er was far more likely to be produced. Our patient H.J. read 12 highly frequent monosyllabic adjectives correctly and with ease. The comparative and superlative forms of these adjectives, presented in a different session, were never read as such. Eleven of the com-

---

[2] This assumption is extensively discussed for the German language by De Bleser and Bayer (1986). Neurolinguistic data are also offered there on the lexical status of the productive s-plural: Patients practically lacking syntactic abilities were still capable of productively deriving this form with their isolated morpho-phonological lexicon. The attribution of German plural forms (with the exception of -s) to level 1 of the lexicon is not contradicted by Köpcke's data (1987). Köpcke offered neologisms to native-speaking German controls to be pluralized, e.g., "das flett." The variety of reactions to the monosyllabic neologisms was remarkable, and agreement on one specific plural form ranged at best between 40 and 66%. The three possible "umlaut" forms (⁻θ, ⁻ə, and ⁻ər) were almost completely ignored.

paratives and eight of the superlatives were read in the positive equivalent. Never did a semantic paraphrase with *mehr* (more) or *meist* (most) occur. One comparative form (*älter*: older) was changed to a noun (*alter*: age). In two cases where the target form was a superlative, the weak congruence form occurred (*kleinst/kleine*, *blindest/blinde*). In another two cases, there was incorrect segmentation so that the noun *Test* (test) (carrying stress unlike the suffix -*est*) occurred as a reaction (*ältest* → *Test*; *ernstest* → *ernst*. . Test). Twenty additional comparatives, all with the "umlaut" form, were mixed with 50 nouns ending on -*er*. The latter were monomorphemic nouns such as *Hocker* (stool) and agentive nouns such as *Drucker* (printer). Even in this condition, no comparative form was read, and the positive form occurred as a reaction in 16 cases. There were three semantic paralexias and one zero reaction.

A comparison of H.J.'s reactions to plural noun forms and graded adjectives shows that, as with the imperfective forms of the verbs, irregular inflections stand a slightly better chance of being read correctly than the regular forms. This finding may imply that Futter and Bub have psycholinguistically misinterpreted the hierarchy of lexical morphology. Instead of being 1 > 2 > 3 (> expressing more prone to disorder), it is actually the opposite, 3 > 2 > 1. This order is also more in line with the "feeding relations" postulated in such layered models, according to which, level 1 can feed into level 2, but 3 cannot (*lice-infested* but not *\*rats-infested*, in other words, irregular plurals precede compounding, but regulars must follow it). For pathology, one would expect it to mean that level 2 could still function well when level 3 is disturbed but not when level 1 is impaired.

In general, however, H.J.'s correct reading of inflected forms is too rare to support or reject such assumptions. What the data clearly express is that H.J.'s morphological errors cannot simply be captured by "omission or substitution of suffixes," as is done frequently in the current literature. Nouns and adjectives are not simply stripped of their suffixes, but the citation form (singular noun, positive adjective) is used as a default form, even if it is based on a different stem (nonumlaut stem) than the inflected form. The substitution of one suffix for another did not occur at all in H.J.'s data for nouns and adjectives.

For verbs, simple suffix deletions would often have been possible, resulting in an imperative. However, H.J. did not produce imperatives. Instead, in over 50% of the cases another form, i.e., the infinitive, was substituted for the inflected form. Other less frequent default forms were the third-person present tense (over 10% of the cases) or a morphologically related noun. A simple subdivision of suffixes in regular and irregular ones is not sufficient for the interpretation of the data, as the regular suffixes are clearly not treated equally with respect to suffix substitution processes. Even if the present tense, the past tense, and the participle are part of a regular paradigm, the imperfective form is never used for substitution and the participle only rarely so. H.J.'s data, rather, indicate that there are lexical marking principles at work in regular paradigms and that the infinitive is the least marked and therefore frequently occurs as a default form.

Some anecdotal data of H.J. may show the strength of this tendency toward the unmarked form. Not only did she read infinitives instead of imperatives (the "stem" forms), but she did so even at the expense of syntactic structure. In German verbs, the verbal particle precedes the infinitive, but it must, due to the verb-second rule, follow the imperative. In 4 of 10 cases, H.J. substituted the lexical citation form with particle-plus-infinitive for an imperative-plus-particle.

| | |
|---|---|
| Lies vor (read aloud) | Lesen...vorlesen (to read...to read aloud) |
| Steig hinauf (go up) | Steigen...hinuntersteigen (to go...to go down) |
| Spring hinunter (jump down) | Springen...hinunterspringen (to jump...to jump down) |
| Such weiter (look further) | Suchen...weitersuchen (to look...to look further) |

A similar pattern with transgression of syntactic structure occurred in another investigation dealing with compound words. Even for verb-noun compound words, in which the verb stem would be the target, the following reading responses were made.

| | |
|---|---|
| Ziehmutter (foster mother) | Mutter...ziehen (mother...to pull) |
| Schießpulver (gun powder) | schießen..pulver (to shoot..powder) |
| Meßbecher (measuring cup) | messen.Glas (to measure.glass) |
| Sprechangst (stage fright) | Angst..sprechen (fright..to speak) |
| Kehrbesen (broom) | kehren Besen (to swipe broom) |
| Klappbett (camp bed) | Bett...zusammenklappen (bed...to fold together) |

These examples may serve to summarize that (1) affix deletion is not the rule and (2) affix substitution was not arbitrary in H.J.'s paralexias to morphologically complex graphemic stimuli.

## MORPHOLOGICAL ERRORS AND SPLIT MORPHOLOGY

An alternative position concerning the lexical representation of morphology was taken up by Anderson (1982) in his split morphology model. According to this view, there is a basic difference between syntax-generated inflectional processes and lexically constructed derivational forms. This position has been adopted in cognitive neuropsychology by Caramazza et al. (1988).

A possible difference between inflection and derivation was investigated using the reading data of H.J. She was given 155 morphologically complex words to read that have a transparent derivation. Of these words, 100 were derived from nouns (20 verbs, 80 adjectives) and 55 from verbs (40 nouns, 15 adjectives). Construction characteristics were the following.

Derivation of nouns (n = 100)
  V (n = 20): nouns ending on *er* + *n*, e.g., pfeffer-n (to pepper)
  A (n = 80): noun + *ig* (n = 35), e.g., witz-ig (funny)
              noun + *lich* (n = 30), e.g., ängst-lich (nervous)
              noun + *isch* (n = 15), e.g., neid-isch (jealous)
Derivations from verbs (n = 55)
  N (n = 40): verb stem + *er*, e.g., druck-er (printer)
  A (n = 15): verb stem + *bar*, e.g., trink-bar (drinkable)

They were compared with 20 simple monomorphemic nouns ending with -*er* (e.g., keller: cellar) and 60 monomorphemic adjectives with the following characteristics.

Highly frequent monosyllabic A (n = 15), e.g., schön (pretty)
Highly frequent bisyllabic A (n = 15), e.g., bequem (easy)
Monomorphemic A ending with -*er* (n = 15), e.g., tapfer (courageous)
Monomorphemic A ending with -*ig* (n = 15), e.g., ledig (single)

For the underived words, no derivational errors were made. Along with correct reactions (46%), mainly semantic paralexias (29%) and zero re-actions (18%) were produced. In contrast, 55% of the stimuli derived from nouns were read with derivational errors, 73% of which consisted of only the noun stem, i.e., the singular noun form, 24% of the plural noun form. The reactions to stimuli derived from verbs contained 38% deri-vational errors, 57% of which were infinitival verbs and 38% the third person singular present tense.

The pattern of the responses to derived forms is qualitatively not dif-ferent from those to inflected forms. As responses to forms with a noun stem, a singular noun form is primarily produced. Here too it makes no difference whether the noun stem in the derived form is the same one as that in the underived one. Stimuli such as *göttlich* (divine) are read as *Gott* (god) as frequently as stimuli such as *weiblich* (female) are read as *Weib* (wife). The plural forms occurred mainly as reactions to derivations on -*lich* without umlaut stem (in 6 of 15 cases, e.g., *kindlich → Kinder*). We have as yet no systematic explanation for this finding. In the derived forms with the verb stem, the substituting form was primarily the infinitive, the second most frequent one a present tense form.

A direct comparison of derived agentive nouns on -*er* and inflected comparative adjectives on -*er* shows some quantitative difference in the patient's ability to produce a correct response (Table 3.4). This overall better performance for agentive nouns, however, may well be due to the different grammatical category of the complex target, nouns leading in general to correct reactions more frequent than adjectives.

In conclusion, it seems that none of the linguistic models of the lexicon is

TABLE 3.4. Comparison of derived agentive nouns and inflected comparative adjectives on -er.

| Words | Correct | 0 | Semantic | Visual | Morphological |
|---|---|---|---|---|---|
| | | | -er | | |
| Comparative (n = 32) | — | 1 | 3 | 1 | 27 |
| Agentive (n = 30) | 8 | 6 | 2 | 3 | 11 |

substantially supported by H.J.'s data—neither the lexical morphology model nor the model of split morphology. For the lexical morphology model, the difference between the processing of regular and irregular forms was not sufficiently outspoken; and with respect to the model of split morphology, no essential difference could be shown to exist between derivation and inflection. In addition, neither of these models is capable of offering an explanation for the systematic patterns evident in the reading errors of H.J.

If one keeps in mind, however, that the patient's lexical abilities are well preserved in other modalities, the psycholinguistic irrelevance of the internal structure of linguistic models comes as less of a surprise.

It need not necessarily be expected that the disturbances in processing graphemic stimuli would follow specific structural aspects of the internal lexicon, given that it is functioning well in other modalities. This case is more likely explained in terms of processing impairments that are specific to graphemic stimuli, whereby markedness hierarchies of the intact lexicon dictate specific compensatory strategies for this impairment.

## Morphological Errors and Information-Processing Models of Reading

We now trace the specific contribution this case may provide to the currently existing psychologically oriented literature regarding the source of morphological errors in information-processing models. As Badecker and Caramazza (1986) have shown, there exist as yet no conclusive arguments that prove that errors considered "morphological" from an operational point of view show a functional difference compared to other errors, either semantic or visual. In other words, there is no conclusive evidence for an independent morphological error source, in contrast to semantic and visual errors, which are clearly differentiated from each other. For example, the English word *thread* has visual similarity but no semantic similarity to *threat*, and *strong* has only semantic but no visual relation to *harder*. In contrast, many so-called morphological errors have morphological as well as semantic and visual affinities to the target word (e.g., *connection/disconnected*).

In the following sections we will discuss some assumptions regarding the source of the morphological error that have appeared in the literature.

## Morphological Errors to Affixed Words, Reflecting a Deficit of GPC

Patterson (1982) proposed as a possible source of morphological errors that the lexical routes would process only stems, whereas affixes (and function words) would be much more dependent on mechanisms of grapheme-phoneme correspondence (GPC). A disturbance of the GPC route, which the standard theory assumes for deep and phonological dyslexia, would therefore lead to morphological errors as well. This assumption has become problematic since Caramazza et al. (1985) reported a patient who was incapable of reading nonwords (i.e., indicating that the GPC was disturbed) yet who did not produce morphological errors.

## Morphological Errors to Affixed Words, Reflecting a Disorder of the Presemantic Morphological Parser

Job and Sartori (1984) argued that the morphological errors performed by their patient Leonardo were caused by a defect of a presemantic morphological parser. In their model of visual word processing, morphologically complex visual words are first parsed into their component morphemes, which then access the orthographic input lexicon in which root morphemes and affixes are distinguished. If there were a deficit in this presemantic parser, it would be predicted that when reading (1) only regularly inflected words should be affected, as irregular words do not undergo morphological parsing; and (2) morphological errors should occur only for truly prefixed words (e.g., *ripreso* in Italian, *repayment* in English) but not for pseudoprefixed words (e.g., *ritardo* in Italian, *religion* in English). Both predictions were met by the patient Leonardo. He read irregularly inflected words better than regular ones (15 of 33 correct versus 6 of 33), and he made only one morphological error among 15 pseudoprefixed words in contrast to 6 of 15 truly prefixed words.

Badecker and Caramazza (1987) offered an alternative solution for this dissociation that is not based on a functional-morphological disturbance. According to these authors, Job and Sartori's data are just as compatible if a visual source of disturbance is assumed as with the adopted morphological source of disorder. Badecker and Caramazza argued as follows: Pseudo-prefixed words such as *religion* have a cohort of visually similar items (e.g., *legion*, *lion*), which, however, are unrelated to each other in the lexical-semantic system. Words with real prefixes such as *repayment* usually have visual cohorts as well, e.g., *payment*, *repay*, *pay*, *repaying*, and *paying*, but these words also have a semantic relation to the target. As a consequence, it is much more likely that morphologically related forms are produced for words with real affixes (having visual-semantic cohorts) than for pseudoaffixed words (with only visual cohorts) even if the source of the disorder is of a visual nature. This effect is called "interface influence." Errors caused by the disturbance of a certain single component, such as the visual input system, may nonetheless reflect organizational traits of another component (such as the semantic component) which is closely connected to the first in a kind of interface relation.

The idea that the source of morphological errors may not be functionally morphological was further elaborated and given empirical support by Funnell (1987).

### MORPHOLOGICAL ERRORS TO AFFIXED WORDS, REFLECTING THE SAME DEFICIT PRINCIPLES THAT UNDERLIE VISUAL-SEMANTIC ERRORS IN NONAFFIXED WORDS

Funnell (1987) took tissue with Job and Sartori's conclusions about the relation between morphological errors and a deficient presemantic parser. These conclusions rested crucially on the differential processing of affixed and pseudoaffixed words. However, as Funnell criticized, the item groups had not been matched for frequency or imageability of either the targets or the "stems" they contained. Frequency is known to play a role for visual recognition, imageability for semantic processing. Therefore if these variables are not controlled in affixed versus pseudoaffixed words, differences in performance may arise that are not related to the affix status, i.e., to morphology. Instead, they might reflect the same visual or semantic constraints that condition the reading of simple monomorphemic words and morphologically complex words alike.

Funnell investigated two patients with material controlled for morphological complexity, frequency, and imageability. One patient, C.J., was a phonological dyslexic and is not discussed here. The other patient, J.G., was a deep dyslexic patient, i.e., he could not read nonwords and made semantic, visual, and morphological paralexias when reading words. Moreover, Funnell demonstrated that his reading of words was strongly influenced by imageability. Highly imageable words were read well, whereas high frequency words with low imageability were rarely read correctly.

Patient J.G. was asked to read 32 pairs of suffixed and pseudosuffixed words matched for mean frequency and imageability. They were presented twice, so that each category contained 64 items, *office-r/corn-er*; *hungr-y/bell-y*. The patient made stem errors for words of both categories. Stem errors were defined as (1) reading of the stem/pseudostem only, e.g., *mastery: master*; *irony: iron*; (2) substituting another ending on the stem, e.g., *speaker: speaking*; *irony: ironing*.

Although the ratio of stem errors to pseudosuffixed words (13 of 64: actually 7 of 32 words) was only half of the ratio of stem errors to suffixed words (30 of 64: actually 19 of 32 words), the results seemed to be clear counter-evidence to a morphological parsing explanation, which would predict no stem errors for pseudosuffixed words as opposed to suffixed ones.

A posthoc analysis seemed to indicate the effect of the relative imageability of the target and stem for the occurrence of stem errors. This point was tested more stringently in another experiment in which 85 items represented three types of words: pseudosuffixed words (e.g., *arm+y*), embedded words (e.g., *grave+l*), and truly affixed words (e.g., *sand+y*). Imageability was varied as follows: highly imageable target and stem (*army, gravel, sandy*); target with low and stem with high imageability (*mouser, wicker, cowl*); target and stem with low imageability (*nicety, tenure, realm*).

The author's predictions were as follows: Words with high imageability on all counts should basically be read correctly, those with low target but high stem imageability should give rise to stem errors, and words low on all counts should lead to visual errors and omissions. These predictions were all borne out for J.G.; in other words, imageability was found to be the determining factor for successful reading of affixed words as well as stems (or pseudoaffixed and embedded words). Therefore morphological errors should be seen only as "apparently morphological" but not functionally so. They do not, Funnell concluded, reflect damage to a presemantic morphological parser; in fact, J.G. did not provide any evidence for existence of such a morphological parser.

To arrive at this conclusion, however, the author used a trick in her data analysis. Remember that the first experiment had shown that J.G. made (at least) double the amount of stem errors on suffixed words as he did on pseudosuffixed ones. Moreover, when the author did a post hoc analysis of the target-versus-stem imageability effect, she found that, in contrast to pseudosuffixed words, the patient made few correct responses to suffixed words with a highly imageable target but a low imageable stem (actually 4 of 7 items times two presentations), and quite a few stem errors occurred in these cases (in fact, 3 of 7 items). Funnell argued that they were not morphological errors but semantic errors; "Since J.G. makes a considerable number of semantic errors when reading unaffixed words, he is likely to make semantic errors when reading affixed words. If such errors share a common root morpheme with the target word, these errors will be indistinguishable from morphological (or stem) errors" (Funnell, 1987, p. 516).

The author used the results of another experiment to decide that those stem errors are in fact semantic. When asked to point to the name of the person when given two morphologically related word cards such as "typist," "typing," J.G. performed at chance. "J.G.'s problem in comprehending suffixed words could be explained as a partial failure to access the meanings of affixes. Since affixes are relatively low in imageability, this failure fits with J.G.'s failure to access the meanings of other word types of low imageability" (Funnell, 1987). Consequently, Funnell gave those suffixed words with a high imageability rating for both stem and target a different treatment in the second reading experiment, which was controlled for imageability. She analyzed them together with the non-

TABLE 3.5. Experiment 2: number of response types (correct, stem errors, visual errors, and omissions) produced by J.G. to 85 words grouped according to predictions based on imageability levels of the target word and stem.

| Target/stem imageability | Word set | Response predicted | Reading response | | | |
|---|---|---|---|---|---|
| | | | No. of words | Correct | Stem errors | Visual errors and omissions |
| High/high[a] | C | Correct | 24 | 19 (+1) | 2 | 2 |
| Low/high[b] | D | Stem errors | 34[c] | 6 (+2) | 17 (+1) | 7 |
| Low/low | E | Visual errors and omissions | 27[d] | 0 (+2) | 4 | 19 |

[a] With the exception of suffixed words.
[b] Including high/high suffixed words.
[c] One unclassified error not included in the analysis.
[d] Two unclassified errors not included in the analysis.
*Note:* Semantic errors, counted as correct responses or stem errors, are given separately in parentheses.
© From Funnell (1987). With permission from Lawrence Erlbaum Assoc. Ltd.

suffixed items which have a low imageable target and a highly imageable stem! The results for J.G. analyzed in this (rather unorthodox) way are shown in Table 3.5. The predicted responses and responses obtained overall were significantly related, $\chi^2 = 50.21$, df = 4, $p < .001$.

However, the prediction that imageability, not morphology, is the principal variable is borne out only if one accepts, with the author, the theoretical bias that morphologically complex words of high imageability are actually low-imageable for the patient, i.e., if one assumes that the cause of the stem errors to suffixed words is semantic rather than morphological—but this point is exactly what the author wanted to prove. She stated: "With one small exception, predicted patterns of performance in this experiment were not based upon distinctions between suffixed, pseudo-suffixed, and embedded words.... The single exception to this recognized the fact that J.G. is likely to make stem errors to suffixed words even when the target word is higher in imageability than the stem" (Funnell, 1987, p. 521). If one reanalyzes the data without this strong assumption in a theory-neutral way, the results no longer speak as convincingly against a morphological parser account and in favor of a unified imageability account.

We took the suffixed words with a highly imageable target and stem out of the category with low imageable targets/high imageable stems (set D) and put them back in set C, so far containing pseudosuffixed and embedded words with overall high imageability. Set E contained words with overall low imageability. The results for J.G. were then as shown in Table 3.6.

The prediction that Hihi would be read correctly was no longer fulfilled. The maximum probability criterion was now .82 (for Pc = .90/.95, at least 30 of 38 or 33 of 38 items should have been read correctly). Furthermore,

TABLE 3.6. Reanalysis of experiment 2 of Funnell (1987).

| Target/stem imageability[a] | Funnell's predicted response | No. of words | Reading responses | | |
|---|---|---|---|---|---|
| | | | Correct | Stem errors | Visual errors/ omissions |
| Hihi | Correct | 38 | 23 (+3) | 10 | 2 |
| Lihi | Stem errors | 20 | 2 (+1) | 10 (+1) | 6 |
| Lili | Visual errors + omissions | 27 | — (+2) | 5 | 20 |

[a] Hihi = high imageability of target and stem. Lihi = low imageability of target, high imageability of stem. Lili = low imageability of target and stem.

using Fischer's exact 2 × 2 table test (PC computer program StatXact 1989), there was no longer any significant difference between the occurrence of stem errors to Hihi and to Lihi items ($p = .1943$, one-sided, n.s.). The number of stem errors in the Hihi category was indeed largely due to the reinclusion of truly affixed words. Again using Fischer's 2 × 2 exact table test, affixed words triggered significantly more ($p = .0019$, one-sided) stem errors (8 of 14) than did nonaffixed words (2 of 24). Although it was no longer the case for the Lihi category, it must be remarked that there were only five truly affixed words (probably with one misclassification: *purser/purse*) of which four triggered a stem error, in contrast to 15 non- or pseudoaffixed words (with the likely misclassification of "signify") with six stem errors. The category Lili was a mixed one, including many function words in both stem and target groups (12 of 27), which are known to provoke zero reactions in deep dyslexic patients.

To test Funnell's prediction with our own patient, H.J., we used the more stringent condition of her test; i.e., the target was of low imageability and the stem of high imageability in pseudoaffixed or embedded words. Funnell here predicted the occurrence of "stem errors." By way of comparison, we gave our patient 40 "stems" to read in isolation, and 12 of them were used in pseudosuffixed words, 28 in embedded words. Examples are shown in Table 3.7. The low-imageable items were given together in a first presentation so as to not bias "stem reading"; the high imageable "stems" were presented later in the same session.

Of the low-imageable items, 15 of 40 were read correctly. In only 2 of 40 cases did the "stem" occur as the only response. In another six cases, the

TABLE 3.7. Stem errors.

| High-imageable stem (n = 40) | Low-imageable pseudosuffix (n = 12) | Low-imageable embedded (n = 28) |
|---|---|---|
| Beton (concrete) | Betonung (emphasis) | |
| Fass (barrel) | Fassung (mounting, composure) | |
| Ei (egg) | | Eile (haste) |
| Klo (toilet) | | Klobig (clumsy) |

highly imageable stem or a semantic paraphase thereof was part of the naming reaction, but additional responses or comments showed that H.J. did not consider this reading response to be adequate.

| | |
|---|---|
| auto-mat (car/automat) | Auto. . .maschine irgendwas (car. . . machine something) |
| strauch-eln (bush/stumble) | Strauch. . .laufen irgendwas (bush. . .run something) |
| ehe-r (marriage/sooner) | Ehe. . hat nichts mit Ehe zu tun (marriage. . has nothing to do with marriage) |

The remaining reactions were as follows.

1. Semantic paralexia to the whole item (n = 7), e.g., Komma-ndo (comma/command, detachment): Soldaten irgendwas, Befehl (soldiers something, command)
2. Morphological paralexia to the whole item (n = 5), e.g., hand-el (hand/ trade): handeln (to trade)
3. Zero-reaction (n = 4)
4. Non-classifiable (n = 1)


Of the 40 high-imageable "stems" presented in isolation, 36 were spontaneously read correctly; there was one zero reaction, one paraphrase, and one semantic paralexia; and in one case the "complex" item was remembered and transferred onto the single one.

This task shows that H.J., like J.G., had a clear imageary effect in reading, but this fact does not override morphological parsing. Words that are pseudocomplex rarely lead to "pseudomorphological errors," which strongly indicates that the morphological errors H.J. made when reading morphologically complex words should not be interpreted as simple semantic errors. The exact nature of the morphological error in H.J., as in J.G., still needs to be explained.

## The Nature of the Morphological Error in H.J.

To appreciate the nature of H.J.'s morphological errors, we compared her performance to the different proposals in the literature.

### H.J.'s MORPHOLOGICAL ERRORS: DO NOT REFLECT THE GPC DEFICIT

The fact that H.J. processed at least some affixes semantically testifies to their lexical status (see above for a report on the diminutives -chen and -lein and the negative un-). Moreover, an analysis of the semantic paralexias to derived adjectives (n = 58) demonstrates that syntactic aspects of suffixation were computed by H.J. Leaving aside the multiword paraphrases (21%), 60% of the semantic paralexias to derived adjectives were also adjectives, indicating that the syntactic category of the suffix had been recognized by the cognitive system. Examples are the following.

| | |
|---|---|
| herrlich (delicious) | froh (happy) |
| niedrig (low) | klein (small) |
| morgig (of tomorrow) | früh (early) |
| herrisch (domineering) | stark (strong) |

These data defeat a purely prelexical account of affixation.

### H.J.'s Morphological Errors: do Not Reflect a Parsing problem

A disorder in the presemantic morphological parser would predict that only regular, not irregular, affixation would be impaired. We showed earlier in the chapter that there was no significant different between these parameters in H.J.'s data. Moreover, the data against GPC also speak against an affix-stripping assumption, as (some) affixes obviously do contact the cognitive system.

### H.J.'s Morphological Errors Reflect a Semantic Variable that Affects both Affixed and Nonaffixed Words

We disagree with Funnell's conclusion that cases such as ours do not provide evidence for morphological parsing in reading. Not only can one see the patient tracing the morphology with her finger, but morphologically complex and pseudo-complex words are treated differently. In the former case, they generally trigger a morphological default system of verbal infinitives, singular nouns, and positive forms of the adjective. The default system even works if the derivation or inflection uses a different stem than the citation form (e.g., *göttlich* (divine), response: *Gott* (god), *kürzer* (shorter), response: *kurz* (short); *tückisch* (whimsical), response: *Tücke* (whim). Reducing morphological errors to the presence of visual-semantic cohorts would ignore this obvious system.

However, we do agree with Funnell that these morphological errors do not result from damage to the morphological parser but, rather, from variables affecting the reading of affixed and nonaffixed words alike, i.e., semantic factors.

If we adopt such a unitary explanation in terms of referential semantics, the following observations can be covered.

1. A strong effect of imageability could be seen for reading morphologically simple words in the partial replication of Funnell reported above.
2. Proper names cannot be read by H.J., as they do not have enough intensional structure (descriptive force) to invoke the semantic system, which is required for phonological realization.
3. Those morphologically complex forms that contain an affix with hardly any referential semantics can be realized only phonologically because the linguistic system offers morphologically unmarked forms as substitutes.

# Conclusion

Marshall and Newcombe (1973) introduced three tasks for future research: (1) formalization of a word recognition and word retrieval model; (2) extension of the interpretive value of such models by considering languages with other writing systems, e.g., syllabic and ideographic ones; and (3) investigation of the relation between dyslexias and dysgraphias. Fifteen years of research on disorders of written language within this paradigm have led to favorable results. In no other area of neuropsychology has the interaction between theory and pathology been so intensive. For each point of the above program, several books have meanwhile been published.

The models available to date have the disadvantage that the internal architecture of the single components have remained largely undetermined. With the elaboration of such models for specific languages, some questions therefore have remained in principle unanswerable. One example is the representation and processing of morphologically complex forms and function words.

With respect to the morphological errors H.J. made in her reading performance, we could show that they were not caused by either semantic or morpholexical defects. The error pattern that emerged was interpreted as a lexical compensation process that made use of markedness principles. We purposely prefer to remain somewhat vague as to exactly what is actually compensated because our knowledge about the internal structure of the orthographic input lexicon is still too unspecific. The existing proposals on these structures clearly cannot explain our data. On the one hand, there is the "addressed morphology model," in which the processing of morphologically complex lexemes involves activation of the word as a single, whole unit from the orthographic lexicon. On the other hand, a "morphological parsing model" has been proposed that assumes a complex word is first decomposed into roots and affixes and that processing then proceeds only according to roots (see Butterworth, 1983, for a comparison of these two views).

Within the context of the first model, it would be difficult to explain H.J.'s reactions—in particular, why there is such a stable pattern of morphological paralexias: One would expect variability in the responses. According to the second, parsing model, the semantic paralexias the patient makes would have to belong to the syntactic category of the word's root only and not to the syntactic category of the entire lexeme. H.J. processes at least the syntactic information of the affix, and wherever possible its semantic contribution as well.

We can hardly claim to have found a general solution for the problems of deep dyslexia or, more specifically, for morphological errors. However, we do believe that we can plausibly infer the symptoms of H.J.'s reading from the assumed disorders. In particular, we have demonstrated in this case study how morphological errors may arise by graphemic presentation without any defect of the visual input system, with a well functioning morphological parser, and with retained morphology in the internal lexicon and the output lexicon. Morphological errors can arise at the interface between the graphemic input lexicon and the semantic system.

The unitary explanation we propose is that referential semantic contents determine what can be read, for content words, function words, and affixes. Our data are irreconcilable with theories starting from a general problem with "little words," as H.J. does not simply ignore function words and even bound morphemes. Our results are consistent, however, with the general observation that deep dyslexics can identify concrete words more easily than abstract ones, and that a word class effect can be recognized when reading.

# Summary

The nature of the morphological error in word reading based on an analysis of the responses of a German patient with "deep dyslexia" has been discussed. The case provides compelling evidence for morphological decomposition in visual word recognition. At the same time, it shows that the occurrence of morphological paralexias does not necessarily presuppose an impairment of the process involved in morphological decomposition during lexical access. The source of such errors may lie in particular properties of the reading system that affect affixed and unaffixed words alike, i.e., low referential semantic content. The pattern of the morphological errors in this case and their dissociation from nongraphemic morphological processing does not reflect a morphological deficit but, rather, the properties of spared morphological representations that provide markedness features used for coping with the deficit of processing morphologically complex graphemic stimuli.

*Acknowledgment.* This chapter is the result of research supported by the DFG (German National Science Foundation) and by the Max Planck Institute for Psycholinguistics. We would like to thank Klaus Willmes for his help with the statistical analysis.

# *References*

Anderson, S.R. (1982). Where's morphology? *Linguistic Inquiry, 13,* 571–613.

Badecker, W., & Caramazza, A. (1987). The analysis of morphological errors in a case of acquired dyslexia. *Brain and Language, 32,* 278–305.

Butterworth, B. (1983). Lexical representation. In B. Butterworth (ed.), *Language Production* (Vol. 2). London: Academic Press.

Caramazza, A. (1986). Reading and lexical processing mechanisms. *Reports of the Cognitive Neuropsychology Laboratory.* Baltimore: The Johns Hopkins University.

Caramazza, A., Laudanna, A., & Romani, C. (1988). Lexical access and inflectional morphology. *Cognition, 28*, 297–332.

Caramazza, A., Miceli, G., Silveri, M.C., & Laudanna, A. (1985). Reading mechanisms and the organisation of the lexicon: evidence from acquired dyslexia. *Cognitive Neuropsychology, 2*, 81–114.

De Bleser, R., & Bayer, J. (1986). German word formation and aphasia. *The Linguistic Review, 5*, 1–40.

Funnell, E. (1987). Morphological errors in acquired dyslexia: a case of mistaken identity. *The Quarterly Journal of Experimental Psychology, 39A*, 497–539.

Futter, C., & Bub, D. (1986). A level-ordered theory of morphological paralexias. Presented at the Academy of Aphasia, Nashville, October 1986.

Job, R., & Sartori, G. (1982). Prelexical decomposition: evidence from acquired dyslexia. *British Journal of Psychology, 74*, 159–180.

Job, R., & Sartori, G. (1984). Morphological decomposition: evidence from crossed phonological dyslexia. *The Quarterly Journal of Experimental Psychology, 36*, 435–458.

Kiparsky, P. (1982). From cyclic phonology to lexical-phonology. In H. van der Hulst & N. Smith (eds.), *The Structure of Phonological Representation. Part I.* Dordrecht: Foris.

Köpcke, K.-M. (1987). Die Beherrschung der deutschen Pluralmorphologie. *Linguistische Berichte, 107*, 23–44.

Marshall, J.C., & Newcombe, F. (1973). Patterns of paralexia: a psycholinguistic approach. *Journal of Psycholinguistic Research, 2*, 175–199.

Patterson, K. (1980). Derivational errors. In M. Coltheart, K. Patterson, & J.C. Marshall (eds.), *Deep Dyslexia*. London: Routledge and Kegan Paul.

Patterson, K.E. (1981). Neuropsychological approaches to the study of reading. *British Journal of Psychology, 72*, 151–174.

Patterson, K.E. (1982). The relation between reading and phonological coding: further neuropsychological observations. In A.W. Ellis (ed.), *Normality and Pathology in Cognitive Functioning*. London: Academic Press.

StatXact (1989). *Statistical Software for Exact Nonparametric Inference*. New York: Cytel Software Corporation.

# 4
# Semic Extraction Behavior in Deep Dyslexia: Morphological Errors

ANDRÉ ROCH LECOURS, SONIA LUPIEN, and DANIEL BUB

As pointed out by Marshall and Newcombe (1980) in their historical per-spective on the conceptual status of deep dyslexia and by Coltheart (1980), clinicians have long been aware that brain-damaged subjects with this par-ticular type of reading disorder can often retrieve semantic information about written open-class words that they cannot read[1] (Benson & Gesch-wind, 1969; Beringer & Stein, 1930; Faust, 1955; Luria, 1970). The status of closed-class items is much less known in this respect, in particular that of bound morphemes (such as *-ion, -ing, -ed* in English). A basic feature of the syndrome is that all deep dyslexic patients delete, add, and substitute bound morphemes (e.g., reading "beautiful" as "beauty" or "beautify"). The level to which the target affix is categorized has not been well docu-mented, however. Theories of affix stripping (see Henderson, 1985, for review) would presumably not consider that morphological paralexias can entail adequate understanding of closed-class bound morphemes, as such units are considered to be removed from the stem prior to lexical ac-cess. There might be other mechanisms behind the production of morpho-logical errors in dyslexic patients, however, including the failure to recover the correct phonology after their grammatical sense has been extracted.

In the present chapter, which one might consider as a complement to the preceding one, we demonstrate that—provided he or she has, to some extent, acquired explicit metalinguistic knowledge—a deep dyslexic can indeed extract at least part and sometimes all of the meaning of the closed-class bound morphemes in words that nevertheless yield morphological paralexias. Evidence in this respect is sought within a corpus of more than 2000 reading responses produced by a patient observed by one us (ARL) at la Salpêtrière in 1966. A number of these responses were accompanied by or restricted to comments of the patient as to the meaning of the stimuli

---

[1] Just as one form of word-finding difficulty has long been known in which, when asked to name objects or images of objects, the aphasic (or sometimes the normal speaker) is capable of providing pertinent circumlocutory information without being able to retrieve the target word itself.

he was requested to read aloud, a phenomenon to which we refer as "semic extraction behavior."

Doctor Adelbêrt, a right-handed francophone obstetrician, was born in 1919. Until the age of 47, he enjoyed good health and devoted a fair part of his time to reading. At the end of June 1966 he consulted for persistent headaches and was diagnosed to have a Foster-Kennedy syndrome. Surgery permitted removal of an apricot-size meningioma from the patient's left olfactory groove but left him with right hemiplegia and speech suppression.

In November of the same year, the patient was transfered to the speech-therapy center of la Salpêtrière. Neurological examination then revealed that severe brachiofacial hemiplegia was still present. Somesthesia was normal or nearly so. There existed no auditory deficit, and visual fields were full. Except for mild buccofacial apraxia, there existed no apraxia or agnosia of any type.

Although the patient indeed remained "talkative" and was an excellent communicator, one who often resorted to prosody, mimicry, and gesture when lexicon failed him, his spontaneous speech production was reduced, with severe word-finding difficulties and mild phonetic disintegration. Prototypical agrammatic behavior was present. The patient's residual language abilities were systematically assessed using the Ducarne Aphasia Battery (1964). Although they were much less obvious than in spontaneous speech, word-finding difficulties were observed in oral naming tasks. Not taking into account the mild arthric disorder, repetition of syllables and isolated words was normal; phonemic paraphasias and verbal deviations, typically closed-class word deletions, were observed in sentence repetition. Written production was entirely dependent on the patient's left hand. Spontaneous writing was reduced to the patient's signature. Single word copy was normal for familiar concrete items (other word types were not tested). Writing to dictation was severely impaired: "Il fait beau" (The weather is nice) was, for instance transcoded as "le bo" (the "bo"). Oral comprehension was considered to be normal; that is, the Ducarne word-picture and sentence-picture matching tasks were executed flawlessly, and Pierre-Marie's test was completed rapidly, without hesitation or error. Written comprehension was normal for word-picture matching, and only a few errors occurred when matching series of written sentences to the drawings of comic-strip-like stimuli.

Reading aloud was strikingly impaired, and prototypical of the behavior then labeled in Paris as *alexie aphasique* and now known everywhere as deep dyslexia (a much better characterized reading disorder since the seminal publication of Marshall and Newcombe in 1966). Isolated letters were frequently misread; nonwords were never read correctly. On the whole, the patient's attempts at reading aloud were limited to single words or locutions. He spontaneously insisted that he could no longer read by decoding letters and syllables, and that written function words had become a mystery to him. Verbal paralexic errors occurred 50% of the time, and a fair proportion of them were of the semantic type.

Further testing of the patient's reading abilities was pursued during the last 2 months of 1966, as Dr. Adelbêrt was undertaking an intensive program of speech therapy. He was then administered a reading test comprising 1400 stimuli, more than 90% of which were single words. Each stimulus was typed in black at the center of a white index card (15 × 10 cm). The order of the cards was randomized, the they were presented successively, in free vision and without temporal constraints. The patient's repsonses were tape recorded and transcribed, eventual comments included. Because the record of the last 94 stimuli was lost, data presented in this chapter bear on the first 1306 items. The list included 1129 French words, 50 nonwords (isolated letters excluded), and 127 other written entities of various types. Word stimuli comprised 904 open-class words (not including 40 interjections): 114 nouns, 240 adjectives, 20 adverbs with a "+*ment*" (+ly) suffix, 250 verbs (50 infinitives, 100 participles, 100 conjugated verbs), and 166 "others." Closed-class items were 50 pronouns, 25 prepositions, 30 conjunctions, 10 determinatives (articles, possessives, demonstratives, and so forth), 40 adverbs without a "+*ment*" suffix, and 10 "others."

Of the 1306 stimuli 43% yielded the expected responses only, 46% yielded one or several inadequate responses, and 11% led to the production of at least one paralexic response and the expected one as well. A total of 2088 behaviors were noted, 1062 (51%) of which corresponded to expected responses and 988 (45%) to paralexic responses; absence of response occurred in 38 cases only (3%).

All of the global linguistic characteristics now considered to be associated with deep dyslexia (Marshall and Newcombe, 1973) were documented to exist in Dr. Adelbêrt's "aphasic alexia": (1) with the exception of two to four letters words, an increase in number of errors was observed with an increase in number of letters in stimuli—*length effect*; (2) independently of word length, an increase in number of errors occurred from nouns (32%) to adjectives (48%), to function words (57%), to infinitives (62%), to participles and conjugated verbs (74%)—the *category effect*: (3) as assessed on a subset of 650 nouns, adjectives, and infinitives of comparable length, error production was greater for "infrequent" than for "frequent" words[2] (28% versu 59%)—the *frequency effect*; and (4) as observed on a subset of 120 nouns of comparable length and frequency, error production was greater for "abstract" than for "concrete" words (23% versus 43%)—the *picturability effect*.

From the descriptive point of view, a large proportion of verbal para-lexias fell into one of the three categories commonly recognized to occur in deep dyslexia. Whatever the type of error, inventory transgression within a same class of words (open-class or closed-class) was not unusual, but class transgression was most exceptional. There existed, in certain cases, immediately obvious formal[3] but no obvious semantic kinship between target and response ("visual errors," "formal paralexias"). It could occur both when the stimulus was an open-class word [see (1) below] and when it was a closed-class word [see (2)]:

(1a) arôme (aroma)      → aumône (charity)
(1b) aminci (thinned)   → amical (friendly)

---

[2] Stimuli with an entry in Gougenheim's (1958) dictionary of fundamental French were considered to be "frequent," the others to be "infrequent."
[3] At least 50% of letters shared by stimulus and response.

(2a) moins (less)        → moi (me)
(2b) quand (when)        → dans (in)

There existed, in other cases, immediately obvious semantic but no obvious formal kinship between target and response (semantic errors, semantic paralexias). It could also occur when the stimulus was an open-class word [see (3)] and when it was a closed-class word [see (4)].

(3a)  chaise (chair)     → table (table)
(3b)  verrat (boar)      → porc (pig)
(4a)  la[4] (the)        → unc (a)
(4b)  car (because)      → donc (therefore)

Moreover, in a large proportion of cases [43.6% of all verbal paralexias (447 instances)[5]], there existed both semantic identity and formal identity or near-identity between the lexical components of the target and response, the error then being restricted to one or several closed-class bound morphemes. Although such paralexias are currently labeled "derivational errors," we avoid this term and, rather, use "morphological error" or "morphological paralexia," the reason for this choice being that, depending on stimuli and responses, such errors can be described by reference to either derivational morphology or inflectional morphology. Most of Dr. Adelbêrt's paralexias thus bore on polymorphemic words and qualified as morphological paralexias in which the error could involve prefixes or suffixes [see prefixes and/or suffixes in (5a), (5b), (6), (8), (9a), and (9b), and prefixes in (5d), (7), and (9d)—*derivational paralexias*] as well as morphological endings [see morphological endings in (5c), (5d), (9c), and (9d)—*inflectional paralexias*]. Moreover, such errors could take the form of affix of morphological ending deletion ["stripping": See (5) and (6)], addition ["filling": see (6) to (8)], or substitution ["swapping": see (8) and (9)].

(5a)  ad-verbe (ad-verb)             → verbe (verb)
(5b)  jardin-ier (garden-er)         → jardin (garden)
(5c)  mange-ant (eat-ing)            → mange (eat)
(5d)  en-gourd-i (be-numb-ed)        → gourd (numb)
(6)   utilc-ment (use-ful-ly)        → in-utile (use-less)
(7)   chant-ant (chant-ing)          → en-chant-ant (en-chant-ing)
(8a)  croy-ance (belief)             → in-croy-able (un-believ-able)
(8b)  en-semble (en-semble)          → as-sembl-ée (as-sembl-y)
(9a)  con-jonc-tion (con-junc-tion)  → in-jonc-tion (in-junc-tion)
(9b)  cert-ainement (cert-ainly)     → cert-itude (certitude)

---

[4] Target and response and marked for feminine gender.
[5] Phenomenologically, therefore, the production of morphological paralexias can be a bona fide semiological feature of deep dyslexia (and, as in the present case, it can even dominate the clinical picture).

(9c)  écriv-ant (writ-ing)          → écriv-ain' (writ-er)
(9d)  dé-riv-ant (de-riv-ing)       → ar-riv-er (to ar-rive)

It seems that the proportion of morphological deviations [such as (5) to (9)] within the Adelbêrt corpus is strongly suggestive that, in line with a number of theories of the mental lexicon (see Henderson, 1985, for a review), polymorphemics with productive affixes, morphological endings, or both—although presented as "single-word" stimuli—can give rise to morpheme-by-morpheme access. One might consider, as an observation further enhancing this suggestion, the fact that on a number of occasions our patient first directly went for the root of such stimuli, and sometimes could not overtly proceed further. Examples cited in (5), above, are potentially illustrative of this point, and examples cited in (10), below, are still more so.

(10a)  dé-riv-ant (drift-ing)           → rive (shore)
(10b)  dé-test-able[6] (de-test-able)   → tête (head)
(10c)  en-cercl-er (to en-circle)       → cercle (circle)
(10d)  en-nobl-i (en-nobl-ed)           → noble (noble)
(10e)  em-bell-issant (em-bell-ishing)  → belle[7] (beautiful)

It is true that, considering stimuli and corresponding responses as wholes, one has to agree that formal and semantic kinship are both inherent to morphological paralexias (see above). Given what we have just said, however, it might be more appropriate to consider that with such deviations formal and semantic kinships are eventually to be sought by comparison of the replaced to the replacing closed-class bound morpheme. Doing it with the Adelbêrt corpus led us to observe bound-Morpheme substitutions in which formal but no semantic kinship was apparent [see (11)], cases in which semantic but no formal kinship was apparent [see (12)], and cases in which both semantic and formal kinships were apparent [see (9c) and (13)]. One has to reckon, however, than in most cases the only kinship between replaced and replacing closed-class bound morphemes was, within the Adelbêrt corpus, their common derivational or flexional potential with regard to the spared lexical root [see (9a), (9b) and (9d)].

(11)  ignor-ait (ignor-ed)       → ignor-ant (ignor-ant)
(12)  recev-ant (receiv-ing)     → recev-eur (receiv-er)
(13)  merc-ier (haberdash-er)    → merc-erie (haberdash-ery)

Our purpose having so far been to illustrate the typology of reading errors within the Adelbêrt corpus, we have restricted the examples that we have cited to presentation of "stimuli" and "responses." It should be

---

[6] Literally "de-head-able.'
[7] Marked for feminine gender.

noted, however, that "semic extraction behavior" (SEB) often accompanied responses, whatever the error type (see above). For instance, in (10c) and (10e) our unexpurgated notations were the following.

(10c) encerler (to encircle)       → Dr. A.: (Makes a circling gesture
                                              with his left hand.)
                                              "cercle"
                                              "No."
                                              "encercler"
(10e) embellissant (embellishing)  → Dr. A.: "belle" (beautiful)
                                              "Beautiful, yes, but
                                              better."
                                              "Ah! yes:"
                                              "embellissement"
                                              (embellishment)

As of this point, one should remember and keep in mind that Dr. Adelbêrt had received university-level education and was to a large extent explicitly aware of morphogrammatical rules, that he was a passionate reader, that he was being reeducated by Blanche Ducarne[8] when tested for his reading abilities, and, above all, that he was then encouraged, as testing went on, to respond even when he felt uncertain and to provide information about his uncertainties, which he did without reluctance in view of the familiar relationship he and the examiner had developed. It was also understood that the latter could challenge his responses whether they were faulty or correct. Had the patient been instructed otherwise or had the testing situation been more constrained, behaviors to be reported below—and maybe interpretations to be proposed as well—might have been appreciably different.

As in (14), below, there were instances when, as observed by pioneers (see above), Dr. Adelbêrt's behavior in front of a given stimulus was limited to SEB.

(14a) quasi (almost)    → Dr. A.: "I can a little, then no."
                           ARL: "Read the word."
                           Dr. A.: "Don't know."
(14b) cracher (to spit) → Dr. A.: "In the handkerchief: to soil."
                           "No. Don't know."
(14) Siméon (Simeon)    → Dr. A.: "A name."
                           "The Apostle."
                           "The Bibles."
                           "Rats! Don't know."
                           "André" (Andrew)
                           "No."

---

[8] That is, reeducated by reference to his specific semiology and taking his cultural background into account.

"Jean" (John)
"No."
"Pierre" (Peter)
"Peter? No."
"Don't know."

There were also instances when SEB would be followed by the production of a full-fledged open-class semantic paralexia as in (3) [see (15a) and (15b)] or—most interestingly, is it not?—would turn out to have been targeted on a word formally similar to the target and be followed by the production of an open-class formal paralexia as in (1) [see (15c) and (15d)].

(15a) tante                    → Dr. A.: "A man: the woman, no, the man
      (aunt; homosexual)                everything."
                                        "homosexual"
                                        "That's it!"

(15b) perdu (lost)             → Dr. A.: "There. To look around
                                        everywhere."
                                        "égaré" (lost)

(15c) décalerons [(we)         → Dr. A.: (Hides the morphological ending
      will unkey]                       "ons" with his left index.)
                                        "There: infinitive."
                                        "On the wall, then..."
                                        "arracher" (to tear out)
                                        "No."
                                        "enlever" (to remove)
                                        "No. Neither."
                                        "décoller" (to unglue)
                                        "That's it."

(15d) "rendrez" [(you)         → Dr. A.: "...la porte"[9]
      will give back]                   "No."
                                        "prendre" (to take)
                                        "...renseignement"[10]
                                        "Neither."
                                        "Don't know."

As in (16), probing from the examiner could also yield information as to the extent of Dr. Adelbêrt's SEB abilities.

(16a) tolérance (tolerance)    → Dr. A: "libéral" (liberal)
                                 ARL: "Look at the word. Do you
                                      really read 'liberal'?"
                                 Dr. A.: "Yes but don't know. To read,
                                      no Tac-tac!"

---

[9] Prendre la porte: to take a leap.
[10] Prendre un renseignement: to ask for an information.

"'Liberal' yes?"
"Ah, no!"
"libéralité" (liberality)
"Not..."
"libre" (free)
"Come on! 'Liberal': yes."

(16b) perroquet (parrot)   → Dr. A.: "There now! On the branch.
Croak. To speak." (With his left
index, the patient draws on the
table the profile of a bird with a
big hooked bill. He insists on the
bird's posture.)
"Beautiful!"
ARL: "Toucan?"
Dr. A.: "No."
ARL: "Eagle?"
Dr. A.: "No."
ARL: "Peacock?"
Dr. A.: "No. In Africa. At home, warm
apartment."
"Perroquet!"

(16c) Grèce (Greece)   → Dr. A.: "Grèce"
ARL: "Lipid?"
Dr. A.: "No. Antique."

(16d) jars (gander)   → Dr. A.: "gander"
ARL: "What is it?"
Dr. A.: "Bird."
ARL: "What is the name of the
female?"
Dr. A.: "Goose."

It is also of interest that, as in (17), Dr. Adelbêrt could and not infrequently did express his capacity for autopriming through nonlinguistic SEB.

(17a) taureau (bull)   → Dr. A.: (Produces a powerful bellowing
onomatopoeia.)
"Like tiger, the same thing: strength."
"taureau"
"Not calf."

(17b) chant (song)   → Dr. A.: (Hums.)
"chant"

(17c) bouc (he-goat)   → Dr. A.: (Pinches his nose.)
"bouc"

Now, getting to the goal of this chapter, one of the most spectacular behaviors of our patient was his capacity to access in part [see (18a) and

(18b)] or in totality [see (18c) and (18d)], the content features of closed-class bound morphemes that he nevertheless remained unable to read aloud.

(18a) indirectement          → Dr. A.: "direction" (direction)
      (indirectly)                    "Direction? No. Ah!"
                                      "nondirection" (nondirection)
                            ARL: "'Nondirection'? Is this what is
                                 written on the card?"
                            Dr. A.: "Nondirection'. Yes. No? Why?"
(18b) tyrannisaient          → Dr. A.: "tyranniser" (to tyrannize)
      (they tyrannized)               "No. Yes, but plural. Third
                                      person. Present."
(18c) agriculteur'           → Dr. A.: "agricole" (agricultural)
      (agriculturist)                 "No."
                                      "agriculture" (agriculture)
                                      "No."
                                      "The gentleman makes
                                      agricultural."
                                      "Rats! Too bad!"
(18d) grandirez              → Dr. A: "grande"[11] (tall)
      [(you) will grow tall]          "'Grande' but..."
                                      "Yes. Again..."
                                      "grand"[12] (tall)
                                      "No."
                                      "Tall, but third person?"
                                      "Future. Second person. Plural."

The Adelbêrt corpus comprised 127 transparent semantic paralexias, which represents 11% of the patient's total paralexic production. This figure regroups three main subtypes: (1) open-class whole-word substitutions [such as (3)], which constitute the prototype; (2) closed-class whole-word substitutions [such as (4)]; and (3) substitutions limited to the lexemic root of polymorphemic word-stimuli [such as (19)].

(19a) bleu-âtre (blu-ish)    → verd-âtre (green-ish)
(19b) six-ième (six-th)      → cinq-uième (fif-th)

However, one might suggest that the typology of the semantically based behaviors of deep dyslexics could be extended to other entities observed within the Adelbêrt corpus, including, for instance, those illustrated in (12), (14), (15c), and (15d), as well as those—of particular interest given the topic of this volume—we have described as representing SEB targeted at closed-class bound morphemes [see (18)].

---

[11] Marked for feminine gender.
[12] Unmarked (masculine).

In addition to 876 clear-cut paralexias (276 formal, 127 semantic, 26 formal-and-semantic, and 447 morphological), 154 instances of SEB were noted within the Adelbêrt corpus,[13] bearing 99 times on open-class [see (15)] and 55 times on closed-class items [once a word (14a) and 54 times a bound morpheme (18)]. Sixty-seven of those bearing on an open-class item were associated with the production of an adequate response [see (16b)]; in this respect, nonverbal priming [see (10c), second quotation, and (17)] appeared to be particularly efficient (it failed only twice among 18). In striking contrast, verbal SEB bearing on a closed-class bound morpheme succeeded only once; as a matter of fact, it failed even in the 12 cases, e.g., (18c) and (18d), when content extraction was apparently exhaustive.

Another attractive property of SEB, one which we are now studying most attentively, is that it can be associated with all three main error types that have been recognized—given current parsing ways and their associated theoretical foundations and resulting terminology—to belong with deep dyslexia. Thus in the Adelbêrt corpus and given our list, SEB, was spontaneously associated eight times with the production of a prototypical "visual error" [as in (15c) and (15d)], 12 times with that of a prototypical "semantic error" [as in (15a) and (15b)], and 51 times with that of a prototypical morphological paralexia [as in (18a) to (18e)].

## Conclusions

The behavior of Dr. Adelbêrt, when he was requested to read aloud isolately presented words, was such (1) that it was often strongly suggestive of morpheme-by-morpheme decoding of polymorphemic single-word stimuli, then usually aiming first at the lexical stem whatever its position from left to right [see (5) and (10); (2) that it was also strongly suggestive that the patient's explicit metalinguistic knowledge, including his knowledge of morphology, permitted him to access at least part of the semic content not only of open-class words or morphemes [see (3), (14) to (17)] but also of closed-class words and bound morphemes [see (11) and (18)]; and (3) that, in the particular case of closed-class bound morphemes, the latter capacity was not sufficient to subserve adequate access to the form of corresponding targets [even when SEB was exhaustive as in (18c) and (18d)]. With regard to the last point (and it seems to us that no statistical analyses are needed in the present context given the above raw data), it might well be that the patient's production of morphological paralexias was, in view of the failure of his attempts at content probing, governed by rules such as those proposed by the authors of Chapter 3. If so, it might indicate that even in a highly educated listener, speaker, writer, and reader of a more or less

---

[13] Not including 14 instances where the patient recognized the possibility of SEB but did not go further.

highly inflected language such as French, overt decoding of written closed-class bound morphemes is naturally done through graphophonemic transcoding rather than through translexical processing. Be this as it may, it seems to us that the reading behavior of Dr. Adelbêrt was compatible with a conception postulating that deep dyslexia is the result of an isolation of translexical semantic reading (Marshall & Newcombe, 1966; Lecours, Lupien, and Belleville, in press). One might insist that the clinical expression of such a disorder supposes that translexical semantic reading was possible prior to brain damage, which obviously is, in turn, to be linked to the subject's cultural background (schooling level, reading habits, type of written code mastered). In other words, one might suggest that deep dyslexia is the result of an interaction between a morbid biological parameter (usually a left sylvian lesion) and a premorbid sociocultural parameter (the mastering of and continued exposure to a given written code). With comparable lesions, a given individual might thus present global alexia, whereas another individual might present spectacular deep dyslexia. (In our experience, which is by and large limited to readers of the French language, the former is far more frequent than the latter.)

One might finally mention that the clinical expression of deep dyslexia might in part be determined not only by factors such as the language of testing (it is apparently easier to obtain a sizeable corpus of morphological paralexias with a patient whose language is French, Italian, or German than with a unilingual native speaker of English), but also by factors such as the nature of the items in the testing lists (had we not included so many participles and conjugated verbs in the Adelbêrt test, the proportion of morphological errors in the corpus would no doubt have been appreciably lower) and, of course, the tester's hypotheses and preconceptions, as well as his or her experimental gadgetry and the constraints it imposes on testing.

## References

Benson, D.F., and Geschwind, N. (1969). The alexias. In P.J. Vinken & G.W. Bruyn (eds.), *Handbook of Clinical Neurology* (Vol. 4). Amsterdam: North Holland, pp. 112–140.

Beringer, K., & Stein, J. (1930). Analyse eines Falles von "Reiner" Alexie. *Z. Ges. Neurol. Psychiatrie, 123*, 473–478.

Coltheart, M. (1980). Deep dyslexia: a review of the syndrome. In M. Coltheart, K.E. Patterson, & J.C. Marshall (eds), *Deep Dyslexia*. London: Routledge & Kegan Paul, pp. 22–47.

Ducarne, B. (1964). *Test pour l'examen de l'aphasie*. Paris: Editions du Centre de Psychologie Appliquée.

Faust, C. (1955). *Die zerebralen Herdstörungen bei Hinterhauptsverletzungen und ihre Beurteilung*. Stuttgart: Thieme.

Gougenheim, G. (1958). Dictionnaire fondamental de la langue française. Paris: Didier.

Henderson, L. (1985). Toward a psychology of morphemes. In A.W. Ellis (Ed.), *Progress in the Psychology of Language* (Vol. 1). London: Erlbaum.

Lecours, A.R., Lupien, S., & Belleville, S. (in press). Lecture analphabète: à propos d'un cas de dyslexie profonde. In M. Nevert (ed.), *Textes et Langages Atypiques*. Montreal: Guérin.

Luria, A.S. (1970). *Traumatic Aphasia*. The Hague: Mouton.

Marshall, J.C., & Newcombe, F. (1966). Syntactic and semantic errors in paralexia. *Neuropsychologia, 4,* 169–176.

Marshall, J.C., & Newcombe, F. (1973). Patterns of paralexia: a psycholinguistic approach. *Journal of Psycholinguistic Research, 2,* 175–199.

Marshall, J.C. & Newcombe, F. (1980). The conceptual status of deep dyslexia: an historical perspective. In M. Coltheart, K.E. Patterson, & J.C. Marshall (eds.), *Deep Dyslexia*, London: Routledge & Kegan Paul, pp. 1–21.

# 5
# Free Use of Derivational Morphology in an Italian Jargonaphasic

Marta Panzeri, Carlo Semenza, Tiziana Ferreri, and Brian Butterworth

One of the ways in which new words are coined to augment the vocabulary of a language is through processes that permit the construction of words from other words, e.g., adjectives from nouns, verbs from adjectives, adverbs from adjectives, and so on. These transformations are performed according to rules, studied under the heading of derivational morphology, that are used for combining bases with one or more of a small number of affixes. Such a set of processes was found to be used creatively by a deeply anomic, neologizing, aphasic patient, R.B., whose case is reported here.

Neologisms uttered by aphasics are known to obey particular rules. For example, they are explicable as legal concatenations of phonemes (Buckingham and Kertesz, 1976), and it has been frequently noted that they are typically correctly inflected (Buckingham and Kertesz, 1976; Butterworth, 1979). Such nuance occurrences are thus particularly interesting because they allow us to study in isolation the operations of rules that are concealed in normal flawless performance. However, neologistic constructions involving the rules of derivational morphology seem to have passed unnoticed in aphasiology. Thus Caplan, Kellar, and Locke's (1972) patient produced the utterance "things that *devorodation* have had." The neologism is composed of a neologistic base "vorod" plus the derivational perfix "de" and the derivational suffix "ation." The authors remarked only that pluralization is absent. How commonly aphasics construct such neologisms is difficult to say. However, R.B. spontaneously produced a fair amount of derivationally compound neolgoisms occurring in a linguistic context that were explicit enough to allow a through analysis of the derivational processes that apply.

## Case report

R.B. was a 66-year-old right-handed Italian businessman with high school education. He spoke Florentine Italian (considered standard Italian).

In June 1986 he suffered an infarction of the left middle cerebral artery. A computed tomography scan revealed a large hypodense temporoparietal area. After a month in a peripheral hospital he was transferred to the Neurology Department of Padova Polyclinic where he came to our attention. At that time he showed a profound linguistic deficit affecting both the receptive and the productive sides of his speech. Apart from linguistic damage, neurological examination showed a right-sided hemianopsia. He was partially anosognosic, and most of the time he displayed an excited mood. He was an uncooperative patient, and formal testing with him was difficult enterprise. On the other hand, he was keen to offer examiners long pieces of uninterrupted jargonaphasic speech. Despite perfect auditory intelligibility, R.B.'s speech was totally incomprehensible owing to the improper use of real words and to the intrusion of neologisms. Several attempts to formal linguistic testing via an Italian version of BDAE and the Token Test failed: His zero scores (word repetition seemed the only partially spared function, scoring 6 of 12, along with word discrimination, 20 of 72) in most cases were probably determined by his poor and inconstant co-operation. However, when testing was rendered less formal and occasional short trials were given, he clearly showed the depth of his anomic defect, although sentence comprehension appeared to be partly sensitive to the context.

His writing, although mechanically correct, was jargonaphasic. He never wanted to write on dictation. His reading was partially preserved when he read a newspaper, whereas on formal testing for reading simple words his score was 1 of 30. "Errors" were confabulations or refusal and could not be classified.

That both emotional behavior and real impairment contributed to his linguistic performance is probably shown by the fact that it was possible to give him nonlinguistic tests, e.g., RAVEN Matrices (the 1947 version, on which he scored 18 of 36 at the time of the our first recording of his speech and 29 of 36 a month later) and Corsi's test, which he performed normally.

## Methods of Data Collection

Conversations between R.B. and various examiners were recorded at 2, 3, 5, and 9 months after onset. A broad phonemic transcription was made with the aid of four independent judges. However, virtually no problems of agreement arose, as the patient's output was clear, and only two or three "words," overlapped by noise, had to be dropped from the analysis. Also, because of the clarity of R.B.'s speech to disagreement was present for segmentation into word-like units even in the few cases in which two or more nonwords occurred in a sequence.

TABLE 5.1. Corpus analyzed: word-like segments and incidence of real words, phonemic paraphasias, derivational neologisms, and other neologisms.

| Months after of set | Real Words | | Phonemic Paraphasias | | Derivational neologisms | | Other neologisms | | Word-like segments (No.) |
|---|---|---|---|---|---|---|---|---|---|
| | No. | % | No. | % | No. | % | No. | % | |
| 2 | 2952 | 94.04 | 69 | 2.20 | 67 | 2.13 | 51 | 1.63 | 3139 |
| 3 | 2332 | 97.13 | 40 | 1.67 | 7 | .29 | 22 | .91 | 2401 |
| 5 | 2328 | 97.57 | 33 | 1.38 | 9 | .38 | 16 | .67 | 2386 |
| 9 | 3427 | 98.54 | 41 | 1.18 | 5 | .14 | 5 | .14 | 3478 |

TABLE 5.2. Distribution of real words according to grammatical categories in R.B. and Italian norms.

| | R.B. | | | | | | | | | |
|---|---|---|---|---|---|---|---|---|---|---|
| | 2 Months After Onset | | 3 Months After Onset | | 5 Months After Onset | | 9 Months After Onset | | Italian Norms | |
| Grammatical Class | N | % | N | % | N | % | N | % | Mean | SD |
| Nouns | 498 | 16.87 | 431 | 18.48 | 358 | 15.38 | 552 | 16.11 | 17.22 | 3.06 |
| Verbs | 565 | 19.14 | 452 | 19.38 | 483 | 20.75 | 754 | 22.00 | 20.47 | 3.13 |
| Adjectives | 339 | 11.48 | 174 | 7.46 | 151 | 6.49 | 261 | 7.61 | 8.52 | 2.02 |
| Adverbs | 415 | 14.06 | 272 | 11.66 | 289 | 12.41 | 474 | 13.83 | 13.92 | 2.40 |
| Articles | 251 | 8.50 | 165 | 7.08 | 162 | 6.96 | 239 | 6.97 | 8.48 | 2.72 |
| Prepositions | 300 | 10.16 | 310 | 13.29 | 309 | 13.27 | 379 | 11.06 | 10.85 | 2.35 |
| Pronouns | 301 | 10.20 | 274 | 11.75 | 274 | 11.77 | 455 | 13.28 | 10.47 | 3.12 |
| Conjunctions | 239 | 8.10 | 227 | 9.74 | 276 | 11.85 | 273 | 7.97 | 9.22 | 2.24 |
| Exclamations | 44 | 1.49 | 27 | 1.16 | 26 | 1.17 | 40 | 1.17 | .79 | .90 |

[a] Semenza, 1986.

## *Analyses*

Appendix 1 provides some information about the characteristics of derivational morphology in Italian.

### WORDS VERSUS NONWORDS

Words and nonwords were counted in each sample. Nonwords were divided into phonemic paraphasias (errors involving one or two phonemes) and neologisms. The data are given in Table 5.1.

### DISTRIBUTION OF REAL WORDS INTO GRAMMATICAL CLASSES AND TYPE/TOKEN RATIO

Real words were divided according to grammatical class. Among verbs, adverbs, and adjectives a distinction has been made between open and closed class items. Among verbs, auxiliaries and copulas were considered closed class. Closed-class adjectives encompassed all adjectives but descriptive ones. Lexically derived adverbs were counted as open class. Percentages over the total are given for each sample in Table 5.2 together with the available normative data for Italian (Semenza, 1986). It can be seen that R.B.'s speech was essentially normal so far as distribution into grammatical classes is concerned. Because the addition of neologisms would alter proportions only negligibly (they were in a small percentage with respect to the overall number of word-like segments and almost always easily classifiable in the open class on the basis of endings and contexts; see below), it was considered legitimate to drop them from this comparison. This first count was performed by token. Unfortunately, at present normative data in Italian by type are not available, although in preparation (Semenza, Panzeri and Pe, in prep.). A count for type was, however, performed with R.B. (Table 5.3), who seemed to master a normally wide vocabulary. Three control subjects matched for age and culture on whose speech a similar count has been made (samples being of the same size as that of R.B.) showed comparable figures.

### TYPES OF NEOLOGISMS

Neologisms were classified according to their morphological composition. They appeared to have been constructed in three ways. First, as in other neologistic jargonaphasics, concatenations of phonemes were used to form bases, which were then inflected correctly in most cases.

### *Example*

(1) *Misecca* italiana—Italian, feminine singular (f.s.) adjective): +*a* in *misecca* is the ending marking an f.s. noun.

TABLE 5.3.  Distribution of Real Word According to Grammatical Categories by Types and by Token in R.B.

| Grammatical Class | 2 Months After Onset | | 3 Months After Onset | | 5 Months After Onset | | 9 Months After Onset | |
|---|---|---|---|---|---|---|---|---|
| | Types | Token | Types | Token | Types | Token | Types | Token |
| Nouns | 228 | 498 | 217 | 431 | 195 | 358 | 253 | 552 |
| Verbs | | | | | | | | |
| Open Class | 238 | 423 | 232 | 374 | 215 | 399 | 320 | 612 |
| Closed Class | 20 | 142 | 20 | 78 | 19 | 84 | 19 | 142 |
| Adjectives | | | | | | | | |
| Open Class | 89 | 147 | 50 | 69 | 50 | 63 | 84 | 128 |
| Closed Class | 64 | 192 | 48 | 105 | 40 | 88 | 59 | 133 |
| Adverbs | | | | | | | | |
| Open Class | 18 | 31 | 15 | 20 | 28 | 45 | 21 | 36 |
| Closed Class | 52 | 384 | 40 | 252 | 43 | 244 | 47 | 438 |
| Articles | 10 | 251 | 11 | 165 | 11 | 162 | 10 | 239 |
| Prepositions | 37 | 300 | 33 | 310 | 40 | 309 | 38 | 379 |
| Pronouns | | | | | | | | |
| Clitics | 14 | 99 | 15 | 97 | 21 | 125 | 19 | 177 |
| Non-Clitics | 45 | 202 | 42 | 177 | 32 | 149 | 45 | 278 |
| Conjunctions | 19 | 239 | 16 | 227 | 24 | 276 | 14 | 273 |
| Exclamations | 14 | 44 | 11 | 27 | 12 | 26 | 10 | 40 |
| Total | 848 | 2952 | 770 | 2332 | 730 | 2328 | 939 | 3427 |
| Open Class | 572 | 1099 | 514 | 894 | 488 | 865 | 678 | 1328 |
| Closed Class | 276 | 1853 | 256 | 1438 | 242 | 1463 | 261 | 2099 |

All neologisms built up with at least one derivational affix (henceforth called *derivational neologisms*) were further divided according to base type ("base" is meant in the natural morphology acception) (Dressler, 1985). A second type of neologism was therefore considered that was composed by a real base with real suffixes, prefixes, or both.

*Examples*

(2) *Fratellismo* is a compound of the real base *fratell(o)* (brother) and the real suffix +*ismo*.
(3) *Affuocato*: the real base *fuoc(o)* (fire) has both a real suffix +*ato* and a real prefix *a*+. The last is especially interesting, as it respects the rule of doubling the first consonant of the base *aff*+, which is perceivable by Italian speakers.
(4) Quel nuovo (that new) ... *macchinarico*: the real base *macchiari(o)* (machinery) and the real suffix +*ico* agree with both the preceding adjectives.

The base was taken as "real where there was at least one real word in the Italian dictionary built up with such a base. This method was necessary because in Italian there is rarely such a clear-cut physical separation between stem and inflexion: Derivations are made in most cases through substitution and not simply through addition, as in English.

Finally, a third type was composed in a neologistic base plus a real derivational suffix, prefix, or both.

*Examples*

(5) Tutto il (all the) *ternessico* che mi aspetta (that waits for me): *terness(o)* is a neologistic base that, coupled with the real suffix +*ico*, perfectly fits in the sentence.
(6) Siamo come ragazzi (we are like boys) *forfitenti* uno dell'altro (one of the other): *forfit(ere)* is a neologistic base, whereas +*enti* is a real plural participal suffix.

A distinction had to be made also in terms of how unambiguously derivational the affix could be. In fact, part of the affixes can be either derivational or inflexional.

(7) Di quelle (of those) *modernate* in Toscana (in Toscana): +*ate* is both a derivational suffix that turns a noun, an adjective, or a verb into a noun, and an inflexional suffix, marking the second plural person of the present indicative and imperative, and the feminine plural past participle of verbs of the first conjugation.

The context could point to the fact that in most cases the affixes were truly derivational, a small proportion being left ambiguous. Table 5.4 reports the number and percentages of the latter types of neologism. It is safe to

TABLE 5.4. Distribution of Derivational Neologisms over time.

| Months After Onset | Neologisms type[a] | Real Base N | %* | neologistic Base | %* | Total | %* |
|---|---|---|---|---|---|---|---|
| 2 | Type 1 | 23 | .73 | 28 | .89 | 51 | 1.62 |
|   | Type 2 | 2 | .06 | 3 | .10 | 5 | .16 |
|   | Type 3 | 3 | .10 | 8 | .25 | 11 | .35 |
|   | Total | 28 | .89 | 39 | 1.24 | 67 | 2.13 |
| 3 | Type 1 | 0 | .00 | 3 | .12 | 3 | .12 |
|   | Type 2 | 0 | .00 | 1 | .05 | 1 | .05 |
|   | Type 3 | 0 | .00 | 3 | .12 | 3 | .12 |
|   | Total | 0 | .00 | 7 | .29 | 7 | .29 |
| 5 | Type 1 | 1 | .04 | 5 | .21 | 6 | .25 |
|   | Type 2 | 0 | .00 | 1 | .04 | 1 | .04 |
|   | Type 3 | 1 | .04 | 1 | .04 | 2 | .08 |
|   | Total | 2 | .08 | 7 | .29 | 9 | .37 |
| 9 | Type 1 | 1 | .03 | 2 | .06 | 3 | .09 |
|   | Type 2 | 1 | .03 | 1 | .03 | 2 | .06 |
|   | Type 3 | 0 | .00 | 0 | .00 | 0 | .00 |
|   | Total | 2 | .06 | 3 | .09 | 5 | .15 |

[a] Type 1 Neologisms are unambiguously derivational, while Type 2 and Type 3 have an affix that can be either derivational or inflectional. In Type 2 the context points to the fact that the affix is truly derivational, while Type 3 are left ambiguous.
[b] As a percent of all word-like segments.

say that R.B. produced a substantial number of what have been termed derivational neologisms whether compounded with a real or a neologistic base.

TYPES OF DERIVATIONAL PROCESSES

The corpus of derivational neologisms thus collected was further analyzed, investigating the type of derivational processes involved in the composition. The complete list of these neologisms, classified according to all possible transformations carried out by affixes, is reported in Appendix 2. The same classification was applied to all derived words from the real words corpus, and all the types of transformation are reported in Appendix 3. The following transformations, including suffixes and prefixes, were identified, which either (1) change the grammatical class of the base or (2) do not change the grammatical class of the base: noun to noun, adjective to noun, verb to noun, noun to adjective, verb to adjective, noun to verb, adjective to adverb, verb to verb, and adjective to adjective. Furthermore, some neologisms consisted of the composition of two bases. Table 5.5 shows the comparison between transformations in real words and in neologisms expressed as a percent of all word-like segments. These data clearly show that R.B. used a vast range of types of transformation in both real words and derivational neologisms.

TABLE 5.5. Types of derivational affixes used by R.B. in real words and in neologisms.

| Derivational processes and examples | Real Words | | | | Neologisms | | | |
|---|---|---|---|---|---|---|---|---|
| | Types | | Tokens | | Types | | Tokens | |
| | N | % | N | % | N | % | N | % |
| *Suffixation* | | | | | | | | |
| Noun → Noun | 23 | .20 | 98 | .86 | 11 | .10 | 34 | .30 |
| Ex. [operaio = oper(a)+aio] [worker = work+er] | | | | | [macchinismo macchin(a)+ismo] [ = machine+ism] | | | |
| Adj. → Noun | 13 | .11 | 63 | .55 | 2 | .02 | 3 | .03 |
| [libertà = liber(o)+tà] [freedom = free+dom] | | | | | [solitismo = solit(o)+ismo] [ = usual +ism] | | | |
| Verb → Noun | 19 | .18 | 109 | .96 | 6 | .05 | 12 | .10 |
| [informazione = inform(are)+zione] [information = to inform+ation] | | | | | [assaggiamento = assaggi(are)+mento] [ ≐ taste+ment] | | | |
| Adj. → Adj. | 4 | .03 | 26 | .23 | 0 | .00 | 0 | .00 |
| [piccolino = piccol(o)+ion] [a little short] | | | | | | | | |
| Noun → Adj. | 14 | .13 | 77 | .67 | 5 | .04 | 5 | .04 |
| [italiano = Itali(a)+ano] [Italian = Italy+an] | | | | | [macchinarico = macchinar(io)+ico] [ = machinery+ic/like] | | | |
| Verb → Adj. | 6 | .05 | 50 | .44 | 1 | .01 | 3 | .03 |
| [resistente = resist(ere)+ente] [resistent = to resist+ent] | | | | | [pissante = neo.+ante] [ = neo.+ant] | | | |
| Noun → Verb | 4 | .03 | 190 | 1.67 | 7 | .06 | 16 | .14 |
| [lavorare = lavor(o)+are] [to work = work+infinitive] | | | | | [sogillare = neo.+are] [ = neo.+infinitive] | | | |
| Adj. > Adv. | 4 | .03 | 104 | .81 | 1 | .01 | 1 | .01 |
| [personalmente = personal(e)+mente] [personally = personal+ly] | | | | | [atamente = neo.+mente] [ = neo.+ly] | | | |
| *Prefixation* | | | | | | | | |
| Noun → Noun | 1 | .01 | 1 | .01 | 2 | .02 | 2 | .02 |
| [disordine = dis+ordine] [disorder = dis+order] | | | | | [concloco = con+neo.] [ = con+neo.] | | | |
| Adj. → Adj. | 4 | .03 | 18 | .16 | 2 | .02 | 2 | .02 |
| [incapace = in+capace] [unable = un+able] | | | | | [derudato = de+neo.] [ = de+neo.] | | | |
| Verb > Verb | 10 | .09 | 56 | .49 | 4 | .03 | 6 | .05 |
| [reagire = re+agire] [to react = re+to act] | | | | | [srende = s+rende] [ = s+to render] | | | |
| *Parasynthetic Processes* | | | | | | | | |
| Noun → Verb | 5 | .04 | 36 | .31 | 2 | .02 | 2 | .02 |
| [accoppiare = a+coppi(a)+are] [to couple = couple+infinitive] | | | | | [affuocato = a+neo.+ato] [ = a+fire+ed] | | | |
| *Composition* | | | | | | | | |
| Base + Base | – | – | 32 | .28 | – | – | 2 | .02 |
| Total | 107 | .93 | 860 | 7.54 | 43 | .38 | 88 | .78 |

## Derivations in Grammatical Context

The appropriateness of the derivational affixes of the neologisms to the grammatical context was then checked. Table 5.6 shows how most derivational neologisms agreed with the grammatical context. Only a small number of them did not agree, clearly matching paragrammatic errors found also elsewhere in R.B.'s speech [see Butterworth, Lauren, Semenza, and Ferreri, 1990) for the paragrammatic aspects of this case]. For example:

(8) Se questo è un (if this is an) *atamente* (adverb) del personale (of the staff): +*mente* is the suffix that turns an adjective into an adverb, whereas here the neologism is clearly in a masculine singular (m.sg.) noun position.

## Productivity

Affixes in both derivational neologisms and derived words were compared in terms of productivity. Because of the lack of a precise list of productivity values from the literature, the incidence of a few affixes generally accepted as highly productive in Italian (Caramazza and Burani, 1987; Dardano, 1978) was checked in these two categories: the group +ismo, +ista, +istico; +ico; +mento; +zione; s+; in+; inter+; con+; a+; de+. The data clearly showed a higher proportion of the more productive affixes in neologisms (Table 5.7).

Table 5.6. The distribution of derivational neologisms according to the appropriateness to the syntactic context. This grammatical category of the neologism is determined by its affix.

| Months after onset | According to the affix | According to the context | | | | Information not sufficient |
|---|---|---|---|---|---|---|
| | | Noun | Adj | Verb | Adverb | |
| 2 | Noun | 37 | 1 | – | – | 7 |
| | Adjectives | – | 5 | – | – | 2 |
| | Verb | – | – | 12 | – | 2 |
| | Adverb | 1 | – | – | – | – |
| 3 | Noun | 2 | – | – | – | 1 |
| | Adjectives | – | 1 | – | – | 1 |
| | Verb | – | – | 2 | – | – |
| | Adverb | – | – | – | – | – |
| 5 | Noun | 3 | – | – | – | – |
| | Adjectives | – | 1 | – | – | – |
| | Verb | – | – | 5 | – | – |
| | Adverb | – | – | – | – | – |
| 9 | Noun | 3 | – | – | – | – |
| | Adjectives | – | 1 | – | – | – |
| | Verb | – | – | 1 | – | – |
| | Adverb | – | – | – | – | – |

TABLE 5.7. Proportions of productive
affixes in derived neologisms and derived
real words.

| Affix | In derived neologisms | | In derived real words | |
|---|---|---|---|---|
| | No. | %[a] | No. | %[b] |
| +ìco | 6 | 6.82 | 9 | 1.08 |
| +ìsmo | 16 | 18.18 | 1 | .12 |
| +ìsta | 1 | 1.14 | 1 | .12 |
| +ìstico | 2 | 2.27 | 0 | 0 |
| +mènto | 5 | 5.68 | 9 | 1.08 |
| +zìone | 2 | 2.27 | 13 | 1.57 |
| a+ | 2 | 2.27 | 2 | .24 |
| con+ | 1 | 1.14 | 3 | .36 |
| de+ | 1 | 1.14 | 7 | .84 |
| in+ | 2 | 2.27 | 7 | .84 |
| inter+ | 1 | 1.14 | 6 | .72 |
| s+ | 1 | 1.14 | 7 | .84 |

[a] As a percent of all derived neologisms (compounded excluded).
[b] As a percent of all derived real words (compounded excluded).

## Discussion

This case appears to be important because it may test major current hypotheses on the retrieval of words including derivational compounds. Three models have been offered so far. According to the first model, words including derivational compounds are retrieved as a whole from the store of words the speaker already knows (Oldfield, 1966). Impairment to such a system would lead to the inaccessibility of word forms. This problem may affect some types of word more than others: perhaps the less frequently used words (Newcombe, Oldfield, and Wingfield, 1965), some specific semantic category (Hart, Berndt, and Caramazza, 1985; Warrington and Shallice, 1984), or perhaps the category of complex derivational words. This situation is not the case with our patient: He showed no loss of particular categories of words and produced novel word-like constructions, which would be unpredicted by this model.

According to the second model, all words that can be analyzed in more than one morpheme are put together at the point of production. The general difficulty with this model is that it fails to discriminate compounds that result in real words, e.g., "fratellanza," from compounds that, although potentially legal, do not, e.g., "fratellismo" (Butterworth, 1983). In normals it appears necessary to postulate a checking mechanism responsible for such discrimination, probably by mapping the constructed word into a lexical store. This process could be disturbed in R.B.

The third possibility is a combination of the two models, such that the second compositional procedure is used just in case the target word is inaccessible. If a patient indeed has an impairment in word retrieval, he or she activates the compositional procedure more often than a normal speaker. This action would lead to a rise in the incidence of both real word and nonword compounds. The activation of the compositional procedure would also probably predict the increment shown by R.B. in the use of more productive affixes. Indeed Aronoff (1976) stated that the most productive classes never have to be listed in the lexicon (Zimmer, 1964) on the assumption that only words that are arbitrary in some way (i.e., phonologically, lexically, or semantically) must be entered in the lexicon. As Stemberger (1985) pointed out, syntax appears to have direct input to productive affixes, which are not prone to loss or incorrect access. However, many if not all aphasics have a word retrieval problem (Goodglass and Geschwind, 1976; Newcombe et al., 1965), so derivational compounds should be a common symptom, yet they have not been previously noted. This lack does not seem to be artifactual, as analysis of published transcripts of such patients, including Italian patients (Panzeri, Semenza, and Butterworth, 1987), shows that these compounds are unremarked in part because they are rare. Why this situation should be is at present unknown.

## Summary

This chapter describes a jargonaphasic whose speech contained neologisms that are legal combinations of meaningful parts of real words and combinations of meaningless (the base) and meaningful (the affix) parts. On the assumption that brain-damaged patients use residual rather than novel abilities, these forms indicate that speakers have a procedure for composing polymorphemic words on-line, but it is employed only when their attempt to find a whole words fails. Such procedure appears to be influenced by the productivity of the endings.

*Acknowledgments.* Livia Tonelli, of the "Centro di Studio per le Ricerche di Fonetica del CNR," made many helpful suggestions on the work and on the drafts of this chapter. The study was supported by grants from NATO to Brian Butterworth, Carlo Semenza, and Marta Panzeri and from the CNR to Unità 14, Scienze del Comportamento, and from Ministero della Pubblica Istruzione to Carlo Semenza. The chapter was written as partial fulfillment of Miss Panzeri's Ph.D. thesis.

# References

Aronoff, M. (1976). *Word Formation in Generative Grammar*. Cambridge, MA: MIT Press.

Buckingham, H.W., & Kertesz, A. (1976). *Neologistic Jargon Aphasia: Neurolinguistics III*. Amsterdam: Swets & Zeitlinger.

Butterworth, B. (1979). Hesitation and the production of verbal paraphasias and neologisms in jargon aphasia. *Brain and Language*, 8, 133–161.

Butterworth, B. (1983). Lexical representation. In B. Butterworth (Ed.), *Language Production Volume 2: Development, Writing and Other Language Processes*. London: Academic Press.

Butterworth, B., Panzeri, M., Semenza, C., & Ferreri, T. (1990). Paragrammatisms: A longitudinal study of an Italian patient. *Language and Cognitive Processes*, in press.

Caplan, D., Kellar, L., & Locke, S. (1972). Inflection of neologisms in aphasia. *Brain*, 95, 169–172.

Caramazza, A. & Burani, C. (1987). Representation and processing of derived words. *Language and Cognitive Processes*, 2, 217–227.

Dardano, M. (1978). *La formazione delle parole nell' italiano di oggi*. Roma: Bulzoni.

Dressler, W. (1985). *Morphonology*. Ann Arbor: Karoma.

Goodglass, H. & Geschwind, N. (1976). Language Disorders (Aphasia). In E.C. Carterette & M. Friedman (Eds.), *Handbook of Perception, Vol. 7*. New York: Academic Press.

Hart, J., Berndt, R.S., & Caramazza, A. (1985). Category-specific naming deficit following cerebral infarction. *Nature*, 316, 439–440.

Newcombe, F., Oldfield, R.C., & Wingfield, A. (1965). Object-naming by dysphasic patients. *Nature*, 207, 1217–1218.

Oldfield, R.C. (1966). Things, words, and the brain. *Quarterly Journal of Experimental Psychology*, 18, 340–353.

Panzeri, M., Semenza, C., & Butterworth, B. (1987). Compensatory processes in the evolution of severe jargon aphasia. *Neuropsychologia*, 25, 919–933.

Semenza, C. (1986). L'esame della produzione afasica spontanea. *Acta Phoniatrica Latina*, 8, 99–112.

Semenza, C. Panzeri, M., & Re, S. (in prep.). Eloquio spontaneo: Categorie grammaticali. Prospettive per la clinica dei deficit lessicali.

Stemberger, J.P. (1985). An Interactive Activation Model of Language Production. In A.W. Ellis (Ed.), *Progress in the Psychology of Language (Vol. 1)*. London: LEA.

Warrington E.K. & Shallice, T. (1984). Category-specific semantic impairment. *Brain*,, 107, 829–851.

Zimmer, K. (1964). Affixal Negation in English and Other Languages: An Investigation of Restricted Productivity, supplement to *Word*, Monograph 5. New York: International Linguistic Association.

# Appendix I: Some Notes on Derivational Morphology in Italian

Some of the peculiarities of Italian derivational morphology are summarized here to help the non-Italian-speaking reader to follow more easily the description of the data.

## Morphological Processes

Word formation is divided into two smaller subfields, of which one is concerned with processes of derivation, (e.g., the derivation of "generazione" (generation) from "generare" (generate), and the other with processes of composition, e.g., "aereoporto" (airport).

The grounds for dividing composition from derivation are sufficiently clear: In the case of *aereoporto* (*airport*) both *aereo* and *porto* (*air* and *port*) can represent words in their own right, whereas with *generazione* (*generation*) the +*zione* (+*ation*) is a purely formative element (a "bound morpheme") that has no status as a "word" on its own (Matthews, 1974).

## Affixation

In Italian, derivation is performed most typically through affixation, whereas no such processes as reduplication, stress change, and tonal modification are found. Vowel modification and subtraction are limited to a few examples, mainly of latinate origin (Scalise, 1984).

Processes of affixation may be divided into prefixation or suffixation, depending on whether the affix is added before the operand or after it. By the same token, the affix itself may be a prefix or a suffix. Infixation is no longer productive and is limited to a few verbal examples of latinate origin.

In Italian there is rarely a clear-cut physical separation between stem and inflection: Derivations are made in most cases through substitution and not simply through addition, as in English. This "rule" is almost always true for suffixation; the processes order is thus: "root + derivational suffix + inflection" (from a formal point of view in Italian every open class root—but foreign loan words—do have an inflectional ending). There are a few exceptions, e.g., the adverbial suffix +mente, which attaches itself to the feminine form of the adjective (Scalise, 1984).

In Italian, as in English, the most common processes are those of suffixation: They are involved in most lexical formations [generare → generare+ zione = generazione (generate → generate+sion = generation); felice → felice+ità = felicità (happy → happy+ness = happiness); and so on] and in all inflectional formation [amo → ama (I love → he/she/it loves); casa → case (house → house+s), etc.]

The main aspect of suffixation processes is transcategorization. Thus a verb can produces a noun (lavorare → lavorazione) or an adjective (lavorare → lavorabile); a noun can produced a verb (scandalo → scandaliz-zare) or an adjective (scandalo → scandaloso); an adjective can produce a noun (veloce → velocità), a verb (veloce → velocizzare), or an adverb (veloce → velocementa). However, in Italian the result of suffixation can be a word of the same category of the base: A noun originates a noun (benzina → benzinaio), an adjective originates an adjective (bianco → biancastro), and a verb originates a verb (lavorare → lavoricchiare). The latter two cases, Adj. → Adj. and Verb → Verb, belong to the peculiar field of alteration, i.e., a derivational process that implies a semantic modification and not a syntactic one, whereas the transformation Noun → Noun is a sort of link between alteration and transcategorization. [For a discussion on the syntactic value of this transformation, see Scalise (1984).]

Although suffixation is the most common process involved in word derivation, examples of prefixation are found in the formation of many derived forms. Usually these kinds of transformation do not imply trans-categorization: Noun → Noun: ordine → dis+ordine (order → dis+order); Adj. → Adj.: felice → in+felice (happy → un+happy); Verb → Verb: costruire → ri+costruire (built → re+build).

In Italian a further phenomenon is present, i.e., parasynthetic deriva-tion. It consists in the simultaneous application of prefixation and suffixa-tion, as with the Noun → Verb, Adj. → Verb transformations +are and +ire: caffeina → de+caffeina+are = decaffeinare; baracca → s+baracca +are = sbaraccare; borghese → in+borghese+ire = imborghesire; biz-zarro → s+bizzarro+ire = sbizzarrire.

## Productivity

Productivity is one of the central mysteries of derivational morphology. The term *productivity* is widely used, but most of the discussion on it is rather vague (Aronoff, 1976).

We list here only some of the most characteristic properties, which seem best to distinguish productivity from nonproductivity.

1. In Italian, as in English, the more a rule is semantically coherent, the more it is productive. A rule is semantically coherent when it adheres closely to the meaning assigned to it by the semantic function of the rule, so that one can predict the meaning of any word formed by that rule.

2. The less an affix has morphological restrictions on the class of basis to which it attaches, the more it is productive. So +ismo in Italian is highly productive, being fairly free morphologically (it can attach even to ad-verbs: pressapoco → pressapochismo).

3. The more a rule is phonologically transparent, the more it is pro-ductive; for example, in Italian, in the transformation Verb → Noun, +sione (less productive than +zione) applies to verbs of the second and third conjugations modifying the base, e.g., discutere → discussione (dis-

cuss → discussion), whereas +zione rarely modifies the base to which it attaches.

4. The more a rule is used in the formation of neologisms (i.e., new words of the language), the more it is productive; for example, in Italian the transformation Noun → Verb +are is highly productive (see below).

5. Productivity cannot be equivalent merely to frequency, so one cannot say that productivity is identified with sheer number (Aronoff, 1976). The possibility of creating neologisms with an affix is far more critical for defining its productivity than the frequency of that affix in the language, which may be due to diachronic borrowings from other languages. Thus +mento, although still productive, is nowadays becoming less productive, for example, with respect to +zione, the latter being used in the formation of modern words such as *ispirazione* (inspiration, which substitutes for *ispiramento*) and *procreazione* (procreation, which substitutes for *procreamento*), even though 1800 Noun +mento and 1300 Noun +zione are listed in the Reverse Index of Italian (Alinei, 1962).

## Transformation Noun → Verb with the Suffixes +are and +ire

One highly productive transformation in Italian is Noun → Verb originating through the suffixes +are and +ire (Dardano, 1978), which have both an inflexional and a derivational function. The suffix +ere, on the other hand, belonging to the second conjugation, has only an inflexional function. One proof in favor of the true derivational value of these suffixes is their use in the formation of neologisms from nouns introduced from other languages, e.g., *stoppare, bluffare,* and *dribblare,* and in new formations such as spintone → spintonare and pupazzetto → pupazzettare. Of course there are many ambiguous cases, e.g, lavoro → lavorare and lavorare → lavoro, in which it is difficult to say which of the two transformations applies. For simplicity's sake (and statistical reasons), in the present work we decided to consider all the ambiguous cases as falling into the first type of transformation: Noun → Verb. This decision was made because it is more iconic to add a new meaning by adding an affix than by subtracting it (as in the transformation lavorare → lavoro) and because of the high productivity of +are and +ire in Italian.

## References

Alinei, M.L. (1962). *Dizionario Inverso Italiano.* The Hague: Mouton & Co.
Aronoff, M. (1976). *Word Formation in Generative Grammar.* Cambridge, MA: MIT Press.
Dardano, M. (1978). *La Formazione delle Parole Nell' Italiano di Oggi.* Rome: Bulzoni.
Matthews, P. (1974). *Morphology.* London: Cambridge University Press.
Scalise, S. (1984). *Generative Morphology.* Dordrecht: Poris Publications.

# Appendix 2: List of Derived Neologisms

Type 1 Neologisms[a]
*Suffixation*

| Morph. transformation | Base | Affix | | Neologism | 2 MONTHS AFTER ONSET Neologism grammatical class according to context | Base grammatical class |
|---|---|---|---|---|---|---|
| **Noun → Noun** | | | | | | |
| +àno | mangiare | +ani | → | *mangiàno* | Noun | Verb |
| | doppio | +ano | → | *doppiàno* | undet. | Adj. |
| | neo. | +ano | → | *medegiàno* | Noun | neo. |
| | neo. | +ano | → | *saddoppiàno* | undet. | neo. |
| | neo. | +ano | → | *saddoppiàno* | undet. | neo. |
| +àro | meta | +ari | → | *metàri* | Noun | Noun |
| +_ico | macchinario | +ico | → | *macchinàrico* | Noun | Noun |
| | luogo | +ica | → | *luógica* | Noun | Noun |
| | neo. | +ico | → | *ternèssico* | Noun | neo. |
| | neo. | +ico | → | *idàldico* | Noun | neo. |
| | neo. | +ici | → | *podèlici* | Noun | neo. |
| +ina | neo. | +ina | → | *calzerìna* | Noun | neo. |
| +ino | neo. | +ino | → | *sostipìdino* | Noun | neo. |
| +ismo | macchina | +ismo | → | *macchinìsmo* | Noun | Noun |
| | fratello | +ismo | → | *fratellìsmo* | Noun | Noun |
| | titolo | +ismo | → | *titolìsmo* | Noun | Noun |
| | realtà | +ismo | → | *realtìsmo* | Noun | Noun |
| | setto | +ismo | → | *settoìsmo* | Noun | Noun |
| | tao | +ismo | → | *taìsmo* | Noun | Noun |
| | tahiti | +ismi | → | *tahitìsmi* | Noun | Noun |
| | fine | +ismi | → | *finìsmi* | Noun | Noun |
| | neo. | +ismo | → | *gratutìsmo* | Noun | neo. |

## 2 MONTHS AFTER ONSET

| Morph. transformation | Base | Affix | | Neologism | Neologism grammatical class according to context | Base grammatical class |
|---|---|---|---|---|---|---|
| | neo. | +ismo | ↑ | segherganismo | Noun | neo. |
| | neo. | +ismo | ↑ | refonismo | Noun | neo. |
| | neo. | +ismo | ↑ | teddoismo | Noun | neo. |
| | neo. | +ismo | ↑ | tettoretismo | Noun | neo. |
| | neo. | +ismo | ↑ | sicoismo | Noun | neo. |
| | neo. | +ismo | ↑ | peditismo | Noun | neo. |
| +ista | gelo | +isti | ↑ | gelisti | Noun | Noun |
| **Adjective → Noun** | | | | | | |
| +èssa: | neo. | +essa | ↑ | lorèssa | Noun | neo. |
| | neo. | +esse | ↑ | lassotèsse | Noun | neo. |
| +ismo: | solito | +ismo | ↑ | solitismo | Noun | Adj. |
| **Verb → Noun** | | | | | | |
| +ita: | neo. | +ita | ↑ | inòscita | Noun | neo. |
| | neo. | +ita | ↑ | òsvita | Noun | neo. |
| +ito: | neo. | +ito | ↑ | sùmito | undet. | neo. |
| +mènto: | assaggiare | +mento | ↑ | assaggiamènto | Noun | Verb |
| | neo. | +mento | ↑ | intossimento | Noun | neo. |
| | neo. | +mento | ↑ | ereddimènto | undet. | neo. |
| | neo. | +mento | ↑ | erendimènto | undet. | neo. |
| | neo. | +menti | ↑ | chiatamenti | Noun | neo. |
| **Noun → Adjective** | | | | | | |
| +istica: | neo. | +istica | ↑ | diermonistica | Adj. | neo. |
| +asco: | fase | +asco | ↑ | fasàsco | Adj. | Noun |
| +ico: | neo. | +ico | ↑ | rumèrico | Adj. | neo. |
| +istico: | eva/evo | +istiche | ↑ | evistiche | undet. | Noun |
| **ADJ. → ADV.** | | | | | | |
| +mènte: | neo. | +mente | ↑ | atamènte | Noun | neo. |

| Process / Rule | Base | Affix | | Result | | |
|---|---|---|---|---|---|---|
| *Preffixation* | | | | | | |
| a+: | a+ | neo. | ↑ | *affrati* | Verb | neo. |
| intra+: | intra+ | tendere | ↑ | *intratendere* | Verb | Verb. |
| *Parasynthetic Processes* | | | | | | |
| a+___+àre | a+fuoco | +ato | ↑ | *affuocàto* | Verb | Noun |
| bi+___+àre | bi+figa | +ano | ↑ | *bifìgano* | Verb | Noun |
| *Composition* | | | | | | |
| ___+___ | auto+neo. | | ↑ | *autoclàsma* | Noun | Noun+neo. |
| ___+___ | neo.+cento | | ↑ | *lentlicènto* | Undet. | Neo+noun |
| *Type 2 Neologisms[b]: Suffixation* | | | | | | |
| Noun → Noun | | | | | | |
| +àta | moderno | +ate[c] | ↑ | *modernàte* | Noun | Noun |
|  | neo. | +ate[c] | ↑ | *laffaràte* | Noun | Neo. |
| Noun → Adjective | | | | | | |
| +àto | vagina | +ata[d] | ↑ | *vaginàta* | Adj. | Noun |
| Verb → Adjective | | | | | | |
| +ènte | neo. | +ente[e] | ↑ | *crènte* | Adj. | Neo. |
|  | neo. | +enti[f] | ↑ | *forfiènti* | Adj. | Neo. |
| *Type 3 Neologisms[a]: Suffixation* | | | | | | |
| Noun → Verb | | | | | | |
| +àre | neo. | +are[h] | ↑ | *soggillàre* | Verb | Neo. |
|  | neo. | +are[h] | ↑ | *tolcàvo* | Verb | Neo. |
| +ere | due | +ere[i] | ↑ | *duère* | Undet. | Noun |
|  | cibo | +ere[i] | ↑ | *cibere* | Verb | Noun |
|  | neo. | +ere[j] | ↑ | *mòggere* | Verb | Neo. |
| +ire | pari | +ire[j] | ↑ | *parire* | Verb | Adj. |
|  | neo. | +ire[j] | ↑ | *sadire* | Verb | Neo. |
|  | neo. | +ire[j] | ↑ | *muccire* | Verb | Neo. |
| Noun → Verb or Verb → Noun | | | | | | |
| +àto | neo. | +ato[k] | ↑ | *fundàto* | Verb | Neo. |
|  | neo. | +ati[l] | ↑ | *fandiàti* | Undet. | Neo. |
| +ènte | neo. | +ente[e] | ↑ | *ricènte* | Undet. | Neo. |

| Morph. transformation | Base | Affix | Neologism | Neologism grammatical class according to context | Base grammatical class |
|---|---|---|---|---|---|
| **2 MONTHS AFTER ONSET** | | | | | |
| **3 MONTHS AFTER ONSET** | | | | | |
| *Type 1 Neologisms[a]: Prefixation* | | | | | |
| con+ | con+ | neo. | → *conclòco* | Noun | Neo. |
| inter+ | inter+ | neo. | → *interinalghisàta* | Undet. | Neo. |
| per+ | per+ | neo. | → *perfitènte* | Adj. | Neo. |
| *Type 2 Neologisms[b]: Suffixation* | | | | | |
| Verb → Noun | | | | | |
| +èndo | neo. | +endo[m] | → *contolèndo* | Noun | Neo. |
| *Type 3 Neologisms[g]: Suffixation* | | | | | |
| Noun → Verb | | | | | |
| +àto | neo. | +ato[k] | → *iposàto* | Verb | Neo. |
| Noun → Verb or Noun → Adjective | | | | | |
| +ànte | neo. | +ante[n] | → *pissànte* | Undet. | Neo. |
| +èse | neo. | +ese[o] | → *anuèse* | Verb | Neo. |
| **5 MONTHS AFTER ONSET** | | | | | |
| *Type 1 Neologisms[a]: Suffixation* | | | | | |
| Verb → Noun | | | | | |
| +siòne | neo. | +sione | → *proforsiòne* | Noun | Neo. |
| +ziòne | neo. | +zioni | → *inogaziòni* | Noun | Neo. |
| | neo. | +zione | → *riziòne* | Noun | Neo. |
| *Type 1 Neologisms[a]: Prefixation* | | | | | |
| s+ | s+rendere | | → *srènde* | Verb | Verb |
| in+ | in+neo. | | → *indevicàrlo* | Verb | Neo. |
| in+ | in+neo. | | → *ingròllano* | Verb | Neo. |
| *Type 2 Neologisms[b]: Suffixation* | | | | | |
| Verb → Adjective | | | | | |
| +ènte | neo. | +ente[e] | → *travacènte* | Adj. | Neo. |

*Type 3 Neologisms[g]: Suffixation*

| Noun → Verb | | | | | | |
|---|---|---|---|---|---|---|
| +ere | peso | +ere[i] | → | pèsere | Verb | Noun |
| | neo. | +ere[i] | → | dièdere | Verb | Neo. |

**9 MONTHS AFTER ONSET**

*Type 1 Neologisms[a]: Suffixation*

| Noun → Noun | | | | | | |
|---|---|---|---|---|---|---|
| +ària | miglia | +arie | → | migliàrie | Noun | Noun |

*Type 1 Neologisms[a]: Prefixation*

| | | | | | | |
|---|---|---|---|---|---|---|
| de+ | de+ neo. | | → | derudàti | Adj. | Neo. |
| in+ | in+ neo. | | → | intimitàre | Verb | Neo. |

*Type 2 Neologisms[b]: Suffixation*

| Noun → Noun | | | | | | |
|---|---|---|---|---|---|---|
| +ènte | neo. | +enti[f] | → | sidènti | Noun | Neo. |
| +ite | lama | +ite[p] | → | lamìte | Noun | Noun |

---

a Type 1 neologisms are unambiguously derivational.

b Type 2 neologisms have a suffix that can be either derivational or inflectional, but the context points to the fact that the suffix is truly derivational.

c +àte is an inflectional suffix, making the second plural person of the present indicative and imperative, and the feminine plural past participle of verbs of the first conjugation.

d +àta is an inflectional affix, marking the feminine singular past participle of verbs of the first conjugation.

e +ènte is an inflectional affix, marking the singular present participle of verbs of the second and third conjugations.

f +ènti is an inflectional suffix, marking the plural present participle of verbs of the second and third conjugations.

g Type 3 neologisms have an affix that can be either derivational or inflectional, whose nature cannot be determined by the context.

h +àre is an inflectional affix, marking the infinitive of verbs of the first conjugation.

i +ere is an inflectional suffix, marking the infinitive of verbs of the second conjugation.

j +ire is an inflectional suffix, marking the infinitive of verbs of the third conjugation.

k +àto is an inflectional suffix, marking the masculine singular past participle of verbs of the first conjugation.

l +àti is an inflectional suffix, marking the plural masculine past participle of verbs of the first conjugation.

m +èndo is an inflectional suffix marking the gerundive of verbs of the second and third conjugations.

n +ànte is an inflectional suffix, marking the present participle of verbs of the first conjugation.

o +èse is an inflectional suffix, marking the third singular person of the past tense of verbs of the second conjugation.

p +ite is an inflectional suffix, marking the second plural person of the present indicative and imperative, and the feminine plural past participle of verbs of the third conjugation.

# Appendix 3: Affixes of Derived Real Words Produced by R.B.

| Morphological transformations | Affix | Occurrence by time after onset | | | | | | | |
|---|---|---|---|---|---|---|---|---|---|
| | | 2 Months | | 3 Months | | 5 Months | | 9 Months | |
| | | No. | % | No. | % | No. | % | No. | % |
| | | Suffixation | | | | | | | |
| Noun → Noun | +àccio | 2 | .06 | 0 | 0 | 0 | 0 | 0 | 0 |
| | +àggio | 1 | .03 | 3 | .12 | 2 | .08 | 4 | .11 |
| | +àia | 2 | .06 | 0 | 0 | 0 | 0 | 0 | 0 |
| | +àio | 1 | .03 | 2 | .08 | 1 | .04 | 1 | .03 |
| | +àle | 0 | 0 | 4 | .17 | 1 | .04 | 4 | .11 |
| | +àme | 1 | .03 | 0 | 0 | 0 | 0 | 0 | 0 |
| | +àno | 5 | .16 | 0 | 0 | 1 | .04 | 4 | .11 |
| | +àrio | 2 | .06 | 0 | 0 | 0 | 0 | 0 | 0 |
| | +àta | 1 | .03 | 3 | .12 | 1 | .04 | 0 | 0 |
| | +ènte | 0 | 0 | 0 | 0 | 0 | 0 | 1 | .03 |
| | +èo | 1 | .03 | 0 | 0 | 0 | 0 | 0 | 0 |
| | +erìa | 0 | 0 | 0 | 0 | 0 | 0 | 2 | .06 |
| | +èro | 0 | 0 | 1 | .04 | 0 | 0 | 0 | 0 |
| | +èse | 0 | 0 | 1 | .04 | 0 | 0 | 3 | .09 |
| | +ètto | 1 | .03 | 1 | .04 | 3 | .13 | 2 | .06 |
| | +ière | 4 | .13 | 7 | .29 | 0 | 0 | 2 | .06 |
| | +ìna | 0 | 0 | 2 | .08 | 1 | .04 | 1 | .03 |
| | +ìno | 1 | .03 | 1 | .04 | 5 | .21 | 6 | .17 |
| | +òlo | 0 | 0 | 0 | 0 | 0 | 0 | 2 | .06 |
| | +òne | 1 | .03 | 0 | 0 | 0 | 0 | 0 | 0 |
| | +òso | 0 | 0 | 0 | 0 | 1 | .04 | 0 | 0 |
| | +òtto | 1 | .03 | 0 | 0 | 0 | 0 | 0 | 0 |
| | +ùncolo | 0 | 0 | 0 | 0 | 1 | .04 | 0 | 0 |
| Adjective → Noun | +ènza | 0 | 0 | 0 | 0 | 0 | 0 | 1 | .03 |
| | +èria | 0 | 0 | 0 | 0 | 1 | .04 | 0 | 0 |
| | +erìa | 0 | 0 | 0 | 0 | 1 | .04 | 0 | 0 |
| | +età | 3 | .10 | 1 | .04 | 1 | .04 | 1 | .03 |
| | +èzza | 1 | .03 | 1 | .04 | 3 | .13 | 2 | .06 |
| | +ìa | 0 | 0 | 0 | 0 | 1 | .04 | 0 | 0 |
| | +ìsmo | 1 | .03 | 0 | 0 | 0 | 0 | 0 | 0 |
| | +ità | 3 | .10 | 8 | .33 | 3 | .13 | 7 | .20 |
| | +izìa | 0 | 0 | 0 | 0 | 2 | .08 | 0 | 0 |
| | +siòne | 0 | 0 | 1 | .04 | 7 | .29 | 2 | .06 |
| | +tà | 4 | .13 | 2 | .08 | 4 | .17 | 1 | .03 |
| | +ùra | 0 | 0 | 0 | 0 | 1 | .04 | 0 | 0 |
| | +ziòne | 0 | 0 | 0 | 0 | 0 | 0 | 0 | 0 |
| Verb → Noun | +ànte | 0 | 0 | 1 | .04 | 0 | 0 | 5 | .14 |
| | +ànza | 0 | 0 | 1 | .04 | 0 | 0 | 1 | .03 |
| | +àta | 0 | 0 | 0 | 0 | 1 | .04 | 0 | 0 |
| | +àto | 0 | 0 | 1 | .04 | 3 | .13 | 7 | .20 |
| | +ènte | 1 | .03 | 1 | .04 | 0 | 0 | 0 | 0 |
| | +ènza | 1 | .03 | 0 | 0 | 11 | .46 | 0 | 0 |
| | +èssa | 1 | .03 | 1 | .04 | 0 | 0 | 0 | 0 |
| | +ièro | 0 | 0 | 1 | .04 | 1 | .04 | 0 | 0 |

| Morphological transformations | Affix | Occurrence by time after onset | | | | | | | |
|---|---|---|---|---|---|---|---|---|---|
| | | 2 Months | | 3 Months | | 5 Months | | 9 Months | |
| | | No. | % | No. | % | No. | % | No. | % |
| | | Suffixation | | | | | | | |
| | +‿io | 0 | 0 | 1 | .04 | 0 | 0 | 0 | 0 |
| | +‿ita | 0 | 0 | 1 | .04 | 1 | .04 | 0 | 0 |
| | +ìto | 0 | 0 | 0 | 0 | 6 | .25 | 0 | 0 |
| | +mènto | 2 | .06 | 1 | .04 | 3 | .13 | 3 | .09 |
| | +siòne | 0 | 0 | 1 | .04 | 0 | 0 | 0 | 0 |
| | +sòre | 0 | 0 | 0 | 0 | 0 | 0 | 7 | .20 |
| | +tòre | 3 | .10 | 6 | .25 | 1 | .04 | 4 | .11 |
| | +ùra | 0 | 0 | 1 | .04 | 0 | 0 | 0 | 0 |
| | +ùta | 0 | 0 | 1 | .04 | 1 | .04 | 1 | .03 |
| | +ziòne | 2 | .06 | 3 | .12 | 3 | .13 | 5 | .14 |
| | ∅ | 2 | .06 | 1 | .04 | 9 | .38 | 2 | .06 |
| Adjective → Adjective | +àrio | 1 | .03 | 0 | 0 | 0 | 0 | 0 | 0 |
| | +ìno | 5 | .16 | 2 | .08 | 1 | .04 | 3 | .09 |
| | +ìssimo | 2 | .06 | 0 | 0 | 4 | .17 | 7 | .20 |
| | +òtto | 1 | .03 | 0 | 0 | 0 | 0 | 0 | 0 |
| Noun → Adjective | +àle | 25 | .80 | 7 | .29 | 1 | .04 | 3 | .09 |
| | +àno | 5 | .16 | 1 | .04 | 0 | 0 | 4 | .12 |
| | +àre | 0 | 0 | 0 | 0 | 1 | .04 | 0 | 0 |
| | +àrio | 1 | .03 | 0 | 0 | 0 | 0 | 0 | 0 |
| | +àto | 1 | .03 | 0 | 0 | 0 | 0 | 3 | .09 |
| | +èo | 2 | .06 | 1 | .04 | 0 | 0 | 0 | 0 |
| | +ése | 0 | 0 | 0 | 0 | 0 | 0 | 2 | .06 |
| | +‿ico | 4 | .13 | 0 | 0 | 0 | 0 | 5 | .14 |
| | +ièro | 0 | 0 | 0 | 0 | 1 | .04 | 0 | 0 |
| | +ìo | 0 | 0 | 0 | 0 | 0 | 0 | 1 | .03 |
| | +ìsta | 0 | 0 | 0 | 0 | 0 | 0 | 1 | .03 |
| | +òne | 0 | 0 | 0 | 0 | 0 | 0 | 1 | .03 |
| | +òso | 3 | .10 | 0 | 0 | 1 | .04 | 0 | 0 |
| | ∅ | 1 | .03 | 0 | 0 | 0 | 0 | 2 | .06 |
| Verb → Adjective | +ànte | 0 | 0 | 1 | .04 | 0 | 0 | 6 | .17 |
| | +àto | 6 | .19 | 1 | .04 | 11 | .46 | 6 | .17 |
| | +‿bile | 2 | .06 | 1 | .04 | 1 | .04 | 0 | 0 |
| | +ènte | 3 | .10 | 2 | .08 | 0 | 0 | 3 | .09 |
| | +ìto | 3 | .10 | 1 | .04 | 0 | 0 | 2 | .06 |
| | ∅ | 0 | 0 | 0 | 0 | 1 | .04 | 0 | 0 |
| Noun → Verb | +àre | 19 | .60 | 36 | 1.50 | 43 | 1.80 | 84 | 2.41 |
| | +ìre | 3 | .10 | 1 | .04 | 0 | 0 | 1 | .03 |
| | +izzàre | 0 | 0 | 2 | .08 | 0 | 0 | 0 | 0 |
| Adjective → Verb | +àre | 0 | 0 | 0 | 0 | 0 | 0 | 1 | .03 |
| Noun → Adverb | ∅ | 7 | .22 | 4 | .17 | 4 | .17 | 4 | .11 |
| Adjective → Adverb | +ièri | 1 | .03 | 2 | .08 | 0 | 0 | 4 | .11 |
| | +mènte | 11 | .35 | 10 | .42 | 27 | 1.13 | 16 | .46 |
| | ∅ | 4 | .13 | 2 | .08 | 4 | .17 | 4 | .11 |
| | | Prefixation | | | | | | | |
| Noun → Noun | ri+ | 1 | .03 | 0 | 0 | 0 | 0 | 0 | 0 |
| Adjective → Adjective | di+ | 6 | .19 | 1 | .04 | 0 | 0 | 0 | 0 |
| | in+ | 1 | .03 | 1 | .04 | 0 | 0 | 2 | .06 |
| | inter+ | 0 | 0 | 6 | .25 | 0 | 0 | 0 | 0 |

| Morphological transformations | Affix | Occurrence by time after onset | | | | | | | |
|---|---|---|---|---|---|---|---|---|---|
| | | 2 Months | | 3 Months | | 5 Months | | 9 Months | |
| | | No. | % | No. | % | No. | % | No. | % |
| | | *Prefixation* | | | | | | | |
| | per+ | 0 | 0 | 1 | .04 | 0 | 0 | 0 | 0 |
| Verb → Verb | con+ | 0 | 0 | 1 | .04 | 2 | .08 | 0 | 0 |
| | de+ | 0 | 0 | 0 | 0 | 1 | .04 | 6 | .17 |
| | di+ | 0 | 0 | 0 | 0 | 0 | 0 | 2 | .06 |
| | dis+ | 0 | 0 | 0 | 0 | 1 | .04 | 0 | 0 |
| | in+ | 0 | 0 | 0 | 0 | 1 | .04 | 1 | .03 |
| | per+ | 1 | .03 | 0 | 0 | 2 | .08 | 0 | 0 |
| | pro+ | 0 | 0 | 1 | .04 | 0 | 0 | 0 | 0 |
| | re+ | 0 | 0 | 1 | .04 | 1 | .04 | 0 | 0 |
| | ri+ | 12 | .38 | 3 | .12 | 6 | .25 | 7 | .20 |
| | s+ | 4 | .13 | 2 | .08 | 1 | .04 | 0 | 0 |
| | | *Parasyntethic Processes* | | | | | | | |
| Noun → Verb | a+____+àre | 2 | .06 | 6 | .25 | 13 | .54 | 11 | .32 |
| | a+____+ìre | 0 | 0 | 1 | .04 | 0 | 0 | 0 | 0 |
| | in+____+ìre | 0 | 0 | 0 | 0 | 1 | .04 | 0 | 0 |
| | pro+____+àre | 0 | 0 | 0 | 0 | 1 | .04 | 0 | 0 |
| | ri+____+àto | 1 | .03 | 0 | 0 | 0 | 0 | 0 | 0 |
| | | *Composition* | | | | | | | |
| | ____+____ | 2 | .06 | 6 | .25 | 13 | .54 | 11 | .32 |

# 6
# A Fluent Morphological Agrammatic in an Inflectional Language?

Jussi Niemi, Matti Laine, and Päivi Koivuselkä-Sallinen

A patient is presented who exhibited an unusual morphological disorder in spontaneous speech and writing. Being initially almost completely speechless she started to exhibit fluent speech coupled with a loss of bound grammatical morphemes in a richly inflected language, viz., in Finnish. Her "agrammatism" was anomalous in two respects. First, she was a fluent speaker, yet she frequently omitted inflectional affixes (cf., however, case 2 of Miceli, Mazzucchi, Menn, and Goodglass, 1983). Second, these omissions took place in a language with rich inflectional (suffixal) morphology, and it has been shown that aphasics in these type of languages typically do not omit but substitute affixes to the degree found in the speech of the present aphasic (Bates and Wulfeck, 1989; for Hebrew: Grodzinsky, 1984; Niemi, Laine, Hänninen, and Koivuselkä-Sallinen, in press; Talay and Slobin, personal communication in Bates, Friederici, and Wulfeck 1987; for Czech: Lehečková, 1988). However, Bhatnagar and Whitaker (1984) have reported a dysfluent Hindi agrammatic who often omitted verb suffixes, producing only the root or the infinitive form of the verb.

It is also noteworthy that our patient did not omit (or substitute) bound morphemes in either repetition or sentence completion tasks. She was thus able to process affixes in contexts and modalities other than spontaneous speech and writing (cf. case 2 of Miceli et al., 1983). Moreover, her syntactic comprehension appeared to be intact. Theoretically, she exhibited an anomaly in terms of the predominant views of agrammatism and of aphasia in general. To sum up, the present aphasic should not have omitted bound grammatical markers to the degree that she did. These omissions (or traditional markers of "agrammatism") are not typically associated with fluent speech output. Moreover, during a 2-week follow-up period she showed relatively fast recovery from the "agrammatic" stage toward language output that resembled a normal speaker's language production. During these weeks her recovery of language output was most notably manifest in inflectional morphology and syntax.

In the following sections we first discuss some general aspects of the present speaker's language output, including complexity of noun phrases as well as word order, word class, and case-marker distribution. After these observations we discuss at length the omissions of inflectional suffixes in her speech, as they are not predictable in Finnish language deficits.

## Procedures

The language of the patient (O.R.) was analyzed on the basis of six audio-taped conversational sessions within a 2-week span in early 1987. The sizes of the corpora are as follows: session 1 (Feb. 3), 3155 words; session 2 (Feb. 4), 746 words; session 3 (Feb. 10), 868 words; session 4 (Feb. 12), 1330 words; session 5 (Feb. 13), 418 words; session 6 (Feb. 16), 573 words (the total numbers of words may differ from these figures in some analyses because some analyses represent sampled data). We compared her language with the two normal Finnish speakers used as controls in the Cross Language Aphasia Study as well as the two Broca agrammatics of the same study (Niemi et al., in press). We will also refer to two Finnish Wernicke speakers (Niemi, Koivuselkä-Sallinen, and Hänninen, 1986; Niemi, Koivuselkä-Sallinen and Laine, in preparation).

## History

O.R. was admitted to hospital because of right peripheral facial paresis, right hemiparesis, and aphasia. Despite extensive neurological examinations, the etiology of her illness remained open. Inconsistencies in symptomatology led later to the conclusion that psychogenic factors (conversion hysteria) were playing a significant role in her prolonged illness. There was some indication, however, of an observable change in brain function. Single photon emission computed tomography (SPECT) by HM-PAO revealed two areas of diminished brain perfusion in the left frontal lobe, although these changes were milder at a follow-up examination.

## General Aspects of O.R.'s Language

### Fluency and Phrase Length

The *fluency* of the patient was analyzed during the six sessions using the traditional word per minute (wpm) count. O.R.'s overall speech rate was 88 wpm, vacillating between 73 and 104 wpm per session with no clear recovery trend. This figure probably lies within the limits of the speech rate of the controls (97 wpm). The overall rate of O.R., however, clearly exceeded the values obtained from the two Broca agrammatics (61 and

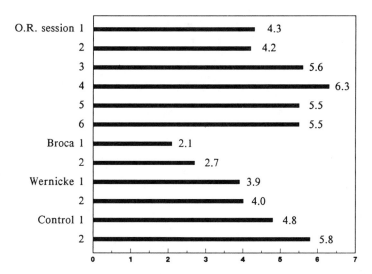

FIGURE 6.1. Average phrase lengths (in words) for O.R., two Broca agrammatics, two Wernicke speakers, and two controls.

55 wpm). We have previously analyzed the words per minute value for Wernicke 1, who had the rate of 110 wpm, which is most probably at the higher end of the normal range (Niemi et al., 1986).

*Phrase* is here defined as a sequence that is signaled either by sentential cues (e.g., structural and intonational) or by such "performance failures" as a long pause or aborted sentence structures. The number of words O.R. produced during a phrase ($\bar{x} = 5.2$) is well within the normal range and well above the values obtained from the narratives of Finnish Broca aphasics analyzed for the Cross Language Aphasia Study (Fig. 6.1). There is some indication of a trend toward an increasing phrase length with time.

Referring to the two quantitative indices and to our impression of her speech output in general, O.R.'s "phonetic" fluency and her sentential and textual fluency are well within normal limits.

## Nominal Phrases

Because Broca agrammatics exhibit a low number of nominal phrases (NPs) with premodifiers as well as genitival NPs (Menn and Obler, in press), we analyzed the frequency of nominal phrases of O.R. carrying a preposed modifier (either an adjective or a noun/pronoun in the genitive). The analysis is based on two sessions that produced the most data (in terms of running words), i.e., sessions 1 and 4. We used the total number of nouns as a point of reference. The results showed that O.R. produced more of these two-member, complex NP phrases during the latter session

TABLE 6.1. Phrase structure complexity in the speech of O.R., Broca agrammatics, Wernicke paragrammatics, and normal controls.

| Subject | Adj+noun | Gen+noun | Total | No. all nouns | % complex NPs out of all nouns |
|---------|----------|----------|-------|---------------|-------------------------------|
| O.R., session 1 | 30 | 17 | 47 | 317 | 14.8 |
| O.R., session 4 | 32 | 17 | 49 | 192 | 25.5 |
| Broca 1 | 5 | 0 | 5 | 105 | 4.8 |
| Broca 2 | 2 | 0 | 2 | 91 | 2.2 |
| Wernicke 1 | 7 | 10 | 17 | 102 | 16.7 |
| Wernicke 2 | 9 | 0 | 9 | 116 | 7.8 |
| Control 1 | 22 | 7 | 29 | 164 | 17.7 |
| Control 2 | 13 | 10 | 23 | 189 | 12.2 |

(Table 6.1). Note, however, that both of these values are close to the control values. The Broca agrammatics had almost floor values, and they also failed to produce any genitival NP constructions of the type here analyzed. In this respect at least, O.R. is unlike a Broca agrammatic. Rather, the frequency of her complex NPs here analyzed is well within the normal range.

## Word Order

The analysis of surface word order was carried out using the minimal three categories that have been frequently used, e.g., in typological studies of word-order change as well as in aphasiology (for aphasia, see Bates, Friederici, Wulfeck, and Juarez, 1988). These three categories are subject (S), verb (V), and any other obligatory NP constituent (X = object, adverbial, or predicative. [See Hakulinen, Karlsson, and Vilkuna (1980), who applied the same categories in a computer analysis of word-order in normal Finnish.]

### OVERALL CONFIGURATION

About half of the clauses O.R. produced during session 1 carried the canonical Finnish SVX surface order (52%). This value clearly exceeds the respective percentages of the Finnish Broca (40%) and Wernicke (38%) speakers as well as those obtained from the controls (41%). At session 4, O.R.'s SVX rate is more normal (42%).

### Position of Subject

The change over time in O.R.'s production of syntax becomes more manifest when the position of the subject is analyzed separately for sessions 1

TABLE 6.2.  Position of subject.

| Subject | % Distribution | | | | | | | |
|---|---|---|---|---|---|---|---|---|
| | O.R., 1 | O.R., 4 | B1 | B2 | W1 | W2 | C1 | C2 |
| S initial | 91.5 | 75.6 | 77.6 | 89.3 | 73.1 | 67.8 | 67.4 | 75.0 |
| S medial | 5.4 | 11.2 | 14.1 | 10.7 | 18.5 | 18.1 | 16.8 | 12.5 |
| S final | 3.1 | 13.2 | 8.2 | 0.0 | 8.4 | 14.1 | 15.8 | 12.5 |

TABLE 6.3.  Word class distribution.

| Word class | Distribution (%) | | | | | | | |
|---|---|---|---|---|---|---|---|---|
| | O.R., 1 | O.R., 4 | B1 | B2 | W1 | W2 | C1 | C2 |
| Adjectives | 3.7 | 5.8 | 2.4 | 0.8 | 2.3 | 2.8 | 5.5 | 3.4 |
| Nouns | 16.3 | 14.5 | 22.4 | 13.8 | 8.1 | 14.0 | 21.1 | 18.9 |
| Pronouns | 23.2 | 20.9 | 3.2 | 15.7 | 24.1 | 23.8 | 13.2 | 14.9 |
| Numerals | 2.0 | 0.4 | 3.0 | 1.8 | 1.4 | 0.9 | 1.0 | 0.7 |
| Verbs | 28.5 | 24.9 | 21.6 | 25.1 | 29.1 | 24.2 | 23.7 | 22.6 |
| Conjunctions | 11.2 | 15.7 | 24.8 | 17.5 | 10.3 | 10.7 | 14.4 | 14.4 |
| P-positions | 0.7 | 0.5 | 0.2 | 0.8 | 0.7 | 0.9 | 1.0 | 1.3 |
| Adverbs | 12.7 | 14.1 | 16.2 | 12.6 | 22.0 | 18.9 | 18.0 | 19.7 |
| Miscellaneous | 1.7 | 3.2 | 6.2 | 12.0 | 2.1 | 3.8 | 2.1 | 4.0 |
| Total | 1955 | 1324 | 468 | 661 | 6140 | 13457 | 778 | 999 |

and 4 (Table 6.2). During session 1 about 90% of her clauses were subject-initial, whereas in session 4 she exhibited about 76% of subject-initial clauses. This change was a drastic one toward the normal distribution of subject placement among the SVX constituents.

## Word Class Distribution

During both sessions 1 and 4, O.R. used a relatively large number of pronouns (Table 6.3). Interestingly enough, this usage was comparable to the frequency of use of pronouns by Finnish Wernicke aphasics. Both O.R. and the Wernicke speakers had a pronoun rate that is about 10 percentage points higher than that of the normal controls. Moreover, as in Wernicke speech, the overuse of pronouns was compensated for by an underuse of nouns. However, the latter observation was not as conspicuous and unambiguous as the overuse of pronouns in O.R.'s speech.

## Case Distribution

To give a brief sketch of Finnish inflection, the most frequent cases of a nominal paradigm are given as an example. In this case the paradigm is simple in that it carries no stem-internal morphophonological alteration, which is rather rare in Finnish. The paradigm is for the *talo* (house) type of words.

| Case | Singular | Plural | Approximate English equivalent of case marker |
|------|----------|--------|-----------------------------------------------|
| Nominative | talo | talo+t | (uninflected stem) |
| Partitive | talo+a | talo+j+a | (uninflected stem) |
| Genitive | talo+n | talo+j+en | of |
| Translative | talo+ksi | talo+i+ksi | (change) into |
| Essive | talo+na | talo+i+na | as |
| Inessive | talo+ssa | talo+i+ssa | in |
| Elative | talo+sta | talo+i+sta | from within |
| Illative | talo+on | talo+i+hin | into (place) |
| Adessive | talo+lla | talo+i+lla | at, possession |
| Ablative | talo+lta | talo+i+lta | from vicinity of |
| Allative | talo+lle | talo+i+lle | to vicinity of |

Session 1 of O.R. carried an exceptionally high percentage of nominative forms (Table 6.4). Nine days later the relative frequency of her nominatives was closer to the normal values. The change in the other crucial category, the genitive, ran also from a highly abnormal to normal or near-normal when we shifted from session 1 to session 4. The paucity of the other cases than the nominative and the genitive during session 1 resembled the output characteristics of the Broca agrammatics. In fact, O.R.'s output even exceeded the abnormality of the Broca speakers. However, during session 4 she closely resembled the normals so far as the relative use of the various cases was concerned. Hence using the present linguistic characteristic, she changed from the abnormal (Broca-like) end of the spectrum toward the normal end within the 9-day period that separated sessions 1 and 4.

TABLE 6.4. Distribution of surface cases in nouns and adjectives.

| Case | Distribution (%) | | | | | | |
|------|-------|--------|------|------|------|------|------|
|      | O.R., 1 | O.R., 4 | B1 | B2 | W2 | C1 | C2 |
| Nominative | 79.3 | 50.0 | 50.0 | 46.2 | 54.2 | 44.4 | 45.7 |
| Partitive | 12.0 | 18.6 | 16.7 | 24.2 | 14.4 | 15.0 | 13.6 |
| Genitive | 3.0 | 10.9 | 4.4 | 8.8 | 7.2 | 14.0 | 13.1 |
| Translative | 0.5 | 0 | 0 | 0 | 0.2 | 0.5 | 1.4 |
| Essive | 0.3 | 0.8 | 2.6 | 0 | 4.1 | 0.5 | 2.7 |
| Inessive | 2.4 | 7.0 | 13.2 | 8.8 | 7.0 | 5.3 | 6.3 |
| Elative | 0.3 | 5.4 | 0 | 1.1 | 3.7 | 2.4 | 1.8 |
| Illative | 1.4 | 2.7 | 3.5 | 4.4 | 2.1 | 3.4 | 4.1 |
| Adessive | 0.8 | 3.9 | 9.6 | 3.3 | 4.4 | 4.8 | 6.3 |
| Ablative | 0 | 0.4 | 0 | 1.1 | 0.7 | 0.5 | 1.4 |
| Allative | 0 | 0.4 | 0 | 2.2 | 1.7 | 9.2 | 3.6 |
| Other | 0 | 0 | 0 | 0 | 0.3 | 0 | 0 |
| Total | 368 | 258 | 114 | 91 | 2102 | 207 | 221 |

## Formal Properties of Inflected Words

The interviews with O.R. yielded the auditory impression that, although being fluent, she often omitted inflectional endings and especially case markers. The analysis of the case marker omissions dealt with nouns, adjectives, pronouns, and numerals. Furthermore, because case markers are copied from the noun head by the adjectival premodifiers in nearly all instances in Finnish, we analyzed the two-member NPs separately. This decision was made *a posteriori* because we wanted to test the end-clipping hypothesis as a major explanation of the omissions that tapped endings in nouns. The omissions in simple NPs are discussed first through observations pooled over the six sessions, after which a brief discussion follows on the time course of these marking errors from sessions 1 through 6. The single-word NPs are dealt with first, followed by the complex (two-member) NPs.

### *Simple NPs*

The 51 case marker errors in the simple NPs produced by O.R. were divided into the following groups: (1) case marker substitutions; (2) case marker omissions with an inflectional stem as the sole marker of case relations; (3) words that carry separate inflectional stems in their paradigms but that occur in the present errors in their base forms; and (4) words with no morphophonological alteration (i.e., words with one stem) in their inflectional paradigms (see the examples below).

SUBSTITUTIONS

The relative infrequency of case marker substitutions (n = 3) in comparison to the omissions is atypical of Finnish Broca agrammatism, where omissions of bound grammatical morphemes are practically nonexistent (Kukkonen, 1983; Niemi et al., in press). Moreover, both fluent and nonfluent speakers would be expected to show substitutions of these morphemes.

As is the case with most substitutions in fluent aphasia, the three instances of substitution in O.R.'s speech could equally well be understood as sentence blends, where two or more structures are incorrectly amalgamated into one [see Butterworth (1985) for use of sentence blends in Wernicke's syntax].

(1) he    ottivat *si+tä*            tode+ksi          (pro *se+n*)
    they took   it+PARTITIVE true+TRANSLATIVE it+ACCUSA-
                                                        TIVE/GEN.

    they took it for granted

In (1) the incorrect *sitä* (it) could be the object of *ottaa* (take) but not in this idiomatic construction, and *todeksi* (as true) is incorrect too. The correct expression with *ottaa* would be *ottaa sen todesta*. The sentence blend hypothesis becomes more plausible when we note that a common expression for "think as true" in Finnish would require the translative in "true" (viz., *luulla todeksi*, where also *sitä* could occur, i.e., *luulla sitä todeksi*).

## OMISSIONS

The 15 instances where the word was incorrectly represented by its inflectional stem without the case marker that triggers the choice between the stems (or the morphophonological alteration within the stem) indicated that affixes can be omitted or deleted in the actual speech processes. Somewhat modifying the terminology of Garrett (1980), these instances are referred to as *stranded inflectional stems*. The relatively frequent use of the stranded inflectional stems suggests that the full listing hypothesis (Butterworth, 1983) of lexical representation of words is not the most parsimonious one in this case, as it would be difficult to see why and how the fully inflected forms would lose their syntactic markers. The full listing hypothesis becomes less explanatory still when we note the priority of inflectional markers in that speech errors of normals usually retain the affixes when the stems are misplaced and that the neologistic forms of jargon aphasics usually have blurred stems but have the affixes unaffected [for normal slips, see Garrett (1980); for criticism, see Stemberger (1985); for Wernicke language output, see Butterworth (1985]. In sentence (2) the form *tytö+i+lle* (of *tyttö*—note the degemination triggered by affixation) is produced as *tytö*, an inflectional stem that does not appear as an independent word in Finnish.

(2) mä jutteli *tytö* (for *tytö+i   +lle*)
    I    talked  girl         girl+PL+ALLATIVE
    I talked to the girls
    (The context disambiguates the choice between the singular and plural of "girl.")

## BASE FORMS FOR INFLECTIONAL STEMS

The nine errors that produce base word forms and that have no required morphophonological changes in the stem are here interpreted as *substitutions* of the base form for the inflectional stem rather than instances of *omissions*.

(3) ja   sit  ei  toise  ymmärrä  *se*      (for *si+tä*)
    and then not others understand it             it+PARTITIVE
    and then the others won't understand it

BASE FORMS FOR INVARIANT PARADIGMS

O.R. produced 24 inflectional errors that dealt with paradigms with no stem-internal morphophonological alteration between the form produced and the (presumed) target form [see sentence (4)]. As an alternative to treating these cases as instances of bound morpheme omissions, these errors could also be explained as arising from lexical look-up, *if* we first assume that inflected forms are represented as separate items in the mental lexicon.

(4) mut jos sä   olet *Espanja* ja   kysy missää on+ko
    but if  you are Spain   and ask where is+QUESTION
    but if  you are in Spain and ask where

    se   talo   tai osote...   (for *Espanja+ssa*)
    that house or address...   Spain +INESSIVE
    that house or address is...


TIME COURSE OF INFLECTIONAL ERRORS IN SIMPLE NPS

The change in the inflectional marker errors of O.R. during the 2-week period was clearly toward more normal language (Table 6.5). When the number of case marker errors was calculated relative to the total number of words produced by O.R. during each session, a distinct decrease of the error rate (in percent) was observed. The error rates session by session, ranging from session 1 to session 6, were 1.1, 0.8, 0.9, 0.1, 0.2, and 0. Although the number of instances is too low to allow for anything but tentative conclusions on the relative persistence of error types, the figures in Table 6.5 suggest that the stranded inflectional stems were dropped out of use earlier than the errors that produced actual Finnish word forms (however incorrect they may be in their present contexts). These observations thus corroborated the view that the nominative is the psycholo-

TABLE 6.5. Case marker errors in single NPs (nouns, adjectives, pronouns, numerals) for each session.

| Errors | Errors, by session | | | | | | |
|---|---|---|---|---|---|---|---|
| | 1 | 2 | 3 | 4 | 5 | 6 | Total |
| Substitutions (e.g., *sitä* for *sen*) | — | 2 | 1 | — | — | — | 3 |
| Stranded inflectional stems (e.g., *tytö* for *tytöille*) | 13 | 1 | 1 | — | — | — | 15 |
| Base forms for inflectional stems (e.g., *se* for *sitä*) | 4 | 1 | 4 | — | — | — | 9 |
| Base forms for invariant paradigms (e.g., *Espanja* for *Espanjassa*) | 19 | 1 | 2 | 1 | 1 | — | 24 |
| *Total* | 36 | 5 | 8 | 1 | 1 | — | 51 |
| *Error percentage* (per no. of words) | 1.1 | 0.8 | 0.9 | 0.1 | 0.2 | 0.0 | 0.7 |

gically real (or more real) form in the Finnish inflectional paradigms of nouns and related word classes (the so-called nominals) (Karlsson, 1982).

## Complex NPs

The 38 case marker errors in the two-member NPs were analyzed in the same four error categories as the simple NPs above. However, because both the preposed modifier and the head noun may carry inflectional errors, the modifier was used as the classifier. Therefore there has to be a fifth category in use, one with a correct modifier but with a head noun that is incorrectly inflected. The five error categories are given in tabular form only, as the basic rationale of the classification was explained in connection with the simple NPs above (Table 6.6). Examples for each category are the following.

Substitution in modifier (n = 2).

(5) mää pese tuka *vasemm+in*    *käde* (for *vasemma+lla käde+llä*)
    I    wash hair left    +with hand    left+ADESSIVE hand+
                                                    ADESSIVE
    I wash my hair with my left hand

Stranded inflectional stem in modifier (n = 1).

(6) mu+1 on ollu *semmos*  kuumejuttu+i (for *semmos+i    +a*)
    I +at has been that-kind fever spell+s    kind    +PL+
                                                    PARTITIVE
    I have had kind of fever spells

Base form instead of an inflectional stem in modifier (n = 21).

TABLE 6.6. Case marker errors in complex NPs (nouns, adjectives, pronouns, numerals) for each session.

| Errors | Errors, by session | | | | | | |
|---|---|---|---|---|---|---|---|
| | 1 | 2 | 3 | 4 | 5 | 6 | Total |
| Substitutions (e.g., *vasemmin käde* for *vasemmalla kädellä*) | 1 | — | 1 | — | — | — | 2 |
| Stranded inflectional stems (e.g., *semmos kuumejuttui* for *semmo(i)sia kuumejuttui*) | 1 | — | — | — | — | — | 1 |
| Base forms for inflectional stems (e.g., *yks lenkin* for *yhden lenkin*) | 15 | 3 | 3 | — | — | — | 21 |
| Base forms of invariant paradigms (e.g., *hullu suomalaisjuoppojen* for *hullujen suomalaisjuoppojen*) | 4 | — | — | — | — | — | 4 |
| Modifier correct, head incorrect (e.g., *vuotavi maha* for *vuotavi(a) mahoja*) | 5 | 1 | 3 | 1 | — | — | 10 |
| Total | 26 | 4 | 7 | 1 | — | — | 38 |

The genitival modifiers (which do not copy the case of the heads) are excluded. The errors are classified in reference to the modifiers.

(7) tee+n nyt *yks* lenki+n                                  (for *yhde+n*)
 do +I nowone run  +ACCUSATIVE/GENITIVE one +ACC./
                                                                                GEN.
 I will now jog one round

Invariant inflectional stem in modifier (n = 4).

(8) *hullus* suomalaisjuoppo+j  +en        kans (for *hullu+j*  +en)
 crazy  Finnish-drunk  +PL+GEN. with        crazy+PL+GEN.
 with crazy Finnish drunks

Modifier correct, head noun incorrect (n = 10).

(9) mä olen vuotavi  *maha* löytäny (for *maho+j*  +a)
 I    have bleeding belly  found        belly+PL+PARTITIVE
 I have found bleeding bellies

Of these types, *b* and *d* (e.g., *semmos* and *hullu*) suggest that the omissions of case markers and other suffixes are not always due to peripheral or phonetic clipping of the final morpheme in the prosodic phrase, as these omissions also take place inside the fluent NP.

## Conclusion

We have summarized our major points in tabular form (Table 6.7) and have contrasted O.R. with two Finnish Broca and two Wernicke aphasics analyzed by us. It appears that O.R. was ambivalent in regard to the three-way classification (Broca–Wernicke–control). In terms of fluency, phrase length, and the use of NP modifiers (NP complexity), she was similar to the controls during sessions 1 and 4. However, her word order developed

TABLE 6.7. Summary of O.R.'s speech production and language characteristics during sessions 1 and 4 compared to Finnish Broca and Wernicke speakers and controls.

| Characteristic | Session 1 | | | Session 4 | | |
|---|---|---|---|---|---|---|
| | B | W | C | B | W | C |
| Fluency | − | − | + | − | − | + |
| Phrase length | − | − | + | − | − | + |
| NP modifiers | − | − | + | − | − | + |
| Word order | + | − | − | ? | ? | ? |
| Word class distribution | − | + | − | − | + | − |
| Case marker distribution | + | − | − | − | − | + |
| Inflectional omissions | Atypical of all | | | Atypical of all | | |
| | Finnish aphasics | | | Finnish aphasics | | |

B = Broca; W = Wernicke; C = controls.
The pluses indicate the closest impressionistic matches, the question marks the undecided ones between groups.

from a state resembling Broca agrammatism toward more normal, whereas her word class distribution was like that of Wernicke narratives during both sessions. The case marker distribution showed a drastic change from a Broca-like pattern to a normal pattern. The most striking observation was, of course, the numerous omissions of bound grammatical morphemes, a feature rarely seen in a richly inflected language. The cases most closely resembling O.R. in this respect are the Italian case 2 of Miceli et al. (1983) and the Hindi agrammatic of Bhatnagar and Whitaker (1984). The Hindi speaker was somewhat dysfluent, whereas the Italian patient of Miceli et al. was fluent.

It must be emphasized that O.R. was certainly not a conclusive case because of her obscure medical background. In any case, her omissions of the bound grammatical morphemes that violated the structure of Finnish language, which led her to come up with illegal word forms, arouse some serious and fundamental problems. Did O.R. exhibit a morphological deficit of organic origin or a hysterical language disorder? It has been observed that morphophonologically marked stranded word stems are rare in aphasic speech (Menn and Obler, in press). Leaving these questions unanswered, future cross-linguistic aphasia studies will hopefully give us a better picture of the spectrum of morphosyntactic deviations in aphasia and related disorders.

*Acknowledgments.* We thank Leila Sarajärvi for her assistance in the preparation of this report as well as the Academy of Finland and the University of Joensuu for their financial support to the Aphasia Research Group.

## References

Bates, E., & Wulfeck, B. (1989). Comparative aphasiology: a cross-linguistic approach to language breakdown. *Aphasiology*, *3*, 111–142.

Bates, E., Friederici, A., & Wulfeck, B. (1987). Comprehension in aphasia: a cross-linguistic study. *Brain and Language*, *32*, 19–67.

Bates, E., Friederici, A., Wulfeck, B., & Juarez, A. (1988). On the preservation of word order in aphasia: cross-linguistic evidence. *Brain and Language*, *33*, 323–364.

Bhatnagar, S., & Whitaker, H.A. (1984). Agrammatism on inflectional bound morphemes: a case study of a Hindi-speaking aphasic patient. *Cortex*, *20*, 295–301.

Butterworth, B. (1983). Lexical representation. In B. Butterworth (ed.), *Language Production* (Vol. 2). London: Academic Press.

Butterworth, B. (1985). Jargon aphasia: processes and strategies. In S. Newman & R. Epstein (eds.), *Current Perspectives in Dysphasia*. Edinburgh: Churchill Livingstone.

Garrett, M. (1980). Levels of processing in sentence production. In B. Butterworth (ed.), *Language Production* (Vol. 1). London: Academic Press.

Grodzinsky, Y. (1984). The syntactic characterization of agrammatism. *Cognition*, *16*, 99–120.

Hakulinen, A., Karlsson, F., & Vilkuna, M. (1980). *Suomen tekstilauseiden piirteitä: kvantitatiivinen tutkimus*. Publications of the Department of General Linguistics, University of Helsinki, No. 6.

Karlsson, F. (1982). *Suomen kielen äänne- ja muotorakenne*. Porvoo: Söderström.

Kukkonen, P. (1983). Motorisen afasian lingvistisiä erityispiirteitä. *Virittäjä*, *87*, 462–481 [English summary: Linguistic characteristics of motor aphasia].

Lehečková, H. (1988). The influence of language type on the manifestation of agrammatism. In P. Koivuselkä-Sallinen & L. Sarajärvi (eds.), *Proceedings of the 3rd Finnish Conference of Neurolinguistics, Joensuu 1987*. Studies in Languages 12, University of Joensuu.

Menn, L., & Obler, L. (eds.). (in press). *Agrammatic Aphasia: A Cross-Language Narrative Sourcebook*. Amsterdam: Benjamins.

Miceli, G., Mazzucchi, A., Menn, L., & Goodglass, H. (1983). Contrasting cases of Italian agrammatic aphasia without comprehension disorder. *Brain and Language*, *19*, 65–97.

Niemi, J., Koivuselkä-Sallinen, P., & Hänninen, R. (1986). Lexical and morphosyntactic patterns in posterior aphasia. In J. Niemi & P. Koivuselkä-Sallinen (eds.), *Joensuu Papers in Neuropsychology and Neurolinguistics* (Vol. 2). University of Joensuu, No. 5.

Niemi, J., Laine, M., Hänninen, R., & Koivuselkä-Sallinen, P. (in press). Agrammatic narrative in Finnish. In L. Menn & L. Obler (eds.), *Agrammatic Aphasia: A Cross-Language Narrative Sourcebook*. Amsterdam: Benjamins.

Niemi, J., Koivuselkä-Sallinen, P. & Laine, M., (in preparation). Syntax and inflectional morphology in aphasia: narratives of Wernicke speakers.

Stemberger, J.P. (1985). An interactive activation model of language production. In A.W. Ellis (ed.), *Progress in the Psychology of Language* (Vol. 1). London: Lawrence Erlbaum Associates.

# 7
# Grammatical Gender in Aphasia

Hubert Guyard, Attie Duval-Gombert, and
Marie-Claude Le Bot

The goal of this chapter is to explain data resulting from linguistic tasks proposed to seven agrammatic and seven paragrammatic patients concerning the masculine and feminine gender in French. Given that the tests we used focus on the specific grammatical domain of gender, two important, and somehow related, notions in studying aphasia from a linguistic point of view have to be addressed: i.e., grammatical analysis and morphology.

## Grammatical Analysis

Many linguistic theories are based on grammatical analysis, even though the true nature of the facts to be considered remains controversial. At the risk of simplifying, we can nevertheless distinguish a linguistic approach based on statistical characteristics (experimental linguistics) from one based on formal characteristics (structural linguistics). Most studies dealing with clinical facts of aphasia are statistical. Patients' performances are quantified, behavioral patterns are defined through more or less significant percentages, and clinical symptoms correspond to exact linguistic "frontiers" that separate acceptable items from unacceptable ones.

For instance, one of our agrammatic patients gave 87% correct answers (from a total of 120) when he had to determine the gender of "simple" words like "timbre" (stamp), but he gave only 64% correct answers when he had to determine the gender of "polymorphemic" words, i.e., words formed by a stem and at least one affix, "timbrage" (stamping), for example, is formed by the radical "timbr" and the suffix "age". However, even when these data point to significant differences, they do not provide information about the nature of the logical defect underlying the patients' impairment. Rather, they tend to show that if we rely on such evidence derivational words do not belong to the same registers as the so-called simple words, and they appear to be more precarious than the latter.

These results are inconclusive because they merely reflect the more or less common use of these words, rather than the pathological formalization that underlies the patients' performances. Chances are that the relative regularity of practices may be taken for the grammatical formalization itself to the point of confusing the normal speaker's categories, which are fixed by usage, and the logical procedure of categorization.

This approach supposes that the normal speaker's categories are the same as those of the patients' as the analysis of correct or wrong answers directly depends on whatever set of categories is determined beforehand. One may consider the traditional categories (nouns, verbs, adjectives, articles, pronouns, adverbs, prepositions, conjunctions) and establish a scoreboard that shows that a particular category is relatively preserved in comparison to any others. The analysis reveals differential percentages of successful or unsuccessful uses regarding each predefined category. With this approach the patient is considered to be a normal speaker who is making mistakes. There is no "reorganization" of the grammar in the context of aphasia, and symptoms are viewed as failures.

There are only a few studies that pay particular attention to the formal characteristics of the items, specifying other linguistic "frontiers" that separate items that can be systematized from those that cannot. When formal characteristics are preferred, it is necessary to determine every linguistic category based on formal criteria. A theoretical consideration is inevitable. Let us, for instance, consider an article in French. What is it? Is it an entire word? What is its relation to the noun? Is there a formal link between article and grammatical gender? Let us consider an adjective: Is it morphologically different from the noun category? Nothing indicates this difference, as adjectives can be nominalized (e.g., un "bavard"), and nouns can be adjectivized (un papa gâteau). *The point is to consider not socially acceptable utterances, but, rather, logically deductive utterances.* This structural approach of aphasic performances is not concerned with each linguistic item per se but emphasizes instead the relations between them. We do not need to know whether an aphasic omits or substitutes articles, for example; but we do need to define as exactly as possible what is an article formally, in comparison with the specific formalization procedure of the patient. Instead of considering one-to-one correspondences between each aphasic answer and the answer normally expected, we take the patient's answers together, as a whole, and we study the internal relation of these answers. There are no longer correct or wrong answers but only answers produced by an underlying abstract system and a pathological system determined on the one hand by a partial adherence to the items proposed at the beginning of the exercise and on the other by an exaggerated generalization on the remaining logical procedures of deduction. The adherence and exaggeration in question thus constitute the patholinguistic conditions of the system.

Our research adopts the latter approach. Therefore no statistical data are to be found hereunder! This choice, however, does not mean that we are satisfied by pinpoint, nearly casual, observations. On the contrary,

we try to determine a strictly qualitative approach of aphasic performances and to identify both the distinctive answerstrategies of the aphasic
patients and the testing situation that makes possible the instigation of
those strategies. In our study, there is no lack of quantitative control of
the results, but it is shifted. We try to go from one stage of observation
where errors are simply noted down to another where errors are systematically induced. These errors may be induced because the test meets the
two patholinguistic conditions mentioned above. The patient's performances depend not only on a lack of abstraction but also on an "excess" of
"grammaticality" (Gagnepain, 1982). The aphasic symptoms thus result
from both a reduction and an excess of grammatical procedures.

The data examined below are drawn from a much larger set of observations. In fact, we have selected among this collection what appeared
to be a significant and appropriate sample with the idea of shedding light
on some underlying linguistic aspects of so-called agrammatism and paragrammatism, as they necessarily also give indications on the functioning
of nonpathological systems (CARAMAZZA, 1986a,b). Once again, but
in other terms, the prototypical nature of the answers is in the present
study to take place of the only seemingly unveiling properties of precise
statistics.

## Morphology

Traditionally, morphology studies word forms. This definition is difficult
to control because it raises the problem of the "word." What is a word?
Is it a sequence of letters between two blanks? Is it a "minimal differential element," or a "monème" in the terminology of Martinet (1957)?
Alternatively, could this notion of "word" refer to a strictly quantitative
segmental element, thus uneasily identifiable with a combination of differential values but more appropriately warrantable by some criterion of
cohesion? We assume here that such a principle is indeed necessary and
that it stipulates that a set of interdependent fragmentary values is assigned to every word as a formal unit (Gagnepain, 1982). This assumption
straightforwardly implies considering articles, prepositions, and pronouns
not as words but as fragments of words. As these fragments relate to noun
or verb sets in obvious way, a similar assertion can be made about grammatical gender, at least with regard to languages such as French. As a
corollary to the above stipulation, we believe, for instance, that similar
relations of formal cohesion hold between a nounset and each of its fragments, whether any considered fragment of a nounset is the formalization
of values alluded to the article, the preposition, or the grammatical gender.
Thus the "noun set," the "verb set," and the adverb constitute three
matrices within which an effect of formal cohesion must be proved as a
relation of segmental order (Urien, 1987; Pergnier, 1986). Our first hypothesis is that agrammatic patients lose this formal cohesion but keep

the differential capacity that allows them to discriminate minimal opposing values. We believe that morphology disappears in the case of agrammatism because it cannot rely on the quantitative invariability of a closed network of interrelated items, wich, however, are not differential paradigms. Agrammatic patients cannot produce but differences; and every value classification is possible (Guyard, 1987), as the sets determined in a pin-point way can be opposed one to each other. The differentiation logic is largely generalized, and paradigms are formed in an uncontrolled fashion.

The theoretical assumption that morphology ensures formal cohesion by constraining a network of partial variation does not mean that it can be reduced to this principle or to the mere existence of quantitative limits. Morphology must also be appreciated from a qualitative point of view, as it is also a matter of flexion and derivation. Morphology indeed opposes mutually exclusive sets, as the whole nominal paradigm is opposed to the whole verbal paradigm, even though the set of flexional values determines at the same time, and qualitatively, the set of derivational values. Our second hypothesis is that paragrammatic patients lose control over these qualitative aspects of flexion and derivation. Any obvious partial identity may become a sort of absolute constant on the basis of which the paragrammatic makes various uncontrolled formalizations.

We thus claim that morphology disappears in the case of paragrammatism because it cannot rely on the differential invariability between a noun paradigm and some variation of paradigm. There are no genuine paradigms any more: Nouns may become verbs and verbs nouns. There is, however, a partial variation mechanism that overgeneralizes and may produce any variation. The segmental logic is exceedingly generalized, and qualitatively uncontrolled values are liable to become interdependent.

## Dissociation Between Two Modes of Systematizing Performances

We distinguish a pathological systematization from an abstract or analytical systematization. The first emerges from the immediate data of the test. In contrast, the other systematization supposes that each obvious item of the test is underlain by an abstract value (Saussure, 1915), or by a set of abstract values (Gagnepain, 1982). The loss of this analytical abstraction is proved by "trap tests" based on homophony, allomorphism, amalgam, discontinuous marking, ordering and significant absence (Urien, 1982, 1987).

## Paragrammatism-traps

Paragrammatic patients have lost the differential dimension of grammatical analysis (Fig. 7.1) because they can be influenced by tests based on homophony and allomorphism.

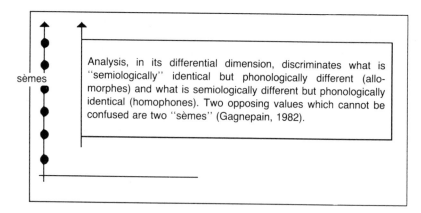

sèmes

Analysis, in its differential dimension, discriminates what is "semiologically" identical but phonologically different (allomorphes) and what is semiologically different but phonologically identical (homophones). Two opposing values which cannot be confused are two "sèmes" (Gagnepain, 1982).

FIGURE 7.1. Differential dimension of grammatical analysis.

## Homophony Trap

We provide three spectacular examples of the homophony trap. They represent the typical answers given by paragrammatic patients.

Example 1: The test consists of a series of dictations (Dubois, 1965). We proposed to the patients a trap based on the homophony between "la" as an article, and "l'a" as the first syllable of certain words ("l'aplomb"). Confronted with "le," these last sequences were interpreted by paragrammatic patients as a combination of the article "la" and the noun. We observed a great number of errors.

l'aplomb/le plomb = la plont*/le plont*
l'assaut/le seau = la seau*/le seau
l'affront/le front = la front*/le front
l'appoint/le point = la point*/le point
l'aplomb/le plomb = la plon*/le plon*
l'accroc/le croc = la craut*/le craut*
l'appuis/le puit = la puis*/le puis*
l'adieu/le Dieu = la Dieu*/le Dieu
l'accroc/le croc = la crot*/le crot*
l'accord/le corps = la cort*/le cort*
*The symbol (*) = wrong answer.*

This test based on the homophony of "la" and "la," allows us to observe false homographies as well as false allographies.

l'affront/le front = la frond*/le front
l'affaire/le fer = la faire*/le fer
l'attrait/le trait = l'attré*/le très*
l'allée/le lait = la lée*/le lait
l'accord/le corps = la core*/le cort*
l'appoint/le point = la point*/le poing

Paragrammatic patients cannot deduce from their grammatical procedure the difference between "l'appuis" and "la puis*." They do not understand the trap. They simply wonder why we present them with identical items. The same protocol also elicits aphasic answers that demonstrate no control of homophony and a blind search for spelling possibilities. The aphasics have systematically made errors because they relied solely on their overgeneralizing segmental logic and neglected the differential values that normally oppose the different spellings to each other. The spelling used by the patients seems to remain within a certain degree of acceptability, though, because the spelling of "frond*," for instance, recalls that of "blond," while "La lée*" that of "la fée." The allography of the homophones is no longer underlaid by lexical differentiation, and the patients answer at random. However, the allography is not totally wild insofar as canonical spelling has been respected to a certain extent.

Example 2: Homophony of the end words "eur" (voleur/lourdeur) and "euse" (voleuse/honteuse) was tested (Mok, 1968). Not all variations were allowed. Flexional sets differed from one another. They couldnot be confused. Thus one can deduce "voleuse" from "voleur" but not "lourdeuse*" from "lourdeur," "voleur" from "voleuse" but not "honteur*" from "honteuse." Therefore we suggest that paragrammatic patients are trapped by these exercises and make erroneous deductions by confusing items that are not different.

We observed exaggerated deductions induced by false conjectures. Patients explored all the possibilities of a partial variations, without limiting its functioning and without distinguishing mutually exclusive derivations. The pattern "visiteuse/visiteur" induced such pathological answers as "honteuse/honteur*." The pattern "patineur/patineuse" induced the pathological answers "fadeur/fadeuse*," "lourdeur/lourdeuse*." The pattern "frileuse/frileux" induced the pathological answers "chomeuse/chomeux*," "patineuse/patineux*," "donneuse/donneux*."

| Frileuse/frileux | Visiteuse/visiteur | Patineur/patineuse |
|---|---|---|
| Honteuse/honteur* | Perceur/perceuse | Fabuleuse/fabuleux |
| Chercheuse/chercheur | Fadeur/fadeuse* | Bricoleuse/bricoleux* |
| Rôtisseuse/rôtisseur | Pécheur/pécheuse | Fumeuse/fumeux |
| Paresseuse/paresseur* | Lourdeur/lourdeuse* | Chômeuse/chômeux |
| Danseuse/danseur | Grandeur/grandeuse* | Patineuse/patineux* |
| Délicieuse/délicieur* | Lutteur/lutteuse | Donneuse/donneux* |
| Semeuse/semeur | Verdeur/verdeuse* | Méticuleuse/méticuleux |

## Allomorphism Trap

Example 1. Paragrammatic patients cannot control the allomorphism of suffixes. In masculine forms the nominal suffix "eur" relates to "eure," "euse" or "(a)trice" in the feminine. Thus the marking of the feminine on this type on noun is done by adding to the stem one of three possible suffixal allomorphs. Paragrammatic patients likely consider every possibility, without being able to select one.

| 1st Time | The same patient.: 2nd Time | The same pat.: 3rd Time |
|---|---|---|
| Un éducateur/ une éducatrice | Un éducateur/ une éducateuse* | Un éducateur/ une éducatrice |
| Un créateur/ une créatrice | Un créateur/une créateuse* | Un créateur/ une créateuse* |
| Un aviateur/ une aviatrice | Un aviateur/une aviateuse* | Un aviateur/ une aviatrice |
| Un flatteur/ une flateresse* | Un flatteur/une flatteuse | Un flatteur/? (unreadable) |
| Un animateur/ une animatrice | Un animateur/ une animatrice | Un animateur/? (unreadable) |
| Un planteur/ une plantatrice* | Un planteur/une plantrice* | Un planteur/? (unreadable) |
| Un acteur/une actrice | Un acteur/une acteure* | Un acteur/une acteure* |
| Un guetteur/ une guetteuse | Un guetteur/une guetteuse | Un guetteur/ une guetteuse |
| Un profiteur/ une profiteuse | Un profiteur/ une profiteure* | Un profiteur/ une profiteuse |
| Un prêteur/ une prêteuse | Un prêteur/une prêteuse | Un prêteur/ une prêteuse |
| Un serviteur/ une serviteuse | Un serviteur/une serviteuse | Un serviteur/ une serviteuse |
| Un porteur/ une porteuse | Un porteur/une porteuse | Un porteur/ une porteuse |
| Un acheteur/ une acheteuse | Un acheteur/une acheteuse | Un acheteur/ une achatrice* |

These patients showed an inability to exclude any number of possible allomorphs in order to single out the appropriate one. They accepted any solution. (This attitude is different from that of the agrammatics'. Agrammatic patients, even when they produced pinpoint identical errors of use, knew that one had to choose one allomorph form and exclude the others). Paragrammatic patients, in contrast, accepted as the feminine form of "éducateur," both "éducateuse*" and "éducatrice*." "Acteur" became "acteure*," "acteuse*," "actrice," and the patients do not find it necessary to exclude one of the allomorphs to select only one. At the same way "profiteur" became "profiteuse" and "profiteure*," even sometimes "profitrice*" and other neologisms. All the solutions coexisted and were considered equivalent, some of them being perhaps more familiar than others.

Example 2: Allomorphism is also important in the feminine form of adjectives, insofar as allomorphs ("t, z, ch, k, s, j, d") are opposed to a significant absence ("o"): (petit/e = o/+t, gris/e = o/+z, blanc/che = o/+ch

franc/que = o/+k, gras/se = o/+s, gentil/le = o/+j, grand/e = o/+d).
Two word series were elaborated based on two constraints: (1) a stage
where the feminine form of the word can be deduced directly from the
spelling of the masculine form (1°Stage: petit/?, grand/?, blanc/?, gris/?,
gras/?, lent/?, sourd/?, gentil/?); and (2) a stage that is not directly morphological and where the spelling of the masculine form does not indicate
the feminine form (2°Stage: peti./peti.e, gran./gran.e, blan./blan.e, gri./
gri.e, gra./gra.e, len./len.e, sour./sour.e, genti./genti.e) (Mok, 1968).

We obtained correct answers when using the first stage whereas the
second stage showed the confusions of the paragrammatic patients, i.e.,
le blan./la ban.e became le bland*/la blande*; le gra./la gra.e became le
grat*/la gratte*; le sour./la sour.e became le sourt*/la sourte*; and finally,
le genti./la genti.e became le gentit*/la gentite*.

| LE BLOND/LA | LE BLOND/ LA blonde | LE BLON./LA | LEBLONd/ LA blonde |
| LE BLANC/LA | LE BLANC/ LA blanche | LE BLAN./LA | LE BLANd*/ LA blande* |
| LE GRIS/LA | LE GRIS/ LA grise | LE GRI./LA | LE GRIs/ LA grise |
| LE GRAS/LA | LE GRAS/ LA grasse | LE GRA./LA | LEGRAt* + LAgratte* |
| LE LENT/LA | LE LENT/ LA lente | LE LEN./LA | LELENt/LAlente |
| LE SOURD/LA | LE SOURD/ LA sourde | LE SOUR./LA | LESOURt*/ LAsourtte* |
| LE GENTIL/LA | LE GENTIL/ LA gentille | LE GENTI./LA | LEGENTIt*/ LA gentite* |

Patient's remarks: "La gratte* Elle a trop mangé! (The fat one...She ate too
much!)

In short, paragrammatic patients, for lack of differentiation between
mutually opposing values, no longer could control the limits of homophony and allomorphism. Gagnepain (1982) called the value produced
by this differentiation procedure "sème." The variation of sonorous sequences were contingent, so patients did not control what phonologically
had been well identified but what semiologically was still to be differentiated (the homophones); and what phonologically had been well differentiated semiologically still had to be identified (allomorphisms).

## Agrammatism Traps

We considered the segmental dimension, where analysis marks bound-
aries, by searching for a minimal cohesion between elements: how far an
element is "one" and how a possible autonomy allowed us to count it
formally as "two" (Fig. 7.2).

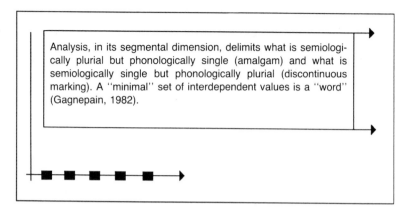

Analysis, in its segmental dimension, delimits what is semiologically plurial but phonologically single (amalgam) and what is
semiologically single but phonologically plurial (discontinuous
marking). A "minimal" set of interdependent values is a "word"
(Gagnepain, 1982).

FIGURE 7.2. Segmental dimension of analysis.

## Amalgam Trap

The same sonorous (or spelled) sequence may contain two grammatical values that are necessarily combined. For instance, one cannot choose "chapeau", or "tête" without selecting its gender. By choosing "le," for example, one selects simultaneously the value definite, as opposed to indefinite ("un"), the value singular, as opposed to plural ("les"), and the value masculine, as opposed to feminine ("la"). This time it is not a matter of logical procedures of exclusion "one without the others", but that of cohesion "not the one without the others." We claim that agrammatic aphasics, although they have lost the ability to segment their utterances into formal units, cannot register several grammatically combined and interdependent values, within a single phonological sequence.

Example 1: We asked severely agrammatic patients to give the appropriate articles for a series of simple words: chapeau," "casquette," "béret," "foulard," "casque," "coiffure," "toque," "bonnet," "képi." The patients were perplexed and gave random answers.

The same items "foulard", "casque", "toque" and "bonnet" were marked (Urien, 1984) by the patients as masculine or feminine, but at a different time during the interview. The random answers showed the patients' lack of confidence. However—and this point is important—when we gave the patients all their own answers together, they were able to indicate the mutual contradictory answers. They did not know if it was "le foulard" or "la foulard," but they were sure that it had to be one or the other. They did not know if "casque" went with "le" or "la," but they knew that one answer excluded the other. Masculine and feminine are always exclusive of each other, even when the formal interdependence between the gender and the stem of the word has been lost.

| *Exercise:* | *First time:* | *Second time:* |
|---|---|---|
| CHAPEAU | le CHAPEAU | le CHAPEAU |
| CASQUETTE | le CASQUETTE* | le CASQUETTE* |
| BERET | la BERET* | la BERET* |
| FOULARD | la FOULARD* | le FOULARD |
| CASQUE | le CASQUE | la CASQUE* |
| COIFFURE | la COIFFURE | la COIFFURE |
| TOQUE | la TOQUE | le TOQUE* |
| BONNET | la BONNET* | le BONNE |
| KEPI | le KEPI | le KEPI |

We proposed his own answers to the patient. He indicated the mutual exclusion answers on his own. He did not know if "foulard" went with "le" or with "la," but he was quite sure that if it was the first answer it couldnot be the other.

| le CHAPEAU | le CHAPEAU |
|---|---|
| le CASQUETTE* | le CASQUETTE* |
| la BERET* | la BERET* |
| la FOULARD* | ○ le FOULARD |
| le CASQUE | ○ la CASQUE* |
| la COIFFURE | la COIFFURE |
| la TOQUE | ○ la TOQUE* |
| la BONNET* | ○ le BONNET |
| le KEPI | le KEPI |

*With the symbol ○ the patient represents incompatible answers.*

Some answers even showed that patients juxtaposed two differential sets that had no relation. Each one had become pathologically independent. We proposed a series of items, and patients selected a masculine ("le") or a feminine ("la") form.

| *Exercise: "le" or "la"?* | *Written answers:* |
|---|---|
| CHEVRE | le CHEVRE |
| POIVRE | la POIVRE* |
| SABRE | le SABRE |
| ZEBRE | la ZEBRE* |
| TIMBRE | le TIMBRE |
| SACRE | la SACRE* |
| SUCRE | le SUCRE |
| CADRE | la CADRE* |
| CENDRE | le CENDRE |
| CIDRE | la CIDRE* |
| POUDRE | le POUDRE* |
| CHIFFRE | la CHIFFRE* |
| VITRE | le VITRE* |
| MONTRE | la MONTRE |
| LUSTRE | le LUSTRE |

*Agrammatic patients were trapped by the amalgam procedure*

Patients, systematically, used "le" and "la" alternatively without considering the existent relations between gender and noun. "Le/la" constitutes a lexical (= differential) opposition that has been treated separately by the patient, aside from the radical oppositions. Patients have two juxtaposed "thoughts" when grammar normally assigns just one. There is no longer and cohesion between the fragments of the noun pattern. The grammatical gender is processed on its own, beyond the other relations of internal solidarity it used to have.

Example 2: The amalgam procedures (Pergnier, 1986) within the same pathological sequence of a determinant value (definite, indefinite, possessive, demonstrative), a number value (singular, plural) and a gender value (masculine, feminine) were tested. Thus when going from "un" to "une" there is only one gender difference, but going from "un" to "cette" we must consider not only the gender opposition but also the difference between an indefinite and a demonstrative determinant. Agrammatic patients cannot face numerous differences simultaneously; they tend to control these differences one by one and to neglect the others. The repeating exercise is as follows.

| *Repeating exercise* | *O = Observer*    *M = Patient* |
|---|---|
| O = SA MAISON/CE GARAGE | M = sa maison/son garage |
| O = CE CHATEAU/LA VOITURE | M = ce château/et la..? C'est "la", mais après? |
| O = LE FROMAGE/CETTE CREME | M = ce fromage/cette crème, mais c'est pas ça! |
| O = LA CLEF/CE BOUTON | M = la clef/ce...ensemble, je peux pas! |
| O = LA CLEF/CE BOUTON | M = la clef/le bouton...avant, c'est pas ça! |
| O = LE JUPON/SA VESTE | M = le jupon/sa... Attends! Je sais!... Veste! |
| O = Encore! | M = le jupon/la veste |
| O = CETTE SOIREE/SON LIVRE | M = son livre/sa quoi? Je sais plus! |
| O = CETTE SOIREE/SON LIVRE | M = soirée..et avant?..cette soirée/ ce livre |
| O = SON SAC/LA MONTRE | M = son sac/sa montre.... Pas encore ça! |
| O = SA GOMME/LE CRAYON | M = sa gomme/son crayon... pas "son"! Je sais plus! |
| O = CETTE BAGUE/LE BIJOU | M = cette... bague/bijou... le bijou? |

*The determinants are differentiated two by two, the differentiation based only on the masculine feminine opposition.*

| | |
|---|---|
| sa/ce | becomes sa/son |
| sa/le | sa/son |
| la/ce | la/ce (but the patient loses the base) |
| la/ce | la/le |

| ce/la | ce/la (but the patient loses the base) |
| le/cette | ce/cette |
| le/sa | le/sa (but the patient loses the base) |
| le/sa | le/la |
| cette/son | son/sa |
| cette/son | cette/ce |
| son/la | son/sa |

The test is a repetition exercise. Patients are asked to repeat several sequences. Agrammatic patients give two kinds of answer. Either they cancel the whole set of relations implied by the use of a particular determinant and give just one relation or they treat all these relation values at the same time but "have forgotten" the nominal nucleus after the determinant. They may say "ce chateau/et la... c'est 'la' mais après?...(I know it is 'la' but what then?)- la clef/ce..? Ensemble je peux pas." Patients show their inability to repeat simultaneously the whole set of formal relations that are required to carry out the test.

## Discontinuous Marking Trap Test

We usually find the gender by using the article ("le/la") or the nominal nucleus ("chapeau bas/tête basse") and even sometimes by using suffixes ("eur/euse"). However, should we count the gender principle three times? Or should we count it formally just once, by stretching it out on three fragments of the nominal pattern?

Agrammatic patients count the gender three times, which is an indication of their pathology because normally the gender is counted just once. Normally we cannot utter the determinant's gender without choosing at the same time the stem gender and the suffix-gender. A normal speaker detects the whole set of gender determinants at once. Agrammatic patients no longer have this ability as the following facts show.

The next exercise is a determination exercise. During the first stage we gave the patients a list of nouns without articles. Patients had to choose between the articles "le" or "la," usually preceding these nouns. Agrammatic patients gave random answers. We then, during the second stage, proposed a second list, which contained the suffixes: "eur/euse." This time patients were sure of their answers. They made no mistakes at all. During a third stage, we proposed the first list of nouns again. This time, patients were able to determine perfectly all the items because they were now aware of the importance of the end-word "euse".

| Observer: stage 1 | Observer: stage 2 | Observer: stage 3 |
|---|---|---|
| vendeuse | vendeur | vendeuse |
| contrôleuse | vendeuse | contrôleuse |
| voleuse | contrôleur | voleuse |
| perceuse | contrôleuse | perceuse |
| menteuse | menteur | menteuse |

| Observer: stage 1 | Observer: stage 2 | Observer: stage 3 |
|---|---|---|
| laveuse | menteuse | laveuse |
| serveuse | | serveuse |
| sauveuse | | sauveuse |
| déménageuse | | déménageuse |
| meneuse | | meneuse |

*Answers of the agrammatic patient:*

| | | |
|---|---|---|
| la vendeuse | le vendeur | la vendeuse |
| le contrôleuse* | la vendeuse | la contrôleuse |
| le voleuse* | le contrôleur | la voleuse |
| le perceuse* | la contrôleuse | la perceuse |
| la menteuse | le menteur | la menteuse |
| la laveuse | la menteuse | la laveuse |
| la serveuse | | la serveuse |
| le sauveuse* | | la sauveuse |
| le déménageuse* | | la déménageuse |
| la meneuse | | la meneuse |

The three stages of this test were carried out during the same session. We noted that the patients systematized the "le/la" opposition as soon as they found the same lexical (or differential) opposition in another place of the sequence ("eur/euse").

That observation proves that Broca aphasics notice only the masculine/feminine opposition, not how many times this opposition is to be marked. The gender distribution is no longer bounded by grammar insofar as there is no more simultaneousness between a set of identical compulsions. The fact that patients have to systematize in a pinpoint manner the "le/la" relation on one hand and the "eur/euse" relation on the other shows that their grammar cannot "grasp" the common necessity of these relations, i.e., their mutual dependence. Patients make an explicit clustering, step by step. The segmental analysis, indicating the interdependence of the internal relations of the network, no longer exists; therefore it cannot indicate the distribution of a unique segmental value of the gender (and not its differential or lexical value). In other words, agrammatism suggests the following, nearly scandalous fact: One segmental gender value may contain at the same time three opportunities for differentiating the masculine from the feminine. In normal speech, segmental and differential values do not coincide. On the contrary, in agrammatic speech, there are as many pathological units as there are opportunities to differentiate.

In the first stage the given sequence "voleuse" does not refer to several imbricated values [(vol/eur − vol/euse) = (stem + suffixes + gender)]. It is here that we test the lack of segmental unit analysis, i.e., the lack of a formal network that makes it possible to count semiologically as one element what would be normally distributed between several phonological sequences.

Conversely, patients may split up this given sequence as soon as they are able to rely on the only grammatical dimension that is still underlying their performances: the differentiation analysis. Thus they are able to add up explicitly the opposing elements: le/la + vendeuse/contrôleuse/voleuse + eur/euse. Not only may they add up the number of opposing elements, but they may establish a correspondence between the masculine value in "le" and the same value in "eur," as well as between the feminine value in "la" and the "euse" suffix.

Agrammatic patients produce an assemblage of isolated differential values. This assemblage is not produced beforehand but depends on the test compulsions. This fact proves that the semiological unit cannot be defined as an assemblage of differential values (Jakobson, 1963) but as a special, formal, strictly segmental network founding the mutual dependence between values (Gagnepain, 1982). In normal speech, the grammatical gender cannot be distributed on the article (le/la) without being distributed at the same time on the nominal nucleus (chapeau/tête) and on the suffix ("eur/euse"), which is not the case with agrammatic speech. Disturbance of this formal interdependence compels agrammatic patients to say one "thing" after another. We understand that this disturbance is characterized by a high level of poor performances.

Conversely, paragrammatic patients are not sure about the exclusion they are supposed to make, as they no longer have differential frontiers. This disturbance is characterized by incoherence.

## The Distinction Between Two Morphological Structures

We distinguish a loss of morphology assignable to the disappearance of a unit of internal variations (this unit establishes a cohesion between several morphological classes) and a loss of morphology assignable to the disappearance of an opposition between the noun and the verb paradigms and between the masculine and feminine paradigms. Lack of cohesion on the one hand and confusion on the other become the real symptoms of the loss of morphology. Therefore morphology supposes the crossing of two logical procedures that may be selectively destroyed in aphasia.

In French, there are two main paradigmatic patterns, the nominal and the verbal; however, the morphemes of the nominal pattern cannot be confused with those of the verbal pattern. They are two patterns that exclude each other qualitatively. In other words, the nominal flexion is not the same as the verbal flexion and vice versa. It seems, however, that agrammatics as well as paragrammatics do not respect the partition between these two kinds of flexion. Agrammatics make the same type of mistake, but for different reasons.

Two subparadigms have to be differentiated within the nominal paradigm of French: the masculine and the feminine. The grammatical gender differentiates two mutually exclusive flexional sets. In other words, a noun necessarily has to be masculine or feminine. Any confusion between the masculine noun set and the feminine noun set is forbidden because of the underlying grammatical analysis, even when the nominal stem seems to be the same ("le voile/la voile"). Both agrammatical and paragrammatics seem to make mistakes when using this grammatical sector. We suggest that agrammatics and paragrammatics do have not the same difficulties.

## Agrammatic Patients and Loss of "Segmental Constancy" Within a Network of Differential Variations

Agrammatic patients master only the differential dimension of analysis. They tend to process only one value at a time. In order to oppose a nominal and a verbal pattern we need to take into account a number of differential values. We suggest that the relation between the noun and the verb worsens because of agrammatic patients' inability to consider all the nominal values together in order to oppose them to all the verbal values.

The cohesion of nominal categories and verbal categories actually disappears. Thus we may say that agrammatic patients have no nouns and no verbs, only isolated differential values.

The first example concerns assessment of noun flexion and verb flexion from a given stem. The stem "bricole" may be included in the noun paradigm ("des bricoles") as well as in the verbal paradigm ("il bricole"). We suggest that agrammatic patients reduce each paradigmatic set to its stem; and if the test artificially isolates the differential value between "il/un" and "elle/une," dthey notice it and treat this value on its own without having it agree with the other noun and verb patterns. The second example contains several stages, and of course we have to consider the succession of these stages. In the first stage the patient was asked to complete an exercise by corresponding a feminine to a masculine form: la pêcheresse/le?—la tigresse/le?. The results showed that agrammatic patients used the material given in the title of the question. They used the simple form of the items; la pêcheresse/le pêcheur, la chanteuse/le chante*. This first stage showed three pinpoint errors, which suggested that agrammatic patients cannot master the relation between nouns and verbs ("le chante," "le bricole," "le surveille").

| Observer | Patient |
|---|---|
| LA PECHERESSE/LE | LA PECHERESSE/LE pêcheur |
| LA TIGRESSE/LE | LA TIGRESSE/LE tigre |
| LA NEGRESSE/LE | LA NEGRESSE/LE nègre |
| LA CHANTEUSE/LE | LA CHANTEUSE/LE chante* ○ verb ? |
| LA BRICOLEUSE/LE | LA BRICOLEUSE/LE bricole* ○ verb ? |
| LA MAITRESSE/LE | LA MAITRESSE/LE maître |
| LA TRAVAILLEUSE/LE | LA TRAVAILLEUSE/LE travail* |
| LA JOURNALIERE/LE | LA JOURNALIERE/LE journal* |
| LA JARDINIERE/LE | LA JARDINIERE/LE jardin* |
| LA LAITIERE/LE | LA LAITIERE/LE lait* |
| LA DROITIERE/LE | LA DROITIERE/LE droit* |

LA PRISONNIERE/LE        LA PRISONNIERE/LE prison*
LA SURVEILLANTE/LE       LA SURVEILLANTE/LE surville* ○ verb ?

A second stage is now possible. From these answers the examiner made a list of items ending with "e"; some of these items accepted the nominal pattern as well as the verbal pattern ("il dépense/une dépense") whereas others accepted only the verbal pattern ("il chavire, il compare"). We asked the following question: "le" or "la"? During this stage, agrammatic patients noticed only the given opposition, i.e., the "le/la" opposition and not the "le/il"—"la/elle" opposition. The third stage asked for special attention by the patients concerning these oppositions: "il, le, elle or la"? Agrammatic patients could then to process what they had forgot ten during stage 2. In other words, the noun/verb opposition was reduced here until a morpheme opposition between "le/il" and "la/elle" was possible. However, we are not certain that patients still have an complete noun paradigm that could be opposed to an complete verb paradigm. If they did so so, the patients would have refused the question we asked them in the second stage.

| Stage 2 (le" or "la"?) | Patient | Stage 3 (il" ou "le", "elle" or "la"?) |
|---|---|---|
| MACHINE | la MACHINE | la MACHINE |
| MELANGE | la MELANGE* | la MELANGE* |
| CONTROLE | le CONTROLE | il-elle CONTROLE |
| BRICOLE | le BRICOLE* | il BRICOLE |
| DISCUTE | la DISCUTE* | elle DISCUTE |
| RECLAME | la RECLAME | il RECLAME |
| COMMENCE | le COMMENCE* | il COMMENCE |
| RENCONTRE | le RENCONTRE* | il RENCONTRE |
| CHAVIRE | le CHAVIRE* | il CHAVIRE |
| DEPENSE | le DEPENSE* | le DEPENSE* |
| REMPLACE | le REMPLACE* | il REMPLACE |
| COMMANDE | la COMMANDE | il COMMANDE |
| SURVEILLE | le SURVEILLE* | il SURVEILLE |
| BATAILLE | la BATAILLE | la BATAILLE |
| COMPARE | le COMPARE* | il-elle COMPARE |

Any opposition was possible—the "le/la" opposition, the "le/il" opposition, and even the "il/elle" opposition—but they were processed by the patients because they take into account the "title" of the exercise and the question of the examiner—not because of an underlying formalization that implicity governs their utterances. Patients processed these oppositions as a whole just because the title of the exercise told them explicitly what to do and not because of an underlying formalization. For agrammatic patients the "le/la" opposition could no longer be related to the whole nominal opposition set, and the "il/elle" opposition could not be related to the whole verbal opposition set.

In a second example the exercise contained two stages. In the first stage; from a given pair of sentences ("un homme qui arbitre est un arbitre/une femme qui arbitre est une arbitre") patients were asked to complete pairs of sentences. The stage focused the patients' attention on only one opposition, the "un/une" opposition; wich is why patients respected it.

| | |
|---|---|
| *Un homme qui arbitre est un arbitre* | *Un homme qui arbitre est un arbitre* |
| *Une femme qui arbitre est une arbitre* | *Une femme qui arbitre est une arbitre* |
| Un homme qui bricole est | Un homme qui bricole est "un bricole*" |
| Une femme qui bricole est | Une femme qui bricole est "une bricole*" |
| Un homme qui guide est | Un homme qui guide est "un guide" |
| Une femme qui guide est | Une femme qui guide est "une guide" |
| Un homme qui explore est | Un homme qui explore est "un explore*" |
| Une femme qui explore est | Une femme qui explore est "une explore*" |
| Un homme qui enseigne est | Un homme qui enseigne est "un enseigne*" |
| Une femme qui enseigne est | Une femme qui enseigne est "une explore*" |

*The agrammatic patient examined one of his answers: "un explore*." He tried to tell us that people say "un explore" for man as well as for woman.*

The patients no longer had at their disposal the grammatical formalization that is needed to reckon all the differential values, which, when taken together, allow us to oppose the noun pattern to the verb pattern. In other words agrammatic patients tend to use the flexional relations given by the examiner because they cannot question them by a real morphological formalization. The following stage of the exercise showed their interpretation. In the second stage, from the given pattern ("un homme qui chante est un chanteur/une femme qui chante est une chanteuse") patients gave the following sentences.

| | |
|---|---|
| *Un homme qui chante est un chanteur* | *Un homme qui chante est un chanteur* |
| *Une femme qui chante est une chanteuse* | *Une femme qui chante est une chanteuse* |
| Un homme qui bricole est | Un homme qui bricole est "un bricoleur" |
| Un femme qui bricole est | Une femme qui bricole est "une bricoleuse" |
| Un homme qui guide est | Un homme qui guide est un "guideur*" |
| Un femme qui guide est | Une femme qui guide est "une guideuse*" |
| Un homme qui explore est | Un homme qui explore est "un exploreur*" |
| Une femme qui explore est | Une femme qui explore est "une exploreuse*" |

| Un homme qui surveille est | Un homme qui surveille est "un surveilleur*" |
| Une femme qui surveille est | Une femme qui surveille est "une surveilleuse*" |

*Agrammatic patients see their morphological system reduced to its base. It agrees with the model given by the examinor.*

The agrammatic patients blindly followed the model. They respected a differential relation which seemed to be enough for them.

Only the differentiation seemed to provide agrammatic patients the possibility of making significant deductions. The differential dimension or the grammatical analysis had hypertrophied. Therefore agrammatic patients accept any value set that can be differentiated from an other value set. An infinity of artificial "paradigms" are possible only because they are not controlled by the "measurement degree" of a segmental unit. The following example is an illustration of this problem. The exercise contains five stages. The example is somewhat long but we believe it is indicative of the agrammatic patients' logical functioning.

During the first stage patients have to choose between several nominal and verbal morphemes (je, moi, il, lui, elle, le, la, son, sa, ce, tu, toi, te, cette, un, une, and the morpheme "zero" has been noted by the symbol <). The list of items to be determined is as follows: poivre, sabre, chambre, and so on.

As a model of possible answers we gave to the patients one complete answer and three partial answers ["il le lui montre, je ≪ poivre, elle ≪ chambre]. The selected items admit a nominal pattern ("la montre") as well as a verbal pattern ("il montre"). Patients then, had to choose a large number of values. Actually, they were dealing with only one value—in this case the value that admits the deduction of a determinant from the nucleus ("timbre"—"son timbre"). They are neglecting all the other values and stop the holes suggested by the layout of the exercise, without giving a real meaning to the items they are writing down. Their answers, e.g., "elle le son sabre*—il la sa chambre*—il le son zèbre*—il le son timbre*" are as follows.

*Question: je, me, moi, il, lui, elle, le, la, son, sa, ce, tu, toi, te, cette, un, une, <*

| IL LE LUI MONTRE | | IL LE LUI MONTRE |
| JE | POIVRE | JE le lui POIVRE |
| ELLE | SABRE | ELLE le son SABRE |
| IL | CHAMBRE | IL la sa CHAMBRE* |
| | ZEBRE | il le son ZEBRE* |
| | TIMBRE | il le son TIMBRE* |
| | SACRE | je le lui SACRE |
| | SUCRE | je le son SUCRE* |
| | CADRE | je le lui CADRE |
| | CENDRE | il la sa CENDRE* |
| | CIDRE | il le son CIDRE* |

| POUDRE | il la sa POUDRE* |
|--------|-----------------|
| CHIFFRE | il la sa CHIFFRE* |
| VITRE | il la sa VITRE* |

In the second stage, the number of determinants was changed (il, le, la, sa, cette, un, son, ce, une, <); at the same time the model inducing the exercise was simplified. This simplification may be enough to allow patients to systematize their answers. This time they are "teaching" us more than in the first stage because they try to systematize the absence or the presence of the pronoun "elle." As a matter of fact, they tended to oppose "son sucre" versus "elle son sucre*." One particular patient made this opposition, arguing that the first utterance meant "the pieces of sugar we put in a sugarbox," and the other "the action of giving sugar, to a dog for instance." In other words, a set of values without any formal cohesion ("elle son sucre*") may have artificially entiired this relation if only this set can be opposed to another. The patient's answers are as follows: "elle le montre, elle son poivre, son poivre, son sabre, elle sa chambre, sa chambre, un zèbre, son timbre, elle son sacre, un sucre, sa cadre, sa cendre, son cidre, sa poudre, son chiffre, sa vitre, elle sa montre, son lustre."

*Question: il, le, la, sa, cette, un, son, ce, une, <,?*

| ELLE LE LUI MONTRE | | ELLE LE LUI MONTRE |
|---|---|---|
| | POIVRE | elle son POIVRE |
| | SABRE | son SABRE |
| | CHAMBRE | elle sa CHAMBRE |
| | ZEBRE | un ZEBRE |
| | TIMBRE | son TIMBRE |
| | SACRE | elle son SACRE |
| | SUCRE | un SUCRE |
| | CADRE | sa CADRE |
| | CENDRE | sa CENDRE |
| | CIDRE | son CIDRE |
| | POUDRE | sa POUDRE |
| | CHIFFRE | son CHIFFRE |
| | VITRE | sa VITRE |

*The patient noted: "elle son sucre = chienne" and "son sucre = boîte" ("she her sugar = female dog" and "his sugar = box"). He explained that there were two answers for "sucre" ("sugar"). The first one say that one gives a piece of sugar to the dog, and the second one indicated the piece of sugar one put in the sugar box.*

The third stage showed that agrammatic patients accept all kinds of value bundles, if only these bundles respect the masculine-feminine difference. We asked patients to decide whether some utterances were correct. If they were correct, patients were to write "yes" that is, or, if not, "no." Thus when talking about "poivre," one particular patient mentioned accepts any masculine bundle ("le son poivre*") and refuses all feminine bundles ("la sa poivre*," "elle la poivre"). We are facing here an exaggerated systematicity that is common to all the examples of this third exercise. The patient considered only the determinant that is close to the "nucleus." The patient's answers were as follows.

| | |
|---|---|
| LE SON POIVRE* = oui | LE CIDRE = oui |
| LE SA POIVRE* = non | LE SON CIDRE* = oui |
| ELLE LE POIVRE = oui | LE SA CIDRE* = non |
| ELLE LA POIVRE = non | CETTE CIDRE* = non |
| | LE CE CIDRE* = oui |
| | |
| SA CHAMBRE = oui | LE SON POIVRE* = oui |
| UNE SA CHAMBRE* = oui | LE SA POIVRE* = non |
| LA SA CHAMBRE* = oui | IL LE POIVRE = oui |
| ELLE LA CHAMBRE = oui | IL LA POIVRE = non |
| ELLE LE CHAMBRE = non | |

*The morphological system of agrammatic patients may be reduced to the masculine/feminine opposition. The patient can constitute artificial paradigmatic sets, only if they are mutually opposing sets. The agrammatic patient still opposes items, but everything has become pathologically opposing.*

Thus the patient carries out "pathological sets" based only on their mutual opposition, which is shown in the fourth stage. We can mislead the patient to such a degree that he accepts the most incongruous sets, if only they can be opposed to each other. For example, note what happens to the following pairs of items: 1 elle la lui montre = oui/elle lui la montre = non; 2 elle sa lui montre = oui/elle lui sa montre = non. This patient has opposed each pair of items by pointing out only the difference between the position of the fragments "la/lui" or "sa/lui."

ELLE LA LUI MONTRE: oui
ELLE LUI LA MONTRE: non
ELLE SA LUI MONTRE: oui
ELLE LUI SA MONTRE: non

A fifth stage shows a conflict between the strategy worked out in the third stage (the account of the grammatical gender of the fragment preceding the nucleus) and the strategy used in the fourth stage (the opposition of two utterances). This time the model is much more complicated, as the patient must correlate the gender opposition, the opposition between the presence or absence of a second determinant, the opposition between an indefinite or a demonstrative determinant, and especially the opposition between the two positions of determinant within the utterance (ce chambre* = non/un chambre* = non/une chambre = oui/cette chambre = oui/une cette chambre* = non/cette une chambre* = oui/un ce chambre* = non/ce un chambre* = oui puis non) The patient does not know to account for all the differential relations suggested by this inducing set, which is why he is separating them into two "subsets." Our patient began to process the first four answers. Then he considered the two following ones ("une cette chambre*"/"cette une chambre*"), and finally he studied the rest. When he had processed all the answers, he was able to compare them and to suppose some incompatibility. That is why he returned to the first strategy, correcting himself and refusing a masculine determinant inappropriate to "chambre"—hence is the reason for the self-correction of "ce un chambre" = yes 1st. = no 2nd.

CE CHAMBRE*: non
UN CHAMBRE*: non
UNE CHAMBRE: oui
CETTE CHAMBRE: oui
UNE CETTE CHAMBRE*: non
CETTE UNE CHAMBRE*: oui
UN CE CHAMBRE*: non
CE UN CHAMBRE*: oui (1) and no (2)

Agrammatic patients use their differential reasoning within the artificial morphological framework offered by the examiner. Patients deduce their answers from this differential dimension, and any given set may be exaggeratedly opposed to another. Agrammatic patients seem to have lost the segmental network authorizing the restriction of the variety of mutually opposing sets.

The hypertrophy of these differential relations is to be found within our noun model between the masculine noun set and the feminine noun set. Agrammatic patients exaggeratedly generalize this way of opposing sets by taking into account the only gender opposition. In other words, the relations between "le voile/la voile"—"un arbitre/une arbitre" have been generalized pathologically to those items that normally have to be realized by considering more differential values together.

In another trap test, patients were asked to cross out the utterances that appeared incorrect or did not occur in usual speech. They had to decide between the following pairs of words.

*Exercise: Agrammatic patients were told to cross out the wrong utterances and then to give the meaning of their answers.*

| | | | |
|---|---|---|---|
| LE GUIDE | LA GUIDE | LE GUIDE | LA GUIDE |
| LE CREPE | LA CREPE | LE SABLE | LA SABLE |
| LE VOILE | LA VOILE | LE CRABE | LA CRABE |
| LE BOITE | LA BOITE | LE NUQUE | LA NUQUE |
| LE SOURCE | LA SOURCE | LE MERLE | LA MERLE |
| LE TOUR | LA TOUR | LE SURVEILLE | LA SURVEILLE |
| LE CLASSE | LA CLASSE | LE SEMOULE | LA SEMOULE |
| LE SIECLE | LA SIECLE | LE TEMPLE | LA TEMPLE |
| LE MOULE | LA MOULE | LE REMPLACE | LA REMPLACE |
| LE VASE | LA VASE | LE DESASTRE | LA DESASTRE |

| | |
|---|---|
| LE GUIDE | LA GUIDE |
| LECARTABLE | LA CARTABLE |
| LE FUME | LA FUME |

| | |
|---|---|
| LE LEGUME | LA LEGUME |
| LE CERCLE | LA CERCLE |
| LE DIRIGE | LA DIRIGE |
| LE GOLFE | LA GOLFE |
| LE SOUPE | LA SOUPE |
| LE SAUVE | LA SAUVE |
| LE PERLE | LA PERLE |

One agrammatic patient extended the gender opposition to all pairs of words based on some analogy with the given model ("le guide/la guide"). The patient accepted "pseudonouns" based upon verbs but indicated a possible meaning "man/woman."

*Exercise; Agrammatic patients were told to cross out the wrong words and then to give the meaning of the correct words.*

| | | | |
|---|---|---|---|
| LE GUIDE | LA GUIDE | LE GUIDE | LA GUIDE |
| LE CREPE | LA CREPE | LE SABLE | xxxxxxxx |
| LE VOILE | LA VOILE | LE CRABE | xxxxxxxx |
| xxxxxxx | LA BOITE | xxxxxxxx | LA NUQUE |
| xxxxxxx | LA SOURCE | LE MERLE | xxxxxxxx |
| LE TOUR | LA TOUR | LE SURVEILLE | LA SURVEILLE |
| xxxxxxx | LA CLASSE | xxxxxxxxxx | LA SEMOULE |
| LE SIECLE | xxxxxxxxx | LE TEMPLE | xxxxxxxxx |
| LE MOULE | LA MOULE | LE REMPLACE | LA REMPLACE |
| LE VASE | LA VASE | xxxxxxxxxxx | LA DESASTRE |

| | |
|---|---|
| LE GUIDE | LA GUIDE |
| LE CARTABLE | xxxxxxxxxxx |
| LE FUME | LA FUME |
| LE LEGUME | xxxxxxxxx |
| LE CERCLE | xxxxxxxxx |
| LE DIRIGE | LA DIRIGE |
| LE GOLFE | xxxxxxxx |
| LE SOUPE | LA SOUPE |
| LE SAUVE | LA SAUVE |
| LE PERLE | LA PERLE |

*The meanings of "correct" words are those we werer waiting for. The items "le guide," "surveille*," "le remplace*," "le fume*," "le dirige*," "le sauve*" refer to men and the items "la guide," "la surveille*," "la remplace*," "la dirige*" and "la sauve*" refer to women. The differential model "le guide/la guide" was wrongly generalized by this agrammatic patient.*

Another patient extended this gender opposition not only to nouns meaning men or women but also to nouns indicating semantic aspects ("le moule/la moule"). This patient accepted the following pairs of words: Le cercle/la cercle, un timbre/une timbre, un grille/une grille, un trèfle/une trèfle. The patient justified his choices: "Le cercle" meant a geometric figure, whereas "la cercle*" meant a group of persons. "Un timbre" meant "a signature stamp" whereas "une timbre*" meant a postage stamp. "Un grille*'' meant "a gril" whereas "une grille" meant something that can be opened or locked. "Le trèfle meant a color of playing cards, whereas "la trèfle*'' meant a little plant: Normally these two meanings are represented by the same differential value ("le trèfle"). This agrammatic patient thus made a differential analysis between two mutually opposing values.

*Exercise: Agrammatic patients were told to cross out the wrong words and then to give the meaning of the correct words.*

| LE GUIDE | LA GUIDE | UN MOUSSE | UNE MOUSSE |
|---|---|---|---|
| LE CARTABLE | xxxxxxxxxx | UN TIMBRE | UNE TIMBRE |
| LE STADE | xxxxxxxx | xxxxxxx | UNE SCIE |
| xxxxxxxxx | LA FUME* | UN POELE | UNE POELE |
| LE LEGUME | LA LEGUME | UN TOUR | UNE TOUR |
| LE CERCLE | LA CERCLE* | UN FLEUVE | xxxxxxxxxx |
| LE DIRIGE | LA DIRIGE | UN MANCHE | UNE MANCHE |
| LE GOLFE | xxxxxxxxxx | UN GRILLE | UNE GRILLE |
| xxxxxxxxx | LA SOUPE | UN VERRE | xxxxxxxx |
| xxxxxxxxx | LA SAUVE | UN VOILE | UNE VOILE |
| xxxxxxxxx | LA PERLE | UN MOULE | UNE MOULE |
| UN TREFLE | UNE TREFLE | | |

LE CERCLE = une figure géométrique    UN TIMBRE = la griffe (tampon?)
LA CERCLE = les gens... ensemble!    UNE TIMBRE = sur la lettre!
LE DIRIGE = lui    UN GRILLE = un steack
LA DIRIGE = elle    UNE GRILLE = fermé... ouvert
UN TREFLE = les cartes
UN TREFLE = les vaches... le pré!
*The hypertrophy between masculine and feminine gender is illustrated.*

Because the exercise required the patients' attention only for the gender opposition and because patients were unable to restrict their deductions by taking into account all morphological relations, they extended their perfect logical reasoning infinitely. During the same test these oppositions were constantly identical. Patients repeated the differences they made at the beginning and did not confuse them. This situation is not the case for paragrammatic patients.

Agrammatic patients have no "semiological unit" able to bundle mutually dependent values. This solidarity normally indicates a segmental dimension that does not take into consideration the differential values simultaneously. Thus, as noted by Gagnepain (1982), by projecting one axis on the other and by crossing the segmental dimension, we observe that a partial variation e.g., ("la voile/sur la voile/sur la voilure/le voilage") may be worked out without multiplying the number of segmental units.

On the contrary, when this simultaneousness disappears, everything can be differentiated (or "opposed"), including artificial sets proposed by "trap tests." Differential logic produces deductions; and pathological reasoning is generalized beyond the patients' control.

## Paragrammatic Patients and Loss of Differentiation Between Mutually Opposing Patterns ("Paradigms")

Paragrammatic patients retain only the segmental dimension of analysis. Thus they are able to make partial variations because they have the formal unit that gives them the network within which the variation can be produced. They are not longer able to differentiate what can still vary. In other words, anything may become a partial variation—but an exaggerated, unlimited variation. The trap tests have only to give to paragrammatic patients a framework of partial variation, and the patients manage and produce every neologism the trap infers, without refusing any of them.

Paragrammatic patients lose the opposition between the noun pattern and the verb pattern. These two flexion sets normally are opposed to each other. Paragrammatic patients tend to confuse them, a point now to be illustrated.

The following exercise shows that, under certain circumstances, paragrammatic patients may "feminize" verbal forms. In the following "trap tests" we asked patients to stop the "gaps". The items are as follows: il vient/elle <, il part/elle < and so on. All our patients have been inferred by the usual specific noun derivation. Some of their answers are "il vient/ elle vienne*, il part/elle parte*," and so on. Under other circumstances they also "masculinized " those verb forms. This time the sense of the induction went from "elle" to "il": "elle soupire/il soupire, elle couvre/il couvre, elle saute/il saute, elle éclate/il éclat*, elle règlemente/il règlement*, elle chante/il chant*, elle prête/il prêt*, elle rejète/il rejète, elle abrite/il abrite, elle récite/il récite, elle monte/il monte, elle coûte/il coût*, elle faute/il faut*." Patients' answers showed this fluctuation between the noun and verb patterns. Moreover, the more they made partial variations, the more they developed confusions.

| | |
|---|---|
| IL VIENT/ELLE vienne* | ELLE SOUPIRE/IL soupire |
| IL PART/ELLE parte* | ELLE COUVRE/IL couvre |
| IL TIENT/ELLE tienne* | ELLE PARLE/IL parle |
| IL MENT/ELLE mente* | ELLE FORCE/IL force |
| IL SORT/ELLE sorte* | ELLE SAUTE/IL saute |
| IL CUIT/ELLE cuite* | ELLE ECLATE/IL éclat* |
| IL SEDUIT/ELLE séduite* | IL FREMIT/ELLE frémite* |
| ELLE REGLEMENTE/IL règlement* | IL SERT/ELLE serte* |
| ELLE CHANTE/IL chant* | |
| IL PLAIT/ELLE plaite* | ELLE PRETE/IL prêt* |
| IL DORT/ELLE dorte* | ELLE REJETE/IL rejet* |
| | ELLE ABRITE/IL abrit* |
| IL ECRIT/ELLE écrite* | ELLE RECITE/IL récite |
| IL BONDIT/ELLE bondite* | ELLE MONTE/IL monte |
| IL RAMOLLIT/ELLE ramollite* | ELLE COUTE/IL coût* |
| IL VOMIT/ELLE vomite* | ELLE FAUTE/IL faute |
| IL INTERDIT/ELLE interdite* | |
| IL TRAHIT/ELLE trahite* | |

*Paragrammatic patients do not respect the differences between nouns and verbs.*

The following shows the reasoning of a paragrammatic patient about three items récite, chante and force: "elle récite? il récite? il récite?... il récit* ou elle récite? Il récite aussi! C'est un récit! Ou une récite*?—elle chante, il chant*, il chante... ou il chant*? On dit un chant! C'est il chant*! (People say "un chant", so.. it must be "il chant*"!)—elle force, il force... elle forte*, il fort*? Je ne pense pas! (I do not think so!) Elle force, il force aussi! Il est fort." We may say paragrammatic patients are subjected to any chance of morphological variation, and nothing (except the dominating common use of speech) stops the use of these variations. "Il récite" or "il récit*" are equivalent, as "une récite* or "un récit." From this point of view there are no more paradigmatic frontiers of the noun and the verb. That is why we obtain the following answers, where the variation of the past participle is unlimited, agreeing with the auxiliary être or avoir: "il a séduit/elle a séduite* & il est séduit/elle est séduite, il a interdit/elle a interdite* & il est interdit/elle est interdite, il a cuit/elle a cuite* & il est cuit/elle est cuite." And also "il a cuit un oeuf/elle a cuite*un oeuf, il a conduit une voiture/elle a conduite* une voiture, il a construit une maison/ elle a construite*une maison."

Patients may also exaggeratedly verbalize nominal forms, so we proposed the next trap test to our patients. They were asked to complete the following couples of words. One of our patients' answers are as follows....

| *Observer, Stg.1* | *Patient* |
| --- | --- |
| IL SECHE | IL SECHE |
| < SECHAGE | il sèchage* |
| ELLE TRICOTE | ELLE TRICOTE |
| < TRICOTTAGE | elle tricottage* |
| IL PLANTE | IL PLANTE |
| < PLANTAGE | il plantage* |
| ELLE NATTE | ELLE NATTE |
| < NATTAGE | elle nattage* |
| IL VISSE | IL VISSE |
| < VISSAGE | il vissage* |

| *Observer, stage 2* | *Patient* |
| --- | --- |
| IL SECHE/ELLE SECHAIT | IL SECHE/ELLE SECHAIT |
| IL SECHAGE*/ | IL SECHAGE*/il sèchait |
| ELLE TRICOTE/ | ELLE TRICOTE/elle tricottait |
| ELLE TRICOTAGE*/ | ELLE TRICOTAGE/elle tricottait |
| IL PLANTE/ | IL PLANTE/IL plantait |
| IL PLANTAGE*/ | IL PLANTAGE*/il plantait |

| *Observer, Stg. 3* | *Patient:* |
| --- | --- |
| ELLE SECHE | ELLE SECHE |
| < SECHAGE | elle sèchage* |
| IL TRICOTE | IL TRICOTE |
| < TRICOTAGE | il tricotage* |
| ELLE PLANTE | ELLE PLANTE |
| < PLANTAGE | elle plantage* |

| *Observer, Stg. 4* | *Patient:* |
|---|---|
| IL SECHE/IL SECHERA | IL SECHE/IL SECHERA |
| IL SECHAGE*/ | IL SECHAGE*/il sèchera |
| ELLE TRICOTE/ | ELLE TRICOTE/elle tricottera |
| ELLE TRICOTAGE*/ | ELLE TRICOTAGE/elle tricottera |
| IL PLANTE/ | IL PLANTE/il plantera |
| IL PLANTAGE*/ | IL PLANTAGE*/il plantera |

*Paragrammatic patients change inflexional forms into derivational ones.*

In these trap tests patients use the determinants as if they were suffixes, which confirms our interpretation of the disorder. Nominal flexion does not exist because it is no longer opposed to the verbal flexion. Everything becomes mutually "derivable" because there are no more differential frontiers between the nominal and the verbal patterns. This kind of patient is victim of the "quatrième proportionnelle." In other words, paragrammatic patients are drawing on their remaining logical ability, i.e., the network of internal variations. This network is functioning like a whirlwind, sweeping away everything it meets; and because the internal variation system is working and expanding without any restriction, it finally may include everything, no matter what it is.

We also observed that paragrammatic patients do not oppose the masculine noun paradigm to the feminine noun paradigm. Everything is possible, no matter which stem may admit the determinant "le" or "la." These determinants are interchangeable, as their substitution is no longer a significant limit. There are numerous confusions and nothing is stable.

The most important example of the disappearance of this differential paradigm frontier is the next one. It contains several stages. In the first stage: we asked paradigmatic patients to place "un" or "une" before a series of items. The list consisted of coiffeur, coiffeure*, coiffe, coiffure, coiffeuse, coiffeutrice*, coiffette*. One patient choses "un" for all the items of this list.

| *Stage 1: "un/une"?* | *Stage 2: "yes/no" oui/non* | *Stage 3: "yes/no"* |
|---|---|---|
| COIFFEUR = un coiffeur | UN COIFFEUR = oui | UN COIFFEUR = oui |
| COIFFEURE* = un coiffeure* | UNE COIFFEURE = oui | UNE COIFFEUR = oui |
| COIFFE = un coiffe* | UNE COIFFE = oui | UN COIFFEURE = oui |
| COIFFURE = un coiffure* | UNE COIFFURE = oui | UNE COIFFEURE = oui |
| COIFFEUSE = un coiffeuse* | UNE COIFFEUSE = oui | UN COIFFEUSE = oui |
| COIFFEUTRICE* = un coiffeutrice* | UNE COIFFEUTRICE* = oui | UNE COIFFEUSE = oui |
| COIFFETTE* = un coiffette* | UNE COIFFETTE* = oui | UN COIFFE = oui |
|  | UNE COIFFEUR* = oui | UNE COIFFE = oui |
|  | UN COIFFEUSE* = oui |  |
|  | UN COIFFEUTRICE* = oui |  |
|  | UN COIFFETTE* = oui |  |

For the second and third stages, we asked patients to make a "lexical decision", they have to answer "yes" if the item is correct, "no" if not.

Here are some of their answers[1]: un coifeur* = oui; une coiffeure* = oui; une coiffe = oui; une coiffure = oui; une coiffeuse = oui; une coiffeutrice* = oui; une coiffette* = oui; une coiffeur* = oui; un coiffe* = oui; un coiffure* = oui; un coiffeuse* = oui; un coiffeutrice* = oui; un coiffette* = oui. Patients accepted any proposition; they excluded nothing.

For the fourth stage, we asked patients to specify the meaning of their answers. The same patient responded as follows.

> UNE COIFFEUR* = "C'est celui qui fait les cheveux" ("the one who cut hair")
> UNE COIFFEURE* = "C'est travailler pour les femmes" ("the one who works for women")
> UNE COIFFE = "C'est une taille bien faîte, bien droite" ("a good hair style, cut straightly")
> UNE COIFFURE = "C'est un dégagement, comme il faut!" ("to cut one's hair short, very neatly")
> UNE COIFFEUSE = "C'est faire une "platte"* (?), une "flatte"* (?)...
> UNE COIFFEUTRICE* = "c'est mettre sous le casque!" ("That is to put somebody under the hair dryer")
> UNE COIFFETTE* = "C'est placer les bigoudis!" ("It is a curling set").
> *Paragrammatic patients confuse masculine nouns with feminine items.*

The patient who gave these answers never seemed to have "meaning trouble", and the meaning was elaborated immediately without any system. The only system he had is the one elaborated by the questions of the examiner during the trap test.

Patients may "synonymize" any pair of items or make them heteronymous. When we asked the same questions again, patients sometimes gave other definitions at random, Thus gender had no flexional value; it constituted one more derived form, allowing partial variation "ad infinitum," and these variations were all equivalent!

One point must be noted. When we asked these patients to choose between "le" or "la," their choices were usually the normal, expected answers. Thus one patient said "la montre, le poivre, le sabre, la chambre, le zèbre, le timbre, le sacre, le sucre, la cadre*, la cendre, le cidre, la poudre, le chiffre, le vitre*, la montre, le lustre." However, with the model "le moule/la moule, le voile/la voile," the same patient as mentioned before accepts the next answers "le montre* et la montre, le chèvre et la chèvre, le poivre et la poivre*, le sabre et la sabre*, le chambre* et la chambre, le timbre et la timbre*" and so on.

| Stage 1: "le/la" | | Stage 2: "oui/non" | Stage 3: "oui/non" |
|---|---|---|---|
| *Observer* | *Patient* | *Observer: Patient* | *Observer: Patient* |
| MONTRE | la montre | LE MONTRE: oui | LE MONTRE: oui |
| POIVRE | le poivre | LA MONTRE: non | LA MONTRE: oui |
| SABRE | le sabre | LE CHEVRE: oui | LE CHEVRE: oui |

---

[1] Of course it is the same patient as mentioned before.

| *Stage 1: "le/la"* | | *Stage 2: "oui/non"* | *Stage 3: "oui/non"* |
|---|---|---|---|
| *Observer* | *Patient* | *Observer: Patient* | *Observer: Patient* |
| CHAMBRE | la chambre | LA CHEVRE: non | LA CHEVRE: oui |
| ZEBRE | le zèbre | LE POIVRE: oui | LE POIVRE: oui |
| TIMBRE | le timbre | LA POIVRE: oui | LA POIVRE: oui |
| SACRE | le sacre | LE SABRE: oui | LE SABRE: oui |
| SUCRE | le sucre | LA SABRE: oui | LA SABRE: non |
| CADRE | la cadre | LE CHAMBRE: oui | LE CHAMBRE: oui |
| CENDRE | la cendre | LA CHAMBRE: oui | LA CHAMBRE: non |
| CIDRE | le cidre | LE TIMBRE: oui | LE TIMBRE: oui |
| POUDRE | la poudre | LA TIMBRE: oui | LA TIMBRE: non |
| CHIFFRE | le chiffre | LE CIDRE: oui | LE CIDRE: oui |
| VITRE | le vitre | LA CIDRE: oui | LA CIDRE: oui |
| MONTRE | la montre | LE SUCRE: oui | LE SUCRE: oui |
| LUSTRE | le lustre | LA SUCRE: oui | LA SUCRE: oui |

Each element of these pseudopairs may mean different things as well as the same extra linguistic "reality": le montre = "C'est une pièce de pistolet" ("It is a piece of a pistol"), la montre = "pour lire l'heure" ("to know what time it is"); le chèvre = "Le chèvre, c'est un animal" ("that is an animal"), la chèvre = "C'est un animal, la chèvre!" ("that is an animal, too!"); le poivre = "C'est du poivre en grain!" ("that is pepper") et la poivre = "C'est mettre du poivre dans une cuisinière, quoi!" ("that is putting pepper into a meal"); le chambre = "C'est..? Ca peut être un chambre dans une maison!" ("It is perhaps a room in a house"), une chambre = "Et la chambre? Je croyais que c'est faire la chambre!" ("I thought it was to clean the room"); le cidre = "C'est le cidre en bouteille" ("It is cider in a bottle"), la cidre = "C'est ce qu'on boit!" ("It is the cider we are drinking"); le sucre = "C'est pour sucrer!" ("It is to sweeten"), la sucre = "C'est le pot où on met le sucre!" ("It is the box where we put the sugar in")]. Here, too, synonymy and heteronymy extend themselves without any real control regarding the pinpoint passing of the same trap test.

*Stage 4*
LE MONTRE = "C'est une pièce de pistolet" ("It is a piece of a pistol")
LA MONTRE = "Pour lire l'heure" ("to know what time it is")
LE CHEVRE = "Le chèvre, c'est un animal!" ("that is an animal!")
LA CHEVRE = "C'est un animal, la chèvre!" ("that is an animal, too!")
LE POIVRE = "C'est du poivre en grain!" ("that is pepper!")
LA POIVRE = "C'est mettre du poivre dans une cuisinière, quoi!" ("that is putting pepper into a meal!")
LE CHAMBRE = "C'est?...Ca peut être une chambre dans une maison!"
LA CHAMBRE = "Je croyais que c'est faire la chambre!"
LE CIDRE = "C'est le cidre en bouteille"
LA CIDRE = "C'est ce qu'on boit!"
LE SUCRE = "C'est pour sucrer!"
LA SUCRE = "C'est le pot où on met le sucre!"

*Stage 5*
IL LE MONTRE = oui = "Il met sa pendule!"
IL LA MONTRE = oui = "...et il est à l'heure!"
IL LE POIVRE = oui = "il fait quelque chose!"
IL LA POIVRE = oui = "...et il met du poivre, donc je mets les deux!"
IL LE CIDRE = oui = "il le cidre; il le met en bouteille!"
IL LA CIDRE = oui = "il la cidre; il peut la boire! On met les deux!"

*Paragrammatic patients do not control the opposition between masculine items and feminine items.*

In other words, so long as the exercise does not include too many partial variations, patients use the "common practice of speech" and answer without noticeable mistakes. Conversely, when the exercise requires management of the trend of partial variations, patients follow these trends and cannot resist.

Thus, agrammatic patients still may oppose morphological sets (Guyard, 1987) but do not control the limits of these sets, by lack of segmental analysis, elaborating the "formal permanence" of an internal variation network.

On the contrary, paragrammatic patients have this internal variation network, but they are its victims: Everything may vary, without limite. The opposition between mutually exclusive paradigms has disappeared, and all items are subjected to a teratological derivation, including those elements that normally have a flexional status.

Theoretically, we cannot add another analysis to the lexical and textual analysis; the morphological analysis. Morphology has no proper existence. It normally results from the intersection of two dimensions of analysis, the differential and segmental dimensions (Fig. 7.3).

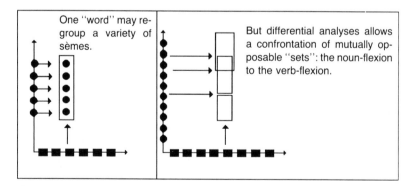

FIGURE 7.3. Morphology supposes a formal setting of internal variation but at the time a differentiation between mutually opposing paradigms.

# Conclusion

The clinical data elaborated here allow us to produce a theory of morphology (Gagnepain, 1982) based on a model that considers the clinical differentiation between agrammatism and paragrammatism. A "normal" analysis produces "abstract reasoning," which can be represented by two "axes": a differentiation axis and a segmentation axis. These two axes are not arranged in a hierarchical order (Jakobson, 1963), one grouping together what the other previously had differentiated. These two axes simply represent the "noncoincidence" (Gagnepain, 1982) of the opposing "element" (= sème) and the segmental "element" (= word). Morphology supposes an abstract relation of each paradigmatic set to its elements, but this relation has proved to be double; there is a qualitative relation and a quantitative relation.

Aphasic patients have only one reasoning dimension and produce exaggerated relations. Trap tests, different for each kind of patient, demonstrate the lost "abstracting capacity." Partial identity traps the two types of patient but in a different way.

Paragrammatic patients retain a segmental network that allows partial variation, but this network can put together any possible value. As a matter of fact, paragrammatic patients cannot maintain the identity of a paradigm; everything may vary with everything. Confusions are numerous. The inductions toward neologisms can easily be systematized.

Agrammatic patients lose this segmental network: They lose the possibility of elaborating a "confined" network of partial variation. This network loses its limits by lack or by excess. When there is a lack, agrammatic patients do not correlate any differential value. These values are considered on their own, without any relation to the others, and so they are juxtaposed. By excess, agrammatic patients will pathologically be inferred by any couple of sets, when a partial opposition allows to differentiate them from one another.

# Summary

Grammatical gender relates to several syntactic and morphological aspects (Champagnol, 1982, 1984, 1987; Desrochers, 1986). Because both Broca's and Wernicke's aphasics make mistakes in the use of grammatical gender, it is possible that we can learn from their aphasia about the nature of grammatical gender.

Paraphasic errors can be approached from two viewpoints. The first takes into account the differences between paraphasic and normal productions and does so for each grammatical class defined beforehand. The results can be recorded as percentages of correct and wrong answers.

The second viewpoint takes into account the aphasic answers according to the specific nature of the proposed linguistic task. The answers can be interpreted within morphological or syntactic "minisystems" included in the tests. In the latter case, the results appeared not to split between correct and wrong answers but between systematic and random answers. We basically adopted the last viewpoint and have presented clinical evidence showing the necessity of dividing this splitting into two phases: (1)-the dissociation between two modes of systematizing performances; and (2)-the dissociation between two modes of controlling morphological structure.

*Acknowledgment.* We thank our colleagues of the University of Rennes II (Laboratoire Interdisciplinaire de Recherches sur le Langage) who have shown the greatest spirit of cooperation and whose expertise has made this study possible. Special thanks go to Professor Sabouraud (Neurology Department, C.H.U. Rennes) who made facilities available for this research and made helpful comments. We also wish to thank many professors and students for their assistance and suggestions especially the members of the C.I.G.A.C. (Centre Interuniversitaire de Glossologie et d'Anthropologie clinique, Louvain). We are grateful to the members of C.R.E.N.O. (Centre de Recherches et d'Etudes en Neuropsychologie de l'Ouest) for their attention and valuable discussion. Last but not least, we gratefully acknowledge the help of Pierre Juban, who revised the chapter.

# References

Caramazza, A. (1986a). On drawing inferences about the structure of normal cognitive systems from the analysis of patterns of impaired performance: The case for single-patient studies. *Brain and Cognition*, *5*, 41–66.

Caramazza, A. (1986b). *On Inferring the Structure of Normal Cognitive Systems from Patterns of Impaired Performances*. Paper given at the 12th Annual Meeting of the Society for Philosophy and Psychology, Baltimore, June (Another version was presented at the Clinical Aphasiology Conference, Jackson Hole, (Wyoming), June 1986).

Champagnol, R. (1987). Recherche sur le genre: temps de classification au masculin et au féminin de substantifs animés. *Année Psychologique*, *87*, 217–236.

Champagnol, R. (1982). Représentation en mémoire de mots et leurs morphèmes de genre et de nombre. *Année Psychologique*, *82*, 401–419.

Champagnol, R. (1984). Représentation lexicale du genre et de ses transformations, *Revue Canadienne de Psychologie*, *38*, 625–644.

Desrochers, A. (1986). Genre grammatical et classification nominale, *Revue Canadienne de Psychologie*, *40*, n°3, 224–250.

Dubois, J. (1965). *Grammaire structurale du français: nom et pronom*, Larousse.

Duval-Gombert, A. (1976). *Les troubles de l'écriture et de la lecture dans les cas d'aphasie*, Thèse, Rennes 2.

Fodor, I. (1959). The origin of grammatical gender, *Lingua*, *8*, 1–41 & 186–214.

Gagnepain, J. (1982). *Du Vouloir Dire. Traité d'épistémologie des sciences de l'homme, T.l, Du Signe, De l'Outil*. Pergamon Press.

Grevisse, M. (1964). *Le bon usage*, Gembloux, Duculot et Paris, Geuthner, 1939; 8°ed.

Guyard, H. (1985). Le test du test, *Tétralogiques*, Presses Universitaires de Rennes 2.

Guyard, H. (1987). *Le concept d'explication en aphasiologie*, Doctorat d'Etat, Rennes 2.

Jakobson, R. (1963). *Deux aspects du langage et deux types d'aphasie*. Essais de Linguistique Générale, Ed. de Minuit.

Le Bot, M.C., Duval-Gombert, A. & Guyard, H. (1984). La syntaxe à l'épreuve de l'aphasie, *Tétralogiques*, Presses Universitaires de Rennes 2.

Le Bot, M.C. (1985). L'aphasie ou le paradoxe du phénomène, *Tétralogiques*, Presses Universitaires de Rennes 2.

Le Bot, M.C. (1987). *Le seuil clinique de l'humain*, Doctorat d'Etat, Rennes 2.

Martinet, A. (1957) Le genre féminin en indo-européen: Examen fonctionnel du problème. *Bulletin de la Société Linguistique de Paris*, *52*, 83–95.

Mok, M.Q.I.M. (1968). *Contribution à l'étude des catégories morphologiques du genre et du nombre dans le français parlé actuel*, La Haye, Mouton.

Nespoulous, J.L., Dordain, M., Perron, C., Ska, B., Bub, D., Caplan, D., Mehler, J. & Lecours, A. (1988). Agrammatism in Sentence Production without Comprehension Deficits: Reduced Availability of Syntactic Structures and/or of Grammatical Morphemes? A Case Study, *Brain and Language*, *33*, 273–295.

Pergnier, M. (1986). *Le Mot*, PUF.

Sabouraud, O., Gagnepain, J. & Sabouraud, A. (1963). Vers une approche linguistique des problèmes de l'aphasie, *Rev. Neuropsychiatr. Ouest*, 1; 2; 3; 4; 6; 3; 3; 3.

Saussure, F. de. (1915). (Cours): *Cours de linguistique générale*, Payot 68, 1°ed.

Urien, J.Y. (1984). Marque et immanence dans la théorie du Signe', *Tétralogiques*, Presses Universitaires de Rennes 2.

Urien, J.Y. (1982). *Le schème syntaxique & sa marque. Application au breton contemporain*, Doctorat d'Etat, Rennes 2, ANRTde Lille III.

Urien, J.Y. (1987). *La trame d'une langue, le Breton. Présentation d'une théorie de la syntaxe et application*, Mouladuriou hor yezh.

Yaguello, M. (1978). *Les mots et les femmes*, Paris, Payot.

# 8
# Cross-Linguistic Study of Morphological Errors in Aphasia: Evidence from English, Greek, and Polish

EVA KEHAYIA, GONIA JAREMA, and DANUTA KĄDZIELAWA

The investigation of errors related to the presence or absence of morphemes found in the speech of aphasics has been the target of research ever since aphasia was described in linguistic terms. The investigations initially examined the occurrence or nonoccurrence of morphological errors alone or in combination with syntactical errors. The performance of patients was mainly characterized by the omission of function words, grammatical inflections and derivations, or both. Studies of morphological errors found in aphasic speech have focused primarily on investigating the origin of these errors, as well as the information they provide about the organization of grammar in the brain.

Badecker and Caramazza (1986) examined whether morphological errors result from a morphological processing deficit or reflect a breakdown of morphological principles in the lexicon. Kehayia, Caplan and Piggott (1984) examined whether morphological errors, found in the speech of agrammatic aphasic patients, reflect a difference between accessing the lexicon or accessing the productive component of morphology where rules apply productively forming the words of the language. They found a clear difference in performance between complex words considered to be listed in the lexicon and those produced by the productive component of morphology. The data also reflected variation in performance on productively produced complex words, thus suggesting a level-ordered representation of the productive component of morphology. Along the same lines, Futter and Bub (1986) reported on data from dyslexic patients that revealed the existence of a level-ordered productive component of morphology. Finally, other studies examined whether morphological errors may be considered as special cases of problems of lexical access either within a single unified lexicon that combines open and closed class items, bound

---

* This chapter is an expanded version of material presented at the Third International Morphology Meeting, Krems, July 1988.

and inflected forms (Bates, Friederici, and Wulfeck, 1987; Stemberger, 1984), or within a "special" grammatical lexicon that has many though perhaps not all of the properties of lexical processing in general (Friederici, 1985; Lapointe, 1985). Regardless of the theoretical or neurolinguistic framework within which each of the above studies is conducted, their major conclusion is that "morphology," i.e., principles of well-formedness of lexical items and rules of word formation, are not lost in aphasia. Rather, brain damage seems to affect the patients' ability to process morphologically complex words and to access the morphemes from the lexicon.

The present study examines, cross-linguistically, the performance of Polish-, Greek-, and English-speaking aphasic patients on repetition, comprehension, and production tasks that require attention to morphological markers such as plural, gender, and case. Our investigation is conducted within the general framework of generative morphology; in this framework, two approaches are current: (1) the Strong Lexicalist Hypothesis assumed by Jackendoff (1975), Lapointe (1985), Lieber (1980), Williams (1981), Selkirk (1982), Walsh (1986), and Di Sciullio and Williams (1987), which requires all morphological relations, both derivational and inflectional, to be expressed in a morphlogical component (Fig. 8.1); and (2) the approach to morphology according to which all words, whether derived presyntactically or built up by the operation of syntax, have a representation at the level of syntax. Within the latter framework, Baker (1985) proposed the existence of a "morphology theory" parallel to other subtheories of the government-binding theory, e.g., the case theory or the government theory. The morphology theory includes principles that determine level ordering effects, principles of strict cyclicity, principles of morphological

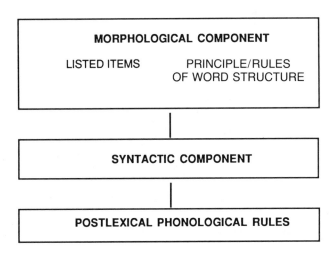

Figure 8.1. Strong Lexicalist Model of Grammar (Walsh, 1986).

subcategorization, and feature percolation. Finally, the morphology theory has access to a simple list of forms so it can deal with phonological exceptions and suppletions of various kinds.

Whether one assumes a "lexicalist" or a "nonlexicalist" framework, one finds that they both presume (1) the existence of word structure—be it expressed in the morphological component or through the principles of a morphology theory operating in the syntactic component—and (2) the existence of a lexicon and a set of principles, specific to the theory of morphology, which determine the well-formedness of complex lexical items.

Presuming the general theoretical framework outlined above, the following issues are of interest in the study of the language systems of Polish, Greek, and English.

1. The three languages differ significantly in the organization and importance of their inflectional systems, Greek and Polish being richly inflected languages and English having a poor inflectional system. Thus in Greek and Polish, nouns and adjectives are always marked for gender, number, and case; and verbs are always marked for voice, tense, person, and number, as well as aspect in Polish. In English, however, nouns and adjectives are marked only for number, whereas verbs are marked for tense and person (in third person singular only).

2. The way lexical items are listed in the lexicon, in the three languages, is also different. More specifically, the English lexicon comprises a set of listed *words* and *affixes* that may undergo morpholexical insertion and thus produce the possible words of the language, as proposed by Walsh (1986). The Greek lexicon is presumed to comprise two sets of words: (1) class I, always consisting of a *root* and an inflectional *affix* and having the subcategorization requirement $(\times)$ root $(+ \cdots Af)$; and (2) class II, always occurring as monomorphemic *words*. For a class I root to occur as a word of the language, it must always be suffixed with an inflectional affix. Class II listings, however, are words that may appear as such in the language. Finally in Polish, the lexicon includes three sets of words: (1) class I, consisting of a set of listed *words* and *affixes*, as the one described above for English; (2) class II, consisting of a *root* and an inflectional *affix* and having the subcategorization requirement of Greek roots, as shown above; and (3) class III, comprising a set of monomorphemic *words*. It must be noted that when roots of class II are affixed with a $\emptyset$ inflectional affix, which may well happen, an epenthesis of a glide and a vowel occurs to preserve the required phonological structure and stress pattern of words in Polish. For example, the root *sportowc-*, when in nominative, receives a $\emptyset$ inflectional affix. However, for the root to surface to the level of the word, the epenthetic *-ie-* is inserted: sportow*ie*c. The stress is thus preserved in penultimate position.

3. As a result of the above described organization of the lexicon in the

three languages, the well-formedness of lexical items is governed by distinct principles specific to each language. Thus inflectional affixes have a different role and importance in a highly inflected language such as Greek because, as was mentioned above, only inflectional affixes allow roots to surface to the level of the word and to be used as words of the language. In Polish, however, even though inflections are important (the language being highly inflected), they are crucial to the surfacing of the root to the level of the word only when class II listed items are considered. Otherwise, inflections have a role similar to that in English.

The present investigation focuses on the following issues.
1. How are the morphological markers of plural, gender, and case affected in aphasic speech in the three languages examined?
2. How are language-specific properties (e.g., form of listed items and subcategorization frames) reflected in morphological errors in aphasia?
3. How do the findings bear on the issues of lexical access and morphological processing discussed in the literature?
4. What are the theoretical implications of our findings, specifically in relation to lexicalist and nonlexicalist approaches to morphology?

## Subjects

The subjects for this study were two Polish-speaking (male, 28 and 34 years old), two Greek-speaking (male, 50 and 55 years old), and two English-speaking (one male 60 years old and one female 78 years old), right-handed, nonfluent aphasics who had suffered a cerebrovascular accident of hemorrhagic origin causing left-hemisphere damage. Their level of education varried from 6 to 12 years. Post onset, except for one Greek-speaking subject, these subjects had undergone speech therapy and were classified as nonfluent Broca's aphasics with agrammatism. At the time of testing, their repetition ability was intact, and their comprehension was good at the simple sentence level. They were all capable of producing simple sentences of the subject-verb (S-V) and subject-verb-object (S-V-O) type. All subjects were matched with controls of the same sex, age, and educational background in each language.

## Methodology

A repetition, a comprehension, and two production tasks requiring attention to the morphological markers of number, case, and gender were used. More specifically, the distinction singular/plural was tested on articles + nouns in subject and object positions, on copulas (Cop) and verbs, and on adjectives. The distinction masculine/feminine/neuter, in Greek, was

TABLE 8.1. Morphological distinctions and types of sentences tested in English.

| | | |
|---|---|---|
| S-V | [-z] | The *dog* is sleeping. |
| | | The *dogs* are sleeping. |
| S-V-O | | The mother feeds the *dog*. |
| | | The mother feeds the *dogs*. |
| S-Cop-A | [-iz] | The *peach* is small. |
| | | The *peaches* are small. |
| S-V-O | | The boy is holding the *peach*. |
| | | The boy is holding the *peaches*. |
| S-V | [-s] | The *cat* is sleeping. |
| | | The *cats* are sleeping. |
| S-V-O | | The mother feeds the *cat*. |
| | | The mother feeds the *cats*. |

tested on articles + nouns and on adjectives (A). The distinction between +/− animate in the masculine, in Polish, was tested on nouns and adjectives. Finally, the distinction between the nominative and accusative cases was examined. Lexical items were matched for frequency and were tested in equal numbers in sentences of the S-V, S-Cop-A, and S-V-O types. Although performance on tasks relevant to the above-mentioned features was examined in all three languages, the choice of stimuli reflects the difference in the manifestation of the morphological markers in each language. For example, in English, the distinction singular/plural was examined in nouns that require the [-s] (cat-cat*s*), [-z] (dog-dog*s*), and [-iz] (peach-peach*es*) plural allomorphs. Nouns were placed in subject and object position in equal numbers (12 of each: six of the S-V or S-Cop-A type and six of the S-V-O type) (Table 8.1).

In Greek, the distinction singular/plural was tested in articles + nouns of masculine, feminine, and neuter gender in the nominative and accusative case. The most representative declensions in terms of frequency were chosen for each gender (see Appendix 1).

In Polish, the distinction singular/plural was tested in class I and class II nouns of masculine (+/− animate), feminine, and neuter gender in the nominative and accusative case (see declensions in Appendix 2). The tasks used were the following.

## Repetition Task

A total of 154 sentences for Greek and English, and 192 sentences for Polish, were tested. The Polish data were increased by 48 sentences (12 in the singular nominative, 12 in the plural nominative, 12 in the singular accusative, and 12 in the plural accusative) to account for the masculine +/− animate distinction. Each sentence included one of the complex lexical items under investigation. Sentences for each language were randomly ordered.

## Comprehension Task

A sentence–picture matching task comprising the same set of stimuli as the ones used in the repetition task was administered. Each stimulus included two line drawings, presented vertically, depicting the singular/plural contrast in the various conditions under investigation.

## Production Task 1

The same set of pictures used for the comprehension task was presented to the subjects in an adaptation of the WUG test. The examiner primed the production of the target sentence (e.g., "the girls are playing") by pointing to the picture corresponding to the sentence "the girl is playing", saying it aloud and then eliciting the production of the target sentence by saying, "and here...." The subject was thus provided with all the necessary lexical items in an attempt to diminish the possibility of word-finding difficulties but had to produce the proper morphological markers in accordance with the picture presented to him.

## Production Task 2

The subjects were told to describe 77 single pictures selected from the stimuli used for the comprehension task and production task 1. The morphological distinctions investigated were tested in equal numbers.

The repetition task was used as a screening measure, whereas the production tasks, which followed the comprehension task, were administered in the following order: production task 2, production task 1.

# Results

## Repetition

A difference in the error pattern of the repetition task was found between Polish and Greek on the one hand and English on the other when nouns had to be inflected for plural. More specifically, although the error rate for Polish and Greek was rather low (9.3% and 15.2%, respectively), it rose in English (37%). These results may reflect the varying importance of the inflectional system between richly inflected (Polish and Greek) and poorly inflected (English) languages. Such a claim may not be unfounded if one considers that in richly inflected languages subjects tend to cling to inflections that play an important role in the interpretation of words and sentences. Bearing on the importance of inflections in Greek, it was noted that in this language errors consisted only of substitutions of one affix for another, whereas the errors found in English consisted only of omissions of affixes. In Polish, where both class I and class II items were tested, both substitutions and omissions were found depending on the class membership of the tested item. For example, if the word belonged to class I, which allows for roots to surface to the level of the word without an added affix, omissions as well as substitutions were found. However, if a word belonged to class II, only substitutions were found. It is interesting to note that the $\emptyset$ inflectional affixed root, which includes the epenthetic vowel, was not produced as a substituting form. A common feature in all three languages is that subjects produced more errors in plural nouns found in the object position than those in the subject position; errors found in the object position rated 77% for Polish, 63.6% for Greek, and 66.7% for English (see Table 8.2 for a detailed outline of the percentage of errors in repetition).

## Comprehension

In the comprehension task, on the distinction of singular/plural in nouns, a dissociation similar to that found in repetition was observed. As can be seen in Table 8.3, the error rate, which is low for both Polish and Greek, rises substantially for the English-speaking subjects.

## Production

In the production task, apart from switches from plural to singular and from plural accusative to singular accusative or nominative, the overall

TABLE 8.2. Repetition task: percentage of errors in the singular/plural distinction on nouns.

| P1 | 8.33% | P2 | 10.4% |
|----|-------|----|-------|
| 77% of the above errors in object position | | | |
| G1 | 13.8% | G2 | 16.6% |
| 63.6% of the above errors in object position | | | |
| E1 | 41.6% | E2 | 30.7% |
| 66.7% of the above errors in object position | | | |

P = Polish subjects; G = Greek subjects; E = English subjects.

TABLE 8.3. Comprehension task: percentage of errors in the singular/plural distinction.

| P1 | 4.1% | P2 | 5.2% |
|----|------|----|------|
| G1 | 11.1% | G2 | 9.7% |
| E1 | 48.6% | E2 | 34.7% |

P = Polish subjects; G = Greek subjects; E = English subjects.

TABLE 8.4. Introduction of numerals in subject and object position in the singular and plural in Polish, Greek, and English.

| Position | Singular | | | Plural | | |
|---|---|---|---|---|---|---|
| | Polish | Greek | English | Polish | Greek | English |
| Subject | 47 | 7 | 24 | 41 | 25 | 27 |
| Object | 28 | 9 | 0 | 31 | 20 | 0 |

TABLE 8.5. Production task 1 (percentage of errors, cumulative results).

| Task | Errors (%) | | |
|---|---|---|---|
| | Polish | Greek | English |
| Nouns, plural → singular | 10 | 40.2 | 44.4 |
| Verbs, plural → singular | 8 | 37.5 | 30.5 |
| Omissions, nouns in the plural | 8 | 15.2 | 0 |
| Omissions, verbs in the plural | 68 | 50.7 | 35.0 |
| Verb-noun agreement | 11 | 34.7 | 27.7 |
| Adjective-noun agreement | 0 | 19.7 | — |
| Numeral-noun agreement | 16 | 0 | 0 |

TABLE 8.6. Production task 2 (percentage of errors, cumulative results).

| Task | Errors (%) | | |
|---|---|---|---|
| | Polish | Greek | English |
| Nouns, plural → singular | 20 | 34.7 | 44.4 |
| Verbs, plural → singular | 0 | 45.0 | 30.5 |

strategy in all three languages and in both tasks was to add numerals in the singular as well as in the plural (Table 8.4). As shown, numerals were produced in both singular and plural, with a higher occurrence when the target structure demanded was in the plural. In Greek, all the numerals produced were properly inflected for number, gender, and case, similarly in Polish most of the numerals (84%) were also properly inflected. It is interesting to note that, in Polish, there were also cases where the subjects produced only the numeral and omitted the noun when the construction elicited was in the plural. This phenomenon was particular to Polish, as in Greek or English there were no cases where the noun following the numeral was dropped. Furthermore, Greek and English had a lower number of occurrences of numerals than Polish. This difference in performance may reflect a language-specific property of Polish (a language that has no articles) or a specific strategy used by the subjects to either gain time or facilitate processing. Whether one or the other explanation is pursued, one must consider the high occurrence of numerals in Polish in relation to the low error rate in nouns inflected for plural, which can be seen in Tables 8.5 and 8.6.

## Discussion

With respect to the distinction singular/plural, in Polish, Greek, and English, the subjects showed a tendency to switch from plural to singular in nouns, articles + nouns, copulas, and verbs in the tasks used. Although no omissions of articles were found in Greek, except when they accompanied a missing noun, there were omissions of verbs and copulas, as well as a small percentage of omissions of nouns in the plural. In English, both subjects tended to omit the inflectional plural marker on nouns with a preference in their omissions for the nonsyllabic [-s] and [-z] plural allomorphs. The syllabic plural allomorph [-iz] was largely retained. This finding coincides with that of Goodglass, Gleason, Bernholz, and Hyde (1972), who attributed the phenomenon to the salience of the syllable. Although we acknowledge the importance of salience in the retention of morphological markers in aphasia, a deeper theoretical explanation is sought here.

According to the lexicalist theoretical framework, the morphological component of grammar consists of a lexicon, which includes all idiosyncratic lexical items in form or meaning, all derivationally or inflectionally formed complex words, and a set of rules and principles that determine the well-formedness of complex lexical items. The output of the morphological component is inserted into the syntactic structures provided by the syntactic component. Finally, the rules of postlexical phonology apply.

Returning to the relative retention of the syllabic plural allomorph, if all +plural nouns are listed in the lexicon, all should be equally accessible or inaccessible, unless there is some feature that differentiates the various allomorphs. Let us hypothesize that the two phonological rules accompanying the affixation of the nonsyllabic plural allomorph on the one hand and of the syllabic plural allomorph on the other occur at two levels. We propose that the rule of epenthesis creating the syllabic allomorph [-iz] takes place lexically, whereas the rule of voicing s → z or devoicing z → s takes place postlexically. Thus in the production of a word such as "buses" the affixation of the plural allomorph and the application of the appropriate phonological rule take place in the morphological component. On the other hand, in the production of a word such as "cats" or "dogs" after accessing such a word from the morphological component, one would have to stop at the postlexical phonology level where rules such as "voicing" or "devoicing" occur, as in the case of the voicing or devoicing of the contracted copula: Contrast "the cat's sleeping" and "the dog's sleeping" where voicing or devoicing of 's occurs depending on the preceding consonant. The consequence of such a proposal is that, in the processing of complex words, although such words can be successfully accessed from the morphological component, a breakdown may occur at the postlexical phonology level, thus creating the differing results on the plural allomorphs found in our data of the English-speaking subjects.

Data from morphological errors produced by French-speaking agrammatic aphasics strongly suggest that breakdown may indeed occur at the surface postlexical phonology level (Jarema and Kehayia, 1988). For example, in cases where "liaison" is required between the article and the noun, as in "les éléphants," although the subjects initially produced the article in the plural, which indicates that they were indeed accessing the plural construction. Breakdown occurred when "liaison" has to apply. Thus they resorted to either an avoidance strategy, which led to the suppression of liaison at all costs and resulted in a switch in gender or number as manifested in what appears as a misselection of the article (*le éléphant*/ lœ elefã/instead of *les éléphants* /lɛzelefã/) or phonological restructuring or phonological distortion of words in cases where substitutions or misselections do not take place (*les l'éléphant*/lɛ lelefã/, *le zéléphants*/lœ zelefã/, *les... z... éléphants*/lɛ z elefã/). We therefore, conclude that, all other things being stable, breakdown may occur at the postlexical phonology level. That is although the subject is accessing the plural morphology from the morphological component, correct production is inhibited at the postlexical phonology level where rules such as the "liaison" apply. This assumption, of course, does not preclude the possibility of an actual deficit in accessing the word with its plural marker as such from the lexicon. Whether the problem lies in accessing the morphological component or in the failure of application of the postlexical phonology rules, in most cases the subjects indicated their awareness of the error or the missing item, which suggests that "morphology" is not lost and that at least basic syntactical structures are available. However, a gap in processing has occurred.

Another interesting feature to be considered is that most of the errors occurred in the plural nouns found in object position. We attribute this phenomenon to a processing deficit for the following reason. In a sentence such as "the woman feeds the goats," the first noun phrase (NP) as well as the verb are in the singular. If we presume a left-to-right nature of the parser as proposed in Cutler (1983) and Segui and Zubizaretta (1985), the processor starts interpreting the sentence marked +singular until it reaches the second NP. At that point, the processor has to assign the thematic role Theme to the second NP as well as take into consideration that this NP is marked -singular or +plural. It is possible, therefore, that at this stage a breakdown in processing occurs and that the feature +singular may be extended and cover the whole sentence. Note that the subjects had no difficulty interpreting S-V-O sentences where both NPs are in the singular. A smaller number of errors were found in sentences where the plural noun occurred in subject position. In such cases, processing starts with the interpretation of an NP marked +plural and is reinforced by the verb, which is also marked +plural. Although some switches of both verbs and nouns into singular were found, these incidents concern only a few errors.

An added factor to be considered here was that of case marking. Although case marking does not appear to be a hindering factor in sentences marked +singular or even in plural nouns in subject position, it certainly adds to the grammatical processing load in sentences where the plural occurs in object position and must therefore be inflected for accusative case. An increased number of errors were found in such sentences. In Greek, in particular, difficulties arose with masculine nouns in -*os* when plural accusative was asked for. Such cases were especially problematic not only because of the object position of the noun in the plural but also because of a stress change specific to this class of nouns according to which stress changes from the antipenultimate position in the nominative to the penultimate position in the accusative. Since this stress change is hypothesized to apply postlexically and, as mentioned above, rules applying at the postlexical phonology level have already been found to be problematic, it is not surprising that the Greek subjects experienced marked difficulty with the production of the plural accusative of masculine nouns in -*os*. Thus switches from accusative plural to nominative plural and from accusative plural to accusative or nominative singular were observed in 70% of the cases. Similar to Greek, in Polish switches from accusative plural to accusative or nominative singular were found.

Finally, the Greek and Polish subjects' performance on gender was not overly problematic. Some errors were found in switches of gender mainly from masculine and feminine to neuter when the noun concerned was in the plural and, furthermore, occcurred in object position. In Polish, in particular, gender switches in numerals, mainly manifested in a move toward the correct uninflected count form, were also observed.

A feature finally to be discussed is that of the types of error found in the three languages, as these errors reflect specific features of the language systems described earlier in the chapter. More specifically, in Greek substitutions rather than omissions of the inflectional affix marking the plural with the one marking the singular were found. Such an observation (see also Grodzinsky, 1982) can be easily explained if one considers the subcategorization frames of words in the lexicon of the languages under investigation. As mentioned earlier, in a language such as Greek, in order for a root to surface at the level of the word it must be affixed with an inflectional affix.

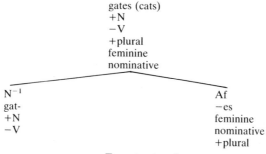

Tree structure 1

Only after the affixation of the inflectional suffix can the root be realized as a word of the language. Thus the production of a bear root would violate the subcategorization requirement of roots in the lexicon.

Unlike Greek, in English a root may surface to the level of the word regardless of the presence or absence of an inflectional affix.

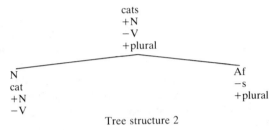

```
            cats
            +N
            −V
            +plural
   ┌──────────────────────┐
   N                      Af
   cat                    −s
   +N                     +plural
   −V
```

Tree structure 2

Taking the above into consideration, it is possible to explain why in English subjects tend to omit affixes, whereas in Greek they tend to substitute one affix for another. Furthermore, what is most interesting is that the subjects do not violate the subcategorization features and principles of well-formedness of words in either language. Similarly, in Polish the subjects were equally sensitive to the subcategorization requirements of the lexical items tested. Thus when a class I item was tested, errors reflected either substitutions or omissions due to the subcategorization requirements of the root shown here:

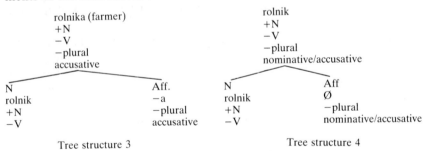

```
   rolnika (farmer)                 rolnik
   +N                               +N
   −V                               −V
   −plural                          −plural
   accusative                       nominative/accusative
 ┌──────────────┐               ┌──────────────┐
 N              Aff.            N              Aff
 rolnik         −a             rolnik          Ø
 +N             −plural        +N              −plural
 −V             accusative     −V              nominative/accusative
```

Tree structure 3                     Tree structure 4

When class II items were tested for, errors consisted only of substitutions because, as in Greek, roots may not surface to the level of the word without the affixation of an affix:

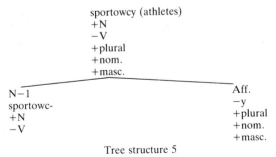

```
            sportowcy (athletes)
            +N
            −V
            +plural
            +nom.
            +masc.
   ┌──────────────────────┐
   N−1                    Aff.
   sportowc-              −y
   +N                     +plural
   −V                     +nom.
                          +masc.
```

Tree structure 5

Similar to Greek, the Polish subjects did not violate the principles of well-formedness of the language by producing bear roots such as *sportowc-* of the class II category.

## Conclusions

The results of this cross-linguistic study investigating the performance of agrammatic aphasic subjects on tasks requiring attention to morphological markers indicate that accessing inflected lexical items can prove to be difficult for aphasic subjects at different levels. Subjects may either have a problem accessing the complex lexical item from the lexicon or encounter difficulties with the application of phonological rules at the surface level of postlexical phonology.

An effect of the role of inflection in the language (rich/poor inflectional systems) was found at least for the repetition and comprehension tasks. Along the same lines, the typology of languages was also found responsible for the type of errors—substitutions versus omissions—found throughout the tasks examined in all three languages. In an attempt to investigate the implications of the data for the two theoretical frameworks outlined earlier, we found that, taking into account the information available up to now, it is difficult to favor an interpretation through one framework over another. Although the data seem to be better explained within the lexicalist framework adopted in this chapter, further testing of the issue is necessary.

Our study, along with the studies mentioned earlier, points toward the generally proposed hypothesis that principles and rules of morphology are not lost in aphasia, as none of the subjects tested produced any such violations; rather, accesss to lexical items is inhibited to varying extents depending on the internal structure of these items, the requirement of the application of postlexical phonological rules, and the effect of the processing load.

*Acknowledgments.* We thank Fanny Rosenoff and Annette Levin, speech-language therapists, for letting us have access to their patients and reporting on their case histories. We have benefited from discussions with David Caplan and Michel Paradis, who also provided us with pictures from the experimental versions of the Michel Paradis Bilingual Aphasia Test (Lawrence Erlbaum Associates, Hillsdale, NJ), which we adapted. We are especially grateful to Glynne Piggott for his comments.

## References

Badecker, W., & Caramazza, A. (1986). The analysis of morphological errors in a case of acquired dyslexia. *Reports of the Cognitive Neuropsychology Laboratory, No. 22.* Baltimore: Johns Hopkins University.

Baker, D.M. (1985). Incorporation: a theory of grammatical function changing. Doctoral dissertation, MIT.

Bates, E., Friederici, A., & Wulfeck, B. (1987). Grammatical morphology in aphasia: evidence from three languages. *Brain and Language, 32*, 19–67.

Cutler, A. (1983) Lexical complexity and sentence processing. In G.B. Flores d'Arcais and R.J. Jarvella (eds.), *The Process of Language Understanding.* New York: Wiley.

Di Sciullio, A.M. & Williams, E., (1987). *On the Definition of Word.* Cambridge, MA: MIT Press.

Friederici, A.D. (1985). Levels of processing and vocabulary types: evidence from online comprehension in normals and agrammatics. *Cognition, 19*, 133–166.

Futter, C. & Bub, D. (1986) A level-ordered theory of morphological paralexias. Presented at the Academy of Aphasia, Nashville, Tennessee.

Goodglass, H., Gleason, J.B., Bernholz, N.A., & Hyde, M.R. (1972). Some linguistic structures in the speech of a Broca's aphasic. *Cortex, 8.* 183–206.

Grodzinsky, Y. (1982). Syntactic representations in agrammatism: evidence from Hebrew. Presented at the Academy of Aphasia, Mohonk, NY.

Jackendoff, R. (1975). Morphological and semantic regularities in the lexicon. *Language, 51*, 639–671.

Jarema, G., & Kehayia, E. (1988). Morphological errors in French-speaking agrammatic aphasics: three case studies. Paper presented at the Academy of Aphasia. Montreal, October 1988.

Kehayia, E., Caplan, D., & Piggott, G.L. (1984). On the repetition of derivational affixes by English agrammatics. *McGill Working Papers in Linguistics*, Vol. 2, No. 1.

Lapointe, S. (1985). A theory of verb from use in the speech of agrammatic aphasics. *Brain and Language, 24*, 100–155.

Lieber, R., (1980). On the organization of the lexicon. Doctoral dissertation, MIT.

Segui, J. & Zubizarreta, M.-L. (1985) Mental representation of morphological complex words and lexical access. *Linguistics* 23, 759–774.

Selkirk, E.O. (1982). *The Syntax of Words. Linguistic Inquiry Monograph No. 7.* Cambridge, MA: MIT Press.

Stemberger, J. (1984). Structural errors in normal and agrammatic speech. *Cognitive Neuropsychology, 1*, 281–313.

Walsh, L. (1986). The nature of morphological representations. Ph.D. thesis, McGill University.

Williams, E. (1981). On the notions "lexically related"and "head of word." *Linguistic Inquiry, 12*, 245–274.

# Appendix 1: Representative Declensions: Greek

| MASCULINE   -os | | |
| --- | --- | --- |
| Nominative | | |
| Singular | **O** pilot**os** | mil**ai** |
| | The pilot | speaks |
| Plural | **Oi** pilot**oi** | mil**oun** |
| | The pilots | speak |

| MASCULINE   -os | | | |
|---|---|---|---|
| **Accusative** | | | |
| Singular | To paidhi | hereta | **ton** piloto |
| | The boy | greets | the pilot |
| Plural | To paidhi | hereta | **tous** pilo**tous** |
| | The boy | greets | the pilots |

| FEMININE   -a | | | |
|---|---|---|---|
| **Nominative** | | | |
| Singular | **I** mathit**ria** | dhiavaz**ei** | to mathima |
| | The student | is reading | the lesson |
| Plural | **Oi** mathit**ries** | dhiavaz**oun** | to mathima |
| | The students | are reading | the lesson |
| **Accusative** | | | |
| Singular | I dhaskala | vlepei | **tin** mathitria |
| | The teacher | looks at | the student |
| Plural | I dhaskala | vlepei | **tis** mathit**ries** |
| | The teacher | looks at | the students |

| NEUTER   -o | | | |
|---|---|---|---|
| **Nominative** | | | |
| Singular | **To** dhendr**o** | einai | psil**o** |
| | The tree | is | tall |
| Plural | **Ta** dhendr**a** | einai | psil**a** |
| | The trees | are | tall |
| **Accusative** | | | |
| Singular | O andras | kovei | **to** dhendr**o** |
| | The man | is cutting | the tree |
| Plural | O andras | kovei | **ta** dhendr**a** |
| | The man | is cutting | the trees |

# Appendix 2: Representative Declensions: Polish

| MASCULINE,   +ANIMATE,   +HUMAN | | |
|---|---|---|
| **Nominative** | | |
| Singular | **Rolnik** | **orze** |
| | The farmer | is ploughing |
| Plural | **Rolnicy** | **orzą** |
| | The farmer | are ploughing |
| **Accusative** | | |
| Singular | **Wołam** | **rolnika** |
| | I am calling | the farmer |
| Plural | **Wołam** | **rolników** |
| | I am calling | the farmer |

| MASCULINE,  -ANIMATE | | | |
|---|---|---|---|
| **Nominative** | | | |
| Singular | **Stół** | **jest** | **okrągły** |
| | The table | is | round |
| Plural | **Stoły** | **są** | **okrągłe** |
| | The tables | are | round |
| **Accusative** | | | |
| Singular | Kupuję | **stół** | |
| | I am buying | the table | |
| Plural | Kupuję | **stoły** | |
| | I am buying | the tables | |

| FEMININE | | | |
|---|---|---|---|
| **Nominative** | | | |
| Singular | **Krowa** | **daje** | mleko |
| | The cow | is giving | milk |
| Plural | **Krowy** | **dają** | mleko |
| | The cows | are giving | milk |
| **Accusative** | | | |
| Singular | Chłop | doi | **krowę** |
| | The farmer | is milking | the cow |
| Plural | Chłop | doi | **krowy** |
| | The farmer | is milking | the cows |

| NEUTER | | | |
|---|---|---|---|
| **Nominative** | | | |
| Singular | **Okno** | **jest** | otwarte |
| | The window | is | open |
| Plural | **Okna** | **są** | otwarte |
| | The windows | are | open |
| **Accusative** | | | |
| Singular | Pani | otwiera | **okno** |
| | The woman | is opening | the window |
| Plural | Pani | otwiera | **okna** |
| | The woman | is opening | the windows |

# 9
# Cross-Linguistic Study of the Agrammatic Impairment in Verb Inflection: Icelandic, Hindi, and Finnish Cases

MARJORIE PERLMAN LORCH

Aspects of verb production in the spontaneous narrative speech of agrammatic aphasics in Icelandic, Hindi, and Finnish are examined in this chapter. Analysis of the pattern of results is framed in linguistic terms capturing morphosyntactic distinctions. The goal of this cross-language analysis is to detail how a deficit in the production of the grammatical morphemes of verb phrases, which has been described as one of the primary features of agrammatism in English, reflects aspects of the Language System.

By comparing the patterns of language breakdown in aphasic production in these three distinct languages, the possible influence of language-specific factors on the Grammar and the Lexicon may be illuminated. Concurrently, these data can contribute to an understanding of the universal aspects of language processing, as reflected in the similarity of aphasic deficits found cross-linguistically.

It must be acknowledged at the outset that this effort cannot be immediately successful given certain inescapable limitations. It seems clear that various other psychological and cognitive factors may also contribute to some of the agrammatics' difficulties in speech production. In order to define the contribution of these factors to the behavior observed initially requires the determination of how these factors interact with the linguistic domain. The lack of detailed models of universal grammar and cognitive processing cause basic limitations in theoretical interpretation. These considerations suggest that the fundamental characterization of agrammatism should begin with a descriptive linguistic approach cast in terms that capture language universal distinctions. In this circumstance, I adopted the stance taken by Jakobson (1971): "I followed Hughlings Jackson's warning against any mixture of different levels in the investigation of aphasia and outlined my typology of aphasic impairments on a strictly linguistic basis."

# Previous Research in Agrammatism

Interest in agrammatism dates from the earliest work in the aphasias. The first description of agrammatism is attributed to Deleuze (1819), in which he noted that "The patient in question used exclusively the infinitive of verbs and never used any pronoun" (Goodglass and Menn, 1985). It is significant that there were numerous early reports of agrammatic aphasia in German-speaking patients. Indeed, Low (1931) pointed out the significant lack of descriptions of agrammatism in English. The fact that both German and French are highly inflected languages may explain why there were a large number of cases documented in these languages and, until recently, few in English. The symptom(s) of agrammatism, as a disorder affecting bound grammatical inflections, would be particularly striking in such languages. Alajouanine (1968) noted that "the richer a language is in distinctions of these types [of grammatical differentiation in inflection], the more glaring agrammatism will appear" (Goodglass and Menn, 1985). The early case studies of agrammatism in German- and French-speaking patients are similar in that the loss of inflections marking person, number, and gender agreement and the predominance of the infinitive form of verbs are evident.

Initial scientific reports in English described agrammatics as having shortened phrase length (Goodglass, Quadfasel, and Timberlake, 1964), a limited word inventory (Goodglass and Hyde, 1969; Jones and Wepman, 1965), and a reduced speaking rate (Howes, 1967; Howes and Geschwind, 1962). Clinically, the term has been used to refer to a simplification of sentence form with an overreliance on content words (Geschwind 1970; Goodglass and Kaplan, 1972).

Although clinical and experimental evidence in English indicates that agrammatic aphasics have difficulty producing bound and free grammatical morphemes, not all grammatical formatives appear to be equally affected. There seems to be some pattern to the spared and impaired inflectional morphology in the spontaneous speech of agrammatics, e.g., the overly frequent use of the verb with the "-ing" inflection in English-speaking agrammatics (Goodglass, 1968).

A number of studies have examined the order of difficulty that agrammatics have in producing noun and verb inflections. Jakobson (1956) characterized the agrammatics' behavior as being due to a dissolution of grammatical rules resulting in the loss of government and concord. The notion of "contiguity" is used to explain the higher degree of difficulty with verb inflections in comparison to noun inflections. It also successfully captures the frequency of occurrence of certain grammatical morphemes (plural "s" is more frequent than possessive "s," which is more frequent than third singular present tense "s") based on the size of the constituent structures over which the government reaches (Jakobson, 1964). However, Jakobson's model cannot be extended to account for the varying degrees of susceptibility in other grammatical forms. Moreover, it would in fact erroneously predict equal vulnerability of all verb inflections, as they all mark government in the clause (de Villiers, 1974).

The choice of verbs, as the focus of a study of agrammatism, may seem less than obvious. Traditionally, agrammatics have been considered to have an impairment affecting closed class items, and it has been generally assumed that open class lexical items were not a problem (Kolk, 1978). There have been a number of new arguments for closer scrutiny of both lexical and inflectional issues with respect to main verbs in agrammatism (Grodzinsky, 1984; Kohn, Lorch, and Pearson, 1989; Kohn, Perlman, and Goodglass, 1984; Marin, Saffran, and Schwartz, 1976; Miceli, Silveri, Villa, and Caramazza, 1984; Saffron, Schwartz, and Marin, 1980a; Wales and Kinsella, 1981).

## English Agrammatic Verb Forms

In clinical descriptions of English-speaking agrammatics, it has been noted that main verbs (V) are typically produced either in the uninflected form (e.g., "walk"), or the V + ing form (e.g., "walking") (Goodglass, 1968; Goodglass & Geschwind, 1976; Jackobson, 1964; Luria, 1970; Myerson and Goodglass, 1972). De Villiers (1974) reported that in her group study the "-ing" form was used twice as often as any other verb form.

These uninflected forms might be described as infinitives, bare stems, or "zero-morph default forms," whereas the -ing form might be considered to be participles (adjectival) or gerundive (nominalized) forms. The difficulty with the syntactic representation of forms such as V + ing and V + O (Object) is due to the existence of numerous homonymous forms in English. Whereas in normal speech they are generally employed in distinct verbal structures, in agrammatic speech the surface structure ambiguities of the reduced sentence constructions produced by English-speaking agrammatics causes confusion as to how these forms should be characterized (Myerson and Goodglass, 1972).

Goodglass and Geschwind (1976) suggested that the agrammatics' production of V + ing forms represented gerundive nominalizations, not present participles or progressives. Saffran, Schwartz, and Marin (1980b) suggested that these ing forms are being used "to name" the action that would normally be expressed as a predicate. The implication is that agrammatics have a deficit in predication (cf. Luria, 1970). That is, when using the -ing form as a nominal, agrammatics are referring to the action without expressing the grammatical relations between sentence constituents. However, Lapointe (1985) argued that gerunds express functional relations that are exactly the same as the relations expressed in sentences containing the corresponding verb form. Thus according to Lapointe, the use of -ing forms as nominals does not imply a deficit in predication.

The English verb system is typified by little use of bound inflection. Instead, there is a general reliance on the use of word order and auxiliary verbs to signal syntactic distinctions. It follows, then, that the questions raised by the difficulties agrammatics have with bound morphemes in verb phrases cannot be easily answered by examining cases in English. The limitations of research into this issue are due to the large number of uninflected forms and the opacity of its underdetermined inflected forms.

One response to this state of affairs has been to turn to a cross-linguistic approach. Most current theorists have expressed the need to consider cross-linguistic data to formulate a more coherent account of agrammatism (Bates, Friederici, and Wulfeck, 1987; Blumstein, 1982; Caplan, 1983; Goodglass and Geschwind, 1976; Lapointe, 1985; Menn, Obler, and Goodglass, 1983).

It is evident that agrammatism is manifest in all languages in the world in which aphasia has been studied. Obviously, these cases of agrammatism vary in certain aspects owing to language-specific distinctions. With regard to bound inflectional morphemes and the potential for impairment in agrammatism, various possibilities exist due to their different phonological, syntactic, and semantic status.

## Form and Function of Predicates

Predicates may be characterized along both formal and functional dimensions. The formal dimension of the degree of "finiteness" involves the number of specified grammatical predicate markings, whereby finite inflection contains more grammatical categories than nonfinite inflection. Nonfinite forms (infinitives and participles) are those that are not marked for tense, whereas finite forms are fully marked.

An alternative formulation, the dimension of degree of "nominalization," pertains to more lexical and semantic aspects of verbs. In the account put forth by Hopper and Thompson (1984), the (universal) prototypical noun is described as referential and static, and the prototypical verb is described as relational and active. The major grammatical classes of Noun and Verb are seen as defining two extremes of the lexical continuum. Many intermediate forms contain relatively more or less of these features. These intermediate forms include the copula, participles, and gerunds, among others. The transitive verb is taken as having the most verb-like qualities, as it expresses relational aspects of activity involving subjects and objects. The copula and participle have more noun-like qualities, expressing more static or referential aspects of the predicate.

Either of these two formulations may be used to interpret the typical pattern of verb phrases found in agrammatism in English, i.e., the use of the uninflected or V + ing form of lexical verbs, and omission of the copula and auxiliary. The uninflected forms have been interpreted as infinitives, or forms lacking grammatical marking. The V + ing form can be taken for the progressive participle, gerund, or inflected default form. The pattern of production in English does not clearly support the interpretation of the operative role of either finiteness or nominalization. Two possible interpretations remain: (1) There is a deficit in predication and a tendency toward nominalization. (2) There is omission of bound and free grammatical morphemes that mark tense and agreement and a tendency toward the use of nonfinite forms.

The intent of this study is to contribute to the resolution of this ambiguity. The nature of this morphosyntactic deficit may be clarified by examining the patterns exhibited by agrammatics who are speakers of highly inflected languages. In the languages under investigation, the formal and functional status of verb inflection is less opaque. Each of the three languages under investigation affords opportunities to test these interpretations by providing distinct morphological forms marking the various grammatical functions. Details of the inflectional systems of Icelandic, Hindi, and Finnish are given below. The specific distinctions that could provide evidence in support of a particular interpretation are identified for each language. (See Lorch, 1986, for more detailed grammatical descriptions.)

# Some Grammatical Details of Icelandic, Hindi, and Finnish

## Icelandic Language

Icelandic is a germanic language that has conserved hundreds of irregular (strong) classes of verbs. Icelandic requires the use of an inflectionally distinct subjunctive mood in a large number of syntactically conditioned contexts. Several of the strong and one of the weak conjugational paradigms have (a zero-morph) form for the first and third singular present tense. The infinitive is an inflected form and requires the use of a free morpheme similar to the English "to." Simple verb forms are generally used for the present and past tense indicative and subjunctive. The compound auxiliary + main verb construction is required for the passive. The present participle is an infrequent form. The progressive is conveyed by using a specific vector verb construction: the auxiliary + past participle form of "go" + the infinitive form of the main verb. The frequently used past participle is inflected for number, gender, and case agreement. However, when used in conjunction with certain auxiliary verbs, the past participle is found in a default form—the singular neuter nominative form.

## Hindi Language

In Hindi, there are elaborate rules determining subject agreement; verbs are marked for gender as well as number. Verb phrases, which are sentence final, typically contain one or two auxiliaries and a main verb. These compound and complex constructions reflect subtle shades of verb meaning that are syntactically conditioned. The Hindi verb stem is an instance of an uninflected, zero-morph form. It frequently functions as the main verb in compound verb phrases. In contrast, the infrequently used infinitive is an inflected form that is used in complex embedded clause constructions. The present tense is a compound construction consisting of the imperfect participle + auxiliary; there is no simple form of this tense. The past tense is a simple verb form; it does not require the use of the auxiliary. The progressive construction employs the uninflected stem form of the main verb with an additional free grammatical morpheme (vector verb) in conjunction with the inflected form of auxiliary. This vector verb is also marked for agreement. There is a default form of agreement inflection in Hindi. The masculine singular is used as the default form for the participle, and the third singular form is used for the auxiliary "to be." This default form is frequently required when the marking of agreement with either the subject or the object nouns is blocked by syntactic conditions.

## Finnish Language

Finnish is an agglutinative language. Individual tense, mood, voice, and number/person morphemes are attached to the verb stem. Morphophonological rules apply to the whole word producing sound changes in both the stem and inflection, forming a synthetic unit. The uninflected verb stem is not a morphologically permissible word form. There are a number of morphological inflections that can attach to the infinitive. The form of the third singular present tense form is similar to the first infinitive, as there is a zero-morph for this number/person category (although morphophonological distinctions occur in many of the conjugational form classes). The weak grade of the infinitive is used in negative constructions with a negative auxiliary. This form carries no agreement inflection. There is also an impersonal passive form of the verb, which is inflected for voice but not for person/number agreement. The simple verb phrase is the most frequently used construction, but compound constructions are required for negation.

## Analysis

The study of agrammatic impairments in verb phrase form and function was carried out on five of the cases and their matched controls included in the Cross-Language Aphasia Study (Menn and Obler, in press), comprising two Icelandic cases (Magnúsdóttir and Thráinsson, in press), one Hindi case (Bhatnagar, in press), and two Finnish cases (Niemi, Laine, Hännannin and Koiruselkä-Sallinen, in press). Texts of several hundred words consisting of four spontaneous narrative speech samples were obtained using identical elicitation materials. Each sample was transcribed by a neurolinguist who was a native speaker of the language in question. Full interlinear morphemic English translations were made of each narrative sample (see Menn and Obler, in press, where complete transcripts can be found). Each patient's language performance was treated as a single case study, and conservative limits were imposed on the use of intersubject comparisons. To identify fine-grained aspects of performance, each individual was examined seperately.

The goal of the data analysis was to construct a profile of quantitative and qualitative performance for each patient compared to the matched normal control in order to determine if verb inflections are differentially affected within each patient and within each language. The examination of the pattern of errors focused on lexical omission, inflectional omission, inflectional substitution, and lexical substitution. Preserved areas of performance were also examined, and the pattern of use of verb forms and verb phrase construction types was described.

The results described the general constitution of the corpus, detailing the number of sentences with obligatory verb phrase slots and the distribution and frequency of correct forms, omitted forms, and errors of the verb phrase constructions. The distribution of verb phrase constructions used by the patients and the controls were compared. For each patient and control, ratios of the distribution of lexical items (nouns and verbs) are reported.

The same general procedure was used to analyze the corpus for each case as follows: (1) the verb phrases were identified within each sentence structure; (2) each verb phrase was categorized according to its structural type; (3) the form of each component verb was identified as either correct or in error; (4) the errors were categorized into one of eight error types; and (5) the produced forms or omissions and the targets for production were coded as to their grammatical form and function.

The coding categories used in each of these steps are detailed for each language: (1) number; (2) person; (3) tense; (4) voice; (5) mood; (6) verb phrase component; (7) negation; (8) gender; (9) case; (10) clitizization; and (11) conjugational form class. A checklist of the grammatical coding categories present in each language is detailed in Appendix 1.

Each verb form in the verb phrase was coded as correct or as an error. The following eight categories were used to differentiate error types: omission, broken off stem form, substitution, lexical selection error, lexical and inflectional selection error, conjugational form class error, derivational form error, and phonological paraphasia. (See Appendix 2 for a detailed description of the error types used in the analysis.) Erroneous productions that resulted in another inflectional form were analyzed as being morphologically based, regardless of whether they were plausible phonological errors, for reasons of consistency. Phonologically based errors were deemed less likely, as the patients included in the study were judged to be relatively free of dysarthria.

Errors were classified using conservative criteria. Both the discourse context and syntactic requirements for grammaticality were used to determine obligatory conditions. Certain anomalous forms occurred that could not be categorized unequivocally as syntactically conditioned errors. These instances are not included in the initial set of analyses as errors but are included in the discussion of the results.

The constituent structure of the verb phrase was also analyzed. Each verb phrase was categorized according to type: simple verb phrase (copula or simple lexical verb) or compound verb phrase (auxiliary verbs and participles, vectors, and main verbs).

For each patient and control, noun/verb ratios are reported. These ratios were based on the number of lexical nouns and verbs occurring in the corpus (pronouns, auxiliary verbs, and copulas were not included). The frequency distribution of nouns and verbs were reported as percentages of the total corpus of the narrative sample for each patient. Token/type ratios were calculated from the number of base forms represented in the inflected forms. Comparisons between the proportions and ratios within and between the patient and control were made by inspection.

# Results

## Case 1, Icelandic: Kiddi

There were 239 verb phrases produced in narrative discourse, with a total of 310 obligatory verb contexts. There were only 8 omissions (2.6%). Of the verbs produced, 291 were correct, and 11 were in error (4%).

### Description of Errors

There were a total of 19 errors: 8 omissions, 3 stems produced without inflections, 6 substitutions, and 2 lexical selection errors. The distribution of error types for each verb category is displayed in Table 9.1.

TABLE 9.1. Performance by verb type: Kiddi.

| Verb form | Correct production | Lexical omission | Inflection substitute | Inflection omission | other |
|---|---|---|---|---|---|
| Auxiliary/copula | 79 | 5 | 3 | — | — |
| Modal | 14 | — | — | — | — |
| Simple finite | 113 | 1 | 3 | 3 | 1 |
| Main verb of comp. | 85 | 2 | — | — | 1 |
| Total | 291 | 8 | 6 | 3 | 2 |

## CHARACTERISTICS OF THE VERB PHRASE STRUCTURES

As the number of (produced) errors was low, the patient appeared to have only a mild deficit. However, inspection of the pattern of the verb forms and verb phrase structures revealed some notable characteristics. Table 9.2 displays the distribution of verb phrase types for the patient and control.

Among the 239 verb phrases produced, 175 were simple verb phrases (73%): 54 copula and 121 simple main verbs. The patient used simple lexical verb phrases significantly less frequently (51%) than the control (61%) (chi-squre 4.00, $p < .05$). These simple lexical verb constructions require morphological inflections that follow complicated form class paradigms. The patient used the copula construction slightly more often (23%) than the control (18%).

The patient produced 64 compound verb phrases (27% of the total verb phrases). Of these compound structures, 32 were auxiliary + infinitive constructions, and 32 were auxiliary + participle constructions. Past participle constructions are relatively more complex in their inflectional morphology when used in conjunction with the auxiliary verb "vera" (to be) than with other auxiliaries. In the constructions with "vera" the past participle must show case, number, and gender agreement with the subject. The patient tended not to produce this type. In the preferred past participle constructions used by the patient, the auxiliary verbs condition the use of a default form—the nominative singular neuter. Of the 32 participle constructions produced, only 10 required the actual marking of agreement of the main verb. The inflections marking the infinitive and the present participle are invariant. Thus in most of the compound verb phrases produced by the patient, the grammatical marking of agreement for number and person is carried solely by the auxiliary; the main verbs require an invariant inflection. The use of these copula and compound verb constructions without main verb agreement represent 45% of all verb phrases produced, which is significantly more than the 31% produced by the control (chi-square 7.83, $p < .01$).

This analysis of the verb phrase types reveals an overreliance on constructions in which number and person, and to a large extent tense, are

TABLE 9.2. Distribution of verb phrases: Kiddi.

| Type of verb phrase | Patient | | Control | |
|---|---|---|---|---|
| | No. | % | No. | % |
| Copula | 54 | 23 | 29 | 18 |
| Auxiliary + infinitive | 32 | 14 | 12 | 7 |
| Auxiliary + participle (−agreement) | 22 | 9 | 10 | 6 |
| Auxiliary + participle (+agreement) | 10 | 4 | 13 | 8 |
| Simple main verb | 121 | 51 | 99 | 61 |
| *Total* | 239 | | 163 | |

represented by the use of free grammatical morphemes rather than bound ones. The limited use of simple lexical verbs also suggests the avoidance of structures that require the production of lexical forms with bound grammatical inflections, which have a great deal of variety and irregularity in Icelandic.

LEXICAL ISSUES

The noun/verb ratio for this patient was 0.48, in contrast to a ratio of 1.23 for the control. This proportion is not due to an excess of verbs. Verbs comprise 18% of the patient's corpus compared with 16.5% of the control corpus. In contrast, it is evident that there is a paucity of nouns in the patient's productions. Lexical nouns comprised only 9% of the patient's corpus compared to 20% of the control corpus. See Table 9.3 for a comparison of the noun/verb ratio and token/type ratios for the major lexical categories represented in the patient and control corpora.

Consideration of the token/type ratios for the nouns and verbs reveals another matter. Whereas the patient used a relatively greater number of verbs in his speech, there was little variety in the verbs used. Of the 242 lexical verbs produced in the patient corpus, only 77 different verbs were represented. The verb token/type ratio of 3.14 is contrasted with the noun token/type ratio of 1.4. The normal control had token/type ratios that indicated variety in both lexical categories: the noun ratio was 1.8 and the verb ratio 1.5.

These results indicate that the patient was able to produce a large number of verb forms correctly. Instances of errors of omission typically occurred in contexts where the subject requiring agreement has also been omitted.

In sum, the verb phrases most frequently produced by this patient tended to be those that marked tense and agreement with auxiliaries rather than inflections on lexical verbs. There was less frequent use of simple lexical verbs or participle forms that required the marking of agreement with bound grammatical inflections. The predominant employment of the copula and compound verb phrases with invariant inflections obviates the

TABLE 9.3. Distribution of major lexical categories: Kiddi.

| Category | Patient | Control |
|---|---|---|
| Noun/verb ratio | 0.48 | 1.23 |
| *Percent of corpus* | | |
| Nouns | 9 | 20 |
| Verbs | 18 | 16 |
| Others | 73 | 64 |
| Token/type ratio | | |
| Nouns | 1.4 | 1.8 |
| Verbs | 3.1 | 1.5 |

necessity of producing inflected forms, which depend on complex and irregular conjugational paradigms in Icelandic. There was also a lack of variety in the actual lexical verbs (base types) being used.

## Case 2, Icelandic: Togga

There were 223 obligatory verb contexts among the 73 verb phrases produced. Of them, 26 (12%) verbs were omitted and 197 (88%) were produced; 145 were produced correctly, and 52 were produced with errors. The total number of errors was 78: 26 omissions and 52 incorrect productions. See Table 9.4 for the distribution of correct, omitted, and incorrect productions by type of verb.

The distribution of correct forms and errors (omissions and erroneous productions) found in this patient's corpus is not evenly distributed among the different types of verbs. There are few errors for modals and vectors. The proportion of correct forms to errors was approximately 2:1 for the auxiliary, copula, and main verb of a compound. For the simple verbs, an error or correct form occurred equally frequently. The distribution of correct forms and errors for simple verbs compared to the other three types was significantly different (chi-square 6.78, $p < .01$). Among the auxiliary, copula, and main verb types, incorrect productions and omissions were equally likely errors. Among the simple verbs, there were three times as many incorrect productions as omissions. The distribution of incorrect productions and omissions for simple lexical verbs was significantly different from the other three types (chi-square 4.84, $p < .05$).

### Description of Errors

The 78 incorrect instances were distributed among the different error types as follows: 26 omissions, 8 broken-off stems without inflections, 29 substitutions, 7 lexical selection errors, 4 lexical and inflectional errors, 3 form class errors, and 1 paraphasia. The distribution of error types for each verb category is displayed in Table 9.5.

TABLE 9.4. Performance by verb type: Togga.

| Verb form | Correct production | Lexical omission | Inflection substitute | Inflection omission | Other |
|---|---|---|---|---|---|
| Auxiliary/copula | 59 | 10 | 11 | — | 1 |
| Modal | 4 | — | 1 | — | — |
| Vector | 7 | — | — | 1 | — |
| Simple finite main | 48 | 11 | 18 | 6 | 7 |
| Main of compound | 27 | 5 | 2 | 2 | 3 |
| *Total* | 145 | 26 | 32 | 9 | 11 |

TABLE 9.5. Verb category by error type: Togga.

| Type of verb | Omission | Broken stem | Substitution | Lexical selection | Lexical + inflectional | Conjugational form class | Paraphasia |
|---|---|---|---|---|---|---|---|
| Auxiliary | 5 | | 4 | | 1 | | |
| Modal | | | 1 | | | | |
| Vector | | 1 | | 1 | | | |
| Copula | 5 | | 6 | | | | |
| Simple lexical | 11 | 6 | 16 | 4 | 3 | 2 | 1 |
| Main verb of compound | 5 | 1 | 2 | 2 | | 1 | |
| *Total* | 26 | 8 | 29 | 7 | 4 | 3 | 1 |

TABLE 9.6. Distribution of verb phrase types: Togga.

| Type of verb phrase | Patient | | Control | |
|---|---|---|---|---|
| | No. | % | No. | % |
| Copula | 50 | 28 | 36 | 16 |
| Simple lexical | 91 | 50 | 152 | 66 |
| Compound | 40 | 22 | 41 | 18 |
| *Total* | 181 | | 229 | |

## CHARACTERISTICS OF VERB PHRASE CONSTRUCTIONS

Among the 181 verb phrases produced by the patient, there were 141 simple main verbs. The copula comprised 28% of the total number of verb phrase constructions in the patient corpus. This proportion is significantly higher than that of the normal control, who used the copula only 16% of the time (chi-square 8.64, $p < .01$) (Table 9.6).

The patient produced simple lexical verb phrases in only 50% of all verb phrases, whereas the control produced simple lexical verbs in 66% of all verb phrases. The use of simple lexical verb phrases in the patient corpus is significantly less frequent than in the control corpus (chi-square 10.85, $p < .01$).

Among the compound constructions, there were only two instances that required agreement of both the lexical verb and the copula. In contrast, there were nine compound constructions in the control corpus that required agreement marking of the lexical verb (see case 1 for further discussion). The number of copula and compound constructions without lexical verb agreement comprised 49% of all verb phrases used by the patient, in contrast to the 30% used by the control. As in the first Icelandic patient, the number of verb phrases that did not require agreement marking of lexical verbs is significantly greater than those used by the control (chi-square 15.36, $p < .001$).

These findings suggest a reliance on structures with a more stative form of predicate (copulas and nonfinite constructions) in which the morphosyntactic representation of agreement is contained in the free grammatical morpheme (the copula or auxiliary verb) in contrast to the bound inflection of a lexical (active, simple, finite) verb.

## LEXICAL ISSUES

The noun/verb ratio for this patient was 0.8, compared to a ratio of 1.0 for the control. In examining the frequency of nouns and verbs in the corpora of the patient and control, it is evident that the patient produced fewer lexical verbs but a similar proportion of nouns. This smaller proportion of lexical verbs in the patient corpus is balanced by the greater use of the

TABLE 9.7. Distribution of major
lexical categories: Togga.

| Category | Patient | Control |
|---|---|---|
| Noun/verb ratio | 0.8 | 1.0 |
| *Percent of corpus* | | |
| Nouns | 15 | 16 |
| Lexical verbs | 15 | 18 |
| Nonlexical verbs | 5 | 2 |
| Other words | 65 | 64 |
| Token/type ratio | | |
| Nouns | 1.6 | 2.2 |
| Verbs | 1.8 | 1.9 |

copula and auxiliary verbs. The proportions of total verbs (20%) for the
two corpora are equivalent (Table 9.7).

The token/type ratio for verbs was 1.8 for the patient and 1.9 for the
control, which suggests that the patient did have a fairly large inventory of
verbs. In contrast, the noun token/type of 1.6 was relatively low for the
patient. (The control corpus showed little variety in noun choice, with a
token/type ratio of 2.2.)

In sum, both the omissions and substitution errors involved finite forms
predominantly. A high percentage of substitutions involved either a nonfinite form being produced instead of a finite form or one inflected finite
form being substituted for another inflected finite form. Although the
copula and auxiliary presented some difficulty (fairly equally), most errors
involved the bound inflections of lexical verbs.

## Case 3, Hindi: Ram

There were 75 obligatory verb phrase contexts in the narrative discourse
produced by the patient Ram. Of them, only 60 verbs were actually produced, and 15 were omitted; 45 were produced correctly and 15 with
errors. The total number of errors is 30: 15 omissions and 15 incorrect
productions. See Table 9.8 for the distribution of correct, omitted, and
erroneously produced verbs.

TABLE 9.8. Performance by verb type: Ram.

| Verb form | Correct production | Lexical omission | Inflection substitute | Inflection omission | Other |
|---|---|---|---|---|---|
| Auxiliary/copula | 22 | 11 | 1 | — | — |
| Vector | 3 | 4 | 1 | 3 | 2 |
| Simple main | 3 | — | 1 | — | — |
| Main of compound | 17 | — | 7 | — | — |
| *Total* | 45 | 15 | 10 | 3 | 2 |

TABLE 9.9. Verb structure by error type: Ram.

| Type of verb | Omission | Broken stem | Substitution | Lexical selection | Lexical + inflectional | Conjugational form class |
|---|---|---|---|---|---|---|
| Auxiliary | 7 | | 1 | | | |
| Vector | 4 | 3 | | 1 | 1 | 1 |
| Copula | 4 | | | | | |
| Simple lexical | | | 1 | | | |
| Main verb of compound | | | 7 | | | |
| *Total* | 15 | 3 | 9 | 1 | 1 | 1 |

## DESCRIPTION OF ERRORS

There were a total of 30 errors, half of which were omissions and the other half production errors. Six of the eight error types are present. The distribution of error types is as follows: 15 omissions, 3 stems produced without inflections, 9 substitutions, 1 lexical selection error, 1 lexical and inflection error, and 1 conjugational form class error. The distribution of error types for each verb structure category is given in Table 9.9.

All of the 15 verb omissions occurred in copula, auxiliaries, or vectors. None of the omissions occurred in lexical main verbs. The copula was omitted in 40% of all obligatory contexts. In compound constructions, the auxiliary was omitted in 29% of obligatory contexts, and vector verbs were omitted in 40% of obligatory contexts.

## CHARACTERISTICS OF VERB PHRASE CONSTRUCTION

The frequency of various types of verb construction contexts produced by the patients was compared with those used by the control. There were nine obligatory contexts for the copula in the patient corpus, which represents 23% of the total verb corpus—similar to the 21% of the verbs used by the control. Only 10% of all the patient's verb phrase constructions consisted of simple verbs. This figure is in contrast to 22% of simple verbs in the control corpus. (Because of the small magnitude of the numbers being compared, chi-square did not reach significance: chi-square 2.45, $p = .12$) (Table 9.10).

Although the patient had difficulty producing the verb "hona" (to be), he frequently (85%) chose verb phrase constructions that required the use of this verb. In contrast, the copula and compound constructions with "hona" comprised only 65% of those produced by the control. The patient used these verb phrase constructions significantly more than the control (chi-square 4.70, $p < .05$).

In Hindi, the expression of tense is reflected in the choice of verb phrase construction type. The present tense is expressed by the imperfect participle + auxiliary construction. There is no simple present tense form. Although the patient chose to use the present tense often, the auxiliary

TABLE 9.10. Distribution of types of verb phrase contexts: Ram.

| Type | Patient | | Control | |
|---|---|---|---|---|
| | No. | % | No. | % |
| Copula | 9 | 23 | 15 | 21 |
| Simple lexical | 4 | 10 | 16 | 22 |
| 2-Verb compound | 19 | 49 | 24 | 33 |
| 3-Verb compound | 7 | 18 | 13 | 18 |
| 4-Verb compound | 0 | | 4 | 6 |
| Total | 39 | | 72 | |

tended to be omitted in these instances. The copular construction was also chosen frequently, but the copula was omitted witha almost equal frequency. The past tense has a simple verb construction in Hindi. The simple past is typically used with verbs of motion, whereas the compound construction—perfect participle + auxiliary—is used to express the habitual past or the past state. The patient rarely used the simple past for expressing the past tense. The present perfect form was often used instead. The use of this tense with verbs of motion gives the verb a somewhat semantically anomalous stative reading.

## LEXICAL ISSUES

The noun/verb ratio for this patient was 1.6, compared to a ratio of 1.25 for the control. Inspection of the frequency distribution of grammatical categories of the patient and control corpora reveals a greater proportion of nouns in the patient's discourse compared to that of the control but a relatively equal proportion of verbs. Verbs comprised 13% of the patient corpus and 16% of the control corpus. In contrast, nouns comprised 30% of the patient corpus and 19% of the control corpus (Table 9.11).

The patient and control differed little in their token/type ratios for verbs (patient 2.1, control 2.7) and for nouns (patient 1.3, control 1.2), in both instances the token/type ratio was higher for the verbs.

To summarize the findings of this corporal analysis, the lexical main verb was never omitted, but many substitutions occurred. The copula was frequently omitted, as was the auxiliary. Vector verbs were involved in most of the errors. There were few errors committed in number and gender agreement. However, the singular masculine inflection, which predominated in the subjects of the narratives, is also a (syntactically conditioned) default form. The compound present perfect construction was used instead of the simple past and was substituted for the imperfect participle in present tense constructions. This use represents a tendency toward a more stative form. The verb stem, which bears no inflection, and the infinitive, which does bear an inflection, appeared in equally few substitution errors.

TABLE 9.11. Distribution of major lexical categories: Ram.

| Category | Patient | Control |
|---|---|---|
| Noun/verb ratio | 1.6 | 1.25 |
| *Percent of corpus* | | |
| Nouns | 30 | 19 |
| Verbs | 13 | 16 |
| Other | 57 | 65 |
| Token/type ratio | | |
| Nouns | 1.3 | 1.2 |
| Verbs | 2.1 | 2.7 |

## *Case 4, Finnish: Peltonen*

For case 4, there were a total of 132 obligatory verb contexts. Of them, 102 verbs were produced, 30 were omitted. Of the 102 verbs were produced, 97 were correct, and only 5 verbs were incorrectly produced. Table 9.12 displays the distribution of correct, omitted, and incorrectly produced verbs by category for the patient Peltonen.

### DESCRIPTION OF ERRORS

Most (30 of 35) errors were omissions. They were distributed among the verb types as follows: auxiliaries 45%, simple verbs 21%, main verb of a compound 5%. Omission occurred for the verb "olla" (to be) as a copula and as an auxiliary with almost equal frequency, but there were no omissions of either negative auxiliary. Lexical verbs were omitted less frequently (17%).

The single inflection substitution, which involved an error in person agreement, occurred in a clause with an omitted subject. Additionally, there were two derivational errors and two phonological paraphasias.

### CHARACTERISTICS OF VERB PHRASE CONSTRUCTION

There were 82 simple verb phrase slots and 20 compound verb phrases in the corpus. There were 55 simple lexical verbs, 25 copulas, and 19 auxiliary + main verb constructions produced. See Table 9.13 for a comparison of the distribution of verb phrase types in the patient and control corpora.

TABLE 9.12. Performance by verb type: Peltonen.

| Verb form | Correct production | Lexical omission | Inflection substitute | Other |
|---|---|---|---|---|
| Auxiliary | 6 | 5 | — | — |
| Negative auxiliary | 10 | — | — | — |
| Modal | 1 | — | — | — |
| Copula | 16 | 11 | — | — |
| Simple main | 45 | 13 | 1 | 4 |
| Main of compound | 19 | 1 | — | — |
| *Total* | 97 | 30 | 1 | 4 |

TABLE 9.13. Distribution of verb phrase types: Peltonen.

| Type of verb phrase | Patient | | Control | |
|---|---|---|---|---|
| | No. | % | No. | % |
| Copula | 27 | 26 | 23 | 17 |
| Simple lexical | 55 | 54 | 92 | 65 |
| Auxiliary + main verb | 19 | 19 | 20 | 14 |
| Auxiliary + auxiliary + main verb | 1 | 1 | 6 | 4 |
| *Total* | 102 | | 141 | |

Twenty-seven of the simple verb phrases consisted of copulas, which represents 26% of all verb phrases. The reliance on the copular construction was significantly less evident (17%) in the control corpus (chi-square 3.74, $p = .05$). There was also relative reduction in the frequency of the use of simple lexical forms by the patient (54%) compared to the control (65%) (chi-square 3.18, $p = .07$).

## LEXICAL ISSUES

The noun/verb ratio for this patient was 1.6 compared to 1.4 for the control, which suggests that there was a paucity of verbs relative to nouns. Coincidentally, there was a high degree of verb omission (39%). Nouns were also affected by omission to a lesser degree (20%).

The token/type ratios for nouns and verbs were the same (1.4) in the patient corpus. These ratios are slightly lower than the ratios found in the control corpus (nouns 1.6, verbs 1.7). Thus this patient seemed to have relatively more difficulty producing verbs than nouns, but there was equal variety in lexical choice for the two categories.

In sum, the overwhelming majority of errors were of omission. Omission of copula and auxiliary verbs occurred with equal frequency. Despite this fact, these forms were both omitted more often than were simple lexical verbs. The copular verb phrase constructions were used with greater frequency by the patient than the control.

## Case 5, Finnish: Aaltonen

In patient Aaltonen's narrative discourse, there were 135 obligatory verb contexts, with 129 verbs produced and 6 omitted. Of the verbs produced, 116 were correct and 12 were incorrect forms. Table 9.14 displays the distribution of correct, omitted, and erroneous verbs by category.

## DESCRIPTION OF ERRORS

There were a total of 18 errors in the corpus. Omission represented 33% of all errors. No errors of either omission or substitution were found for

TABLE 9.14. Performance by verb type: Altonen.

| Verb form | Correct production | Lexical omission | Inflection substitute | Inflection omission | Other |
|---|---|---|---|---|---|
| Auxiliary | 1 | — | — | — | — |
| Negative auxiliary | 10 | — | — | — | — |
| Modal | 9 | — | — | — | — |
| Copula | 23 | 1 | — | — | — |
| Simple main | 58 | 3 | 7 | — | 1 |
| 1st Compound | 11 | 2 | 1 | 1 | 1 |
| 2nd Compound | 4 | — | — | — | 1 |
| *Total* | 116 | 6 | 8 | 1 | 3 |

TABLE 9.15. Distribution of error types: Altonen.

| Type of verb | Omission | Broken stem | Inflection substitution | Lexical selection |
|---|---|---|---|---|
| Copula | 1 | | | |
| Simple lexical | 3 | | 7 | 1 |
| 1st Main verb of compound | 2 | 1 | 1 | 1 |
| 2nd Main verb of compound | | | | 1 |

TABLE 9.16. Distribution of verb phrase constructions: Altonen.

| Type | Patient | | Control | |
|---|---|---|---|---|
| | No. | % | No. | % |
| Copula | 23 | 21 | 28 | 24 |
| Simple lexical | 70 | 64 | 73 | 62 |
| 2-Verb compound | 10 | 9 | 17 | 14 |
| 3-Verb compound | 7 | 6 | 0 | |
| Total | 110 | | 118· | |

the auxiliary, negative auxiliary, or modal verbs. The distribution of error types is shown in Table 9.15. There were eight substitution errors, all of which involved inflections of finite forms. Six of them involved the substitution of plural forms for singular forms within a sequence of six consecutive sentences, and several attempts at self-correction occurred.

VERB PHRASE CONSTRUCTIONS

The distribution of various types of verb construction produced by the patient and the control is presented in Table 9.16. The patient and control showed a similar pattern of verb phrase use. The copula was used in 21% of the verb phrases by the patient and in 24% by the control.

LEXICAL ISSUES

The noun/verb ratio was 0.8 for both patient and control. The patient showed great limitation in the variety of verbs produced. The token/type ratio was 2.5 compared to a verb ratio of 1.5 for the control. These findings suggest that, although the patient produced nouns and verbs in a proportion similar to that of the normal control, there was a reduction in the variety of verbs used. The patient's limited word choice was found to be specific to verbs. The variety of nouns was equivalent to that of the control.

   In summary, the verb "olla" (to be) was used correctly as copula, auxiliary, and negative auxiliary in all but one instance. Although there were few errors in verb production overall, the token/type ratio indicates a specific reduction in the number of different verbs available to the patient.

Three of the errors occurred in a formulaic phrase. Several other verb omissions occurred. Most of the errors produced involved the confusion of opposing pairs of inflectional and lexical forms: singular and plural inflections, present and past tense inflections, and the direction of verbs of motion.

## Discussion

Verb phrases and the requisite grammatical formatives appear to be highly susceptible to impairment in the speech production of agrammatic aphasics. The pattern of agrammatic production includes the overreliance on verb forms that have been characterized alternatively as nonfinite default forms or nominalizations. This clinical finding reflects one of the linguistic aspects of the disorder that has broad theoretical implications. The issue currently under investigation is whether the agrammatic deficit pertains to predicate form or function. Specifically, are these verb forms deficient in the number of grammatial categories marked? Or, instead, do they represent less relational and more static, referential predicates?

Research efforts to clarify the problem in English have been equivocal. This investigation has examined the pattern of agrammatic speech in patients speaking languages in which the grammatical morphology bears distinctive and overt structural marking. It was hoped that this study might lead to a determination of the properties of the bound inflections that are subject to the deficit.

This discussion first focuses on the findings of impairments in bound morphology with respect to the notions of degree of finiteness and nominalization. Differences in the overall pattern of impairment in the five case studies are attributed to language-specific distinctions. Second, the impairment of vector verbs is considered in the light of these language-specific distinctions. This grammatical category is shown to contrast with the third set of findings regarding the auxiliary and copula, which seem to exhibit a similar pattern in all of the cases and languages.

## *Impairments of Bound Grammatical Morphemes*

### ICELANDIC LANGUAGE

In Icelandic, the impaired verbs produced by the agrammatics Kiddi (case 1) and Togga (case 2) clearly involved difficulty in marking grammatical categories in finite forms. Kiddi rarely made errors involving the substitution of inflection but produced discourse composed predominantly of forms that require few inflectional category markings. He produced few simple lexical finite verbs and tended instead to produce copular or compound verb phrase constructions that do not require agreement marking on the lexical main verb. Although Togga did not avoid these finite forms, she committed many errors of inflection when producing them. Substitutions of inflections involved employment of either a nonfinite form when a finite form was required or a finite form that was marked incorrectly for grammatical category. There were very few exceptional instances where Togga produced a finite form when a nonfinite form was required.

In Icelandic, it appears that the complex inflectional requirements of grammatical marking of number, person and gender agreement. tense, voice, and mood, in combination with the difficult conjugational paradigms, describe difficulties with verb forms found in these two agrammatics. The finding that nonfinite forms were significantly more frequent in the corpora of the Icelandic agrammatics than the normal controls supports the interpretation that the deficit in verb production is a result of the inflectional form requirements of this language.

HINDI LANGUAGE

In Hindi, the only two forms that could be considered truly nonfinite are the verb stem and the infinitive. The Hindi verb stem (a zero-morph form) and the infinitive (an inflected form) are equally bare of grammatical marking of tense and agreement, but they occur in different syntactic environments. The verb stem occurs as the main verb in common compound verb phrase constructions, whereas the infinitive is an infrequent form that functions as a gerund. Surprisingly, each of these forms occurred only twice as substitutions for participles in Ram's corpus (case 3). The fact that neither the verb stem nor the infinitive was more often found as a substitution is problematic when trying to determine whether the impairment in Hindi agrammatism can be characterized by notions of finiteness or nominalization.

Unfortunately, the data from the only other published Hindi-speaking agrammatic case study (Bhatnagar and Whitaker, 1984) does not clarify this issue. Their report stated that the patient's errors included "occasional" instances of infinitive or verb stem substitutions, but more specific detail about the relative frequency of the two forms was not provided. No examples of sentences with this type of substitution were cited. Moreover, a category for substitutions that could represent either or both of these forms was not included in their data analysis.

The defective predicates found in Ram's corpus often contained substitutions of the perfective participle for the present tense imperfective participle. This finding cannot be interpreted as a choice of a nonfinitive form for a finite form because the participle in Hindi is marked for tense/aspect as well as gender and number. Both the present tense imperfect participle and the perfect participle are marked for the same number of grammatical categories. Therefore the formal dimension of finiteness cannot be used to draw a distinction between these two forms.

The degree of nominalization appears to capture an important distinction between these two participle forms. The perfective form has a more stative reading when used with action verbs. In this respect, the perfective form can be considered a less active relational predicate than the imperfective in the relation it expresses.

The significance of the notion of nominalization, as it applies to the impairment found in the Hindi-speaking agrammatic, is strengthened by the finding of few errors in agreement marking. However, it must be pointed out that because of the nature of the narratives elicited the singular masculine form was required in most instances. The form is a syntactic default form that is employed frequently. This evidence of intact agreement marking must therefore be taken as tentative. Thus the notion of degree of nominalization rather than finiteness may be more adequate in describing the distinction between predicate types found in Hindi agrammatism.

## FINNISH LANGUAGE

In Finnish, the deficit in the expression of predication seems to be of a different nature entirely. The errors found in Peltonen's corpus (case 4) were almost all those of lexical omission rather than morphologically erroneous productions. Aaltonen's corpus (case 5) showed little if any impairment with respect to verb phrase form. The fact that there were no substitutions of nonfinite for finite forms or incorrect finite forms produced by the Finnish-speaking agrammatics (exceptions are noted) suggests that the realization of a fully inflected word form is produced in a manner that is significantly different than in other languages that have been examined with respect to agrammatism. Indeed, Niemi et al. (in press) stated that none of the 15 Finnish agrammatic cases they had examined produced any morphological errors. As in the present case, the agrammatic deficit in verb phrase production involved errors of omission exclusively.

The explanation for the finding of lexical verb omission in Peltonen's speech may lie in the unusual morphophonemic properties of the language. It appears that the synthetic unit of stem + inflections is a tightly bound phonological form. The representation of the base stem and inflectional forms must be quite abstract phonologically, as there are complex morphophonological patterns that distinguish related conjugational forms. In Finnish, all of the morphemes, both lexical and inflectional, must be selected prior to the possibility of any phonological realization. Therefore a representation that is incompletely inflected cannot be uttered. This may account for the verb omission in Peltonen's speech.

The Finnish infixes for tense and mood appear to be somewhat more phonologically independent. They are unaffected by the complex morphophonemic changes that apply to the stem and the inflections for voice and number/person. In both Finnish-speaking agrammatics some instances of tense anomaly (substitution) were evident, but the substitution of other inflections was rare.

## Impairment of Free Grammatical Morphemes

VECTOR VERBS

In Icelandic and Hindi, there is a class of structurally similar non-main verbs that contain both lexical and grammatical features. The function of these vector verbs is different in the two languages, however. In Icelandic the function of this small group of vector verbs seems to be primarily that of semimodels that are used in conjunction with nonfinite predicates. These forms are similar to the English forms such as "used to X" and "going to X." The Icelandic vector verbs are typically used with the infinitive form of the main verb to express aspectual meanings. These constructions have fewer grammatical morpheme marking requirements. As a result, little impairment was found in the use of these vector verbs in either Icelandic agrammatic case. These vector verbs seemed to be a preferred form of default in the case of Kiddi (case 1), being significantly overrepresented in that corpus compared to the control.

In contrast, Hindi contains a large number of vector verbs, which are (syntactically) required in many verb phrase constructions. These Hindi vector verbs have little semantic content. They play a syntactic role that is similar to that of an auxiliary. These Hindi vectors exhibited the greatest disruption of all the verb phrase components in Ram's speech (case 3). Thus there seems to be little comparability between the pattern of agrammatic impairment found in Icelandic and Hindi with regard to the class of vector verbs, apparently owing to the differences in their syntactic roles.

Note that for both of these languages (and perhaps Finnish as well), modals, which can be considered to carry a fair degree of semantic information, did not attract errors in any of the agrammatic patients. However, it is remarkable that modals were extremely infrequent in all of the patients' corpora. This finding bears further investigation.

The pattern of impairment in the most semantically empty, free grammatical morphemes was similar across cases and languages. The Icelandic, Hindi, and Finnish agrammatics all had relative difficulty with the production of the copula and auxiliary verbs. They seemed to be equally affected in all cases (c.f. Miceli, Mazzuchi, Menn, and Goodglass, 1983). Despite this difficulty, verb phrase constructions requiring these elements were overrepresented in the patients' speech. Stative copulas and nonfinite compound constructions were used more frequently by the patients than the controls, who used more simple active finite lexical verb phrase forms.

## Conclusions

The findings reported here suggest that the impairment of verb forms found in agrammatism is manifest in a distinctly different manner owing to language-specific factors. The status of the grammatical markings of inflections in these languages reflect different semantic, syntactic, and phonological form and functions. These factors determine the manner in which a deficit in predication is manifested. The three languages investigated here contain elaborate systems of grammatical inflection. However, these languages differ as to the formal and functional characteristics in the way in which grammatical distinctions are expressed. Icelandic contains great morphological complexity with fairly limited syntactic variability. Hindi, in contrast, has limited morphological variability but a large component of syntactic complexity. Finnish is distinctive in its morphophonological complexity and textual variety.

Although both the factors of nonfiniteness and nominalization have been implicated in the verb impairment found in English agrammatism, it has been argued that these factors vary in prominence in Hindi compared to Icelandic. Whereas the pattern of performance in Icelandic is best described as tending towards use of nonfinite forms and difficulty in finite inflections, the pattern in Hindi seems to reflect a tendency toward more stative and less active relational predicates. The omission of verbs in Finnish could be inferred to be the result of difficulty with selection of inflections (and/or stems), but a more specific characterization does not seem to be obtainable. It appears that all morphemes must be available for the morphophonemic realization of an articulatable Finnis form.

Although language-specific factors distinguished the expression of the agrammatic impairment in bound grammatical morphology, "semantically empty" free grammatical morphemes were affected similarly in all three languages.

This study described the patterns of agrammatic impairment in inflectional morphology found in aphasic speakers of three highly inflected languages with distinct formal and functional properties. The quality of the agrammatic production of bound grammatical morphemes was found to reflect language-specific differences. The major language-specific factors contributing to the pattern of findings seemed to be the morphological aspects the conservative conjugational paradigms in Icelandic, the syntactic and lexical complexity of the sentence-final verb phrases of Hindi, and the morphophonemic aspects of the agglutinating process of Finnish.

It must be stressed that these conclusions are drawn on the basis of only five case studies. The contribution of the range of individual variation, from premorbid and clinical factors, to the patterns of language deficit is yet to be determined. Distinctions between this intersubject variation and cross-language differences depend on the collection and analysis of additional case studies.

Nevertheless, the interpretation of the present findings may be used as a set of predictions that can inform the investigation of other languages that have similar properties. The goal is to develop a typology that captures the pattern of agrammatic speech disturbance cross-linguistically.

This typology can serve as a model of normal language production framed in terms of language-specific processing requirements. At the same time, the question of what universal factor(s) underlies agrammatism may be addressed.

## References

Alajouanine, Th. (1968). *L'Aphasie et le Langage Pathologique*. Paris: Bailliére et Fils.

Bates, E., Friederici, A., & Wulfeck, B. (1987) Comprehension in aphasia: a cross-linguistic study. *Brain and Language, 32*, 19–67.

Bhatnagar, S. (in press). Hindi. In L. Menn and L. Obler (eds.), *Agrammatic Aphasia: A Cross-Language Narrative Sourcebook*. Amsterdam: John Benjamins.

Bhatnagar, S., & Whitaker, H. (1984). Agrammatism on inflectional bound morphemes: a case study of a Hindi-speaking aphasic patient. *Cortex, 20*, 295–301.

Blumstein, S. (1982). Language dissolution in aphasia: evidence for linguistic theory. In L. Obler and L. Menn (eds.), *Exceptional Language and Linguistics*. New York: Academic Press.

Caplan, D. (1983). A note on the "word-order problem" in agrammatism. *Brain and Language, 21*, 9–20.

De Villiers, J. (1974). Quantitative aspects of agrammatism in aphasia. *Cortex, 10*, 36–54.

Geschwind, N. (1970). The organisation of language in the brain. *Science, 170*, 940–944.

Goodglass, H. (1968). Studies on the grammar of aphasics. In S. Rosenberg and J. Kopin (eds.), *Developments in Applied Psycholinguistics Research*. New York: Macmillan.

Goodglass, H., & Geschwind, N. (1976). Language disorders (aphasia). In E.C. Carterette and M.P. Friedman (eds.), *Handbook of Perception*. Vol. 7. New York: Academic Press.

Goodglass, H., & Hyde, M. (1969). How aphasics begin their utterances. Unpublished Progress Report. USPHS grant NS 07615. Boston Veterans Administration Medical Center.

Goodglass, H., & Kaplan, E. (1972). *The Assessment of Aphasia and Related Disorders*. Philadelphia: Lea & Febiger.

Goodglass, H., & Menn, L. (1985). Is agrammatism a unitary phenomenon? In M-L. Kean (ed.), *Agrammatism*. New York: Academic Press.

Goodglass, H., Quadfasel, F.A., & Timberlake, W.H. (1964). Phrase length and the type and severity of aphasia. *Cortex, 1*, 133–158.

Grodzinsky, Y. (1984). The syntactic characterization of agrammatism. *Cognition, 16*, 99–120.

Hook, P. (1974). *The Compound Verb in Hindi*. Ann Arbor: University of Michigan.

Hopper, P. and Thompson, S. (1984). The discourse basis for lexical categories in universal grammar. *Language, 60*, 703–752.

Howes, D. (1967). Hypotheses concerning the functions of the language mechanism. In S. Salzinger & K. Salzinger (eds.), *Research in Verbal Behaviour and Some Neurophysiological Implications*. New York: Academic Press.

Howes, D., & Geschwind, N. (1962). Statistical properties of aphasic speech. Unpublished Progress Report, USPHS grant M-1802. Veterans Administration Hospital, Boston.

Jakobson, R. (1956). Two aspects of language and two types of aphasic disturbances. In R. Jakobsen & M. Halle (eds.), *Fundamentals of Language*. The Hague; Mouton.

Jakobson, R. (1964). Towards a linguistic typology of aphasic impairments. In A. de Reuck & M. O'Connor (eds.), *Disorders of Language*. London: Churchill.

Jakobson, R. (1971). *Studies on Child Language and Aphasia*. The Hague: Mouton.

Jones, L., & Wepman, J. (1965). Grammatical indicants of speaking styles in normal and aphasic speakers. In K. Salinger & S. Salinger (eds.), *Research in Verbal Behavior and Some Neurophysiological Implications*. New York: Academic Press.

Kohn, S., Lorch, M., & Pearson, D. (1989). Verb finding in aphasia. *Cortex, 25,* 57–69.

Kohn, S., Perlman, M., & Goodglass, H. (1984). The relative specificity of nouns and verbs in agrammatics' circumlocutions. Los Angeles: Academy of Aphasia.

Kolk, H. (1978). The linguistic interpretation of Broca's aphasia: a reply to Marie-Louise Kean. *Cognition, 6,* 353–361.

Lapointe, S. (1985). A theory of verb form use in the speech of agrammatic aphasics. *Brain and Language, 24,* 100–155.

Lorch, M. (1986). *A Cross-Linguistic Study of Verb Inflections in Agrammatism*. Doctoral dissertation, Boston University.

Low, A. (1931). A case of agrammatism in the English language. *Archives of Neurology and Psychiatry, 25,* 556–597.

Luria, A. (1970). *Traumatic Aphasia*. New York: Basic Books.

Magnúsdóttir, S., & Thráinsson, H. (in press). Icelandic. In L. Menn & L. Obler (eds.), *Agrammatic Aphasia: A Cross-Language Narrative Sourcebook*. Amsterdam: John Benjamins.

Marin, O., Saffran, E., & Schwartz, M. (1976). Dissociations of language in aphasia: implications for normal language function. *Annals of the New York Academy of Sciences, 280,* 868–884.

Menn, L., & Obler, L. (in press). *Agrammatic Aphasia: Cross-Linguistic Narrative Sourcebook*. Amsterdam: John Benjamins.

Menn, L., Obler, L., & Goodglass, H. (1983). *Agrammatism: Why Cross-Language Approaches?* Minneapolis: Academy of Aphasia.

Miceli, G., Mazzuchi, A., Menn, L., & Goodglass, H. (1983). Contrasting cases of Italian agrammatic aphasia without comprehension disorder. *Brain and Language, 19,* 65–97.

Miceli, G., Silveri, M., Villa, G., & Caramazza, A. (1984). On the basis for the agrammatics' difficulty producing main verbs. *Cortex, 20,* 207–220.

Myerson, R., & Goodglass, H. (1972). Transformational grammars of three aphasic patients. *Language and Speech, 15,* 40–50.

Niemi, J., Laine, M., Hänninen, R. and Koivuselkä-Sallinen, p. (in press). Finnish. In L. Menn and L. Obler (eds.), *Agrammatic Aphasia: a cross-language narrative sourcebook*. John Benjamins, Philadelphia.

Saffran, E., Schwartz, M., & Martin, O. (1980a). The word order problem in agrammatism: production. *Brain and Language*, *10*, 3–280.

Saffran, E., Schwartz, M., & Martin, O. (1980b). Evidence from aphasia: isolating the components of production. In B. Butterworth (ed.), *Language Production. Vol. 1. Speech and Talk.* New York: Academic Press.

Wales, R., & Kinsella, G. (1981). Syntactic effects in sentence completion by Broca's aphasics. *Brain and Language*, *13*, 301–307.

# Appendix 1:  Language-Specific Grammatical Inflectional Categories Evident in the Verb Phrase Corpora

x = present
— = absent

| Category | Icelandic | Hindi | Finnish |
|---|---|---|---|
| Number | | | |
|   Singular | x | x | x |
|   Plural | x | x | x |
| Person | | | |
|   First | x | x | x |
|   Second | x | x | x |
|   Third | x | x | x |
| Tense | | | |
|   Present | x | x | x |
|   Past | x | x | x |
|   Future | — | x | — |
| Voice | | | |
|   Active | x | x | x |
|   Passive | — | — | x |
|   Middle | x | — | — |
| Mood | | | |
|   Indicative | x | x | x |
|   Subjunctive | x | — | — |
|   Imperative | x | — | x |
|   Conditional | — | — | x |
| Verb phrase component | | | |
|   Infinitive | x | x | x |
|   Verb stem | — | x | |
|   Participle | x | x | x |
|   Finite | x | x | x |
| Negation | — | — | x |
| Gender | | | |
|   Masculine | x | x | — |
|   Neuter | x | — | — |
|   Feminine | x | x | — |
| Case | | | |
|   Nominative | x | — | x |
|   Inessive | — | — | x |
|   Illative | — | — | x |
|   Partitive | — | — | x |

| Category | Icelandic | Hindi | Finnish |
|---|---|---|---|
| Participle number | | | |
| Singular | x | x | — |
| Plural | x | x | — |
| Clitics | x | x | x |
| Conjugational form class | x | x | — |

# Appendix 2:  Error Categories

1. *Omission*. Used for absent verbs that were considered to be obligatory in the linguistic context of the utterance.

2. *Broken-off stem form*. The initial morpheme(s) of a verb produced in an incomplete broken-off form without the required bound inflection(s). For example, in the production "rah-" for the target "raha" the inflection for tense, number, and gender is left off (Hindi).

3. *Substitution*. A verb form was produced, but the morphological inflection was grammatically incorrect. For example, the infinitive form "sona" was produced instead of the masculine singular present participle form "sota" (Hindi).

4. *Lexical selection error*. A semantically incorrect verb form was produced with the correct morphological inflection. This category included both phonologically and semantically based substitutions. For example, the verb "tuli," meaning "came," was used in a context requiring the verb "lahti," meaning "went." The grammatical inflection is correct (Finnish).

5. *Lexical and inflectional error*. There is a semantically incorrect inflectional substitution. For example, the auxiliary verb "var" (was) was produced in the past indicative when "geti"—the present subjunctive of the modal verb "can"—was required (Icelandic).

6. *Conjugational form class error*. A verb was produced in an inflected form that did not correspond to the appropriate conjugational pattern. For example, the strong verb "lata" (to put) was conjugated according to the weak paradigm to produce "latti" but marking the correct grammatical categories. The target was "let" (Finnish). The form produced is roughly equivalent to "put-ed" in English.

7. *Derivational form error*. A verb form was produced with a morphologically incorrect stem but correct grammatical inflection. For example, the verb "liikutin" meaning "to move" was produced with the causative stem form rather than the required intransitive stem "liikun." Note that the bound grammatical inflection is correct (Finnish).

8. *Phonological paraphasia*. A nonexistent form is produced that consists of a phonological distortion of a real word. For example, the production "gau" was a phonological distortion of the verb "ga" (check); it is not interpretable as an error of verb morphology (Icelandic).

# 10
# Agrammatism: Evidence for a Unified Theory of Word, Phrase, and Sentence Formation Processes*

PIERRE VILLIARD

Psycholinguistic theory and grammatical theory, though related in more or less obvious ways, remain different logical constructs for a number of reasons. As summarily indicated below, it may be noted, for instance, that contemporary grammatical theory is elaborated on a closed system of rules that apply in structurally defined contexts, and that this system is largely built on intuitional grounds, i.e., on grammaticality judgments that presumably mirror some steady-state linguistic knowledge.

> *Grammatical theory*
> Closed system
> Intuitional grounds
> Static knowledge

Psycholinguistic theory, on the other hand, is based on empirical facts, i.e., on observed behaviors, necessarily brought about through some open system of strategies or processes that dynamically make use of grammar, among other things. Perhaps the components of the latter system should be thought of as intrinsically adaptive, as linguistic behavior is determined not only by grammatical knowledge but also by general nonlinguistic knowledge. Moreover, it is conditioned by such factors as memory limitations and attentional capacity or availability.

> *Psycholinguistic theory*
> Open system
> Empirical facts
> Dynamic use

Agrammatic behavior, as one of the empirical facts that a psycholinguistic theory should account for, is discussed here mainly in relation to the externalization of hypothetical linguistic deficits. Our suggestion is that

---

* This chapter is a modified version of a communication given in July 1988 at the International Symposium on Phonology. Morphology, and Aphasia held in Krems, Austria.

agrammatism may be conceived as the surface reflection of something other than a linguistic impairment.

## Background

As is well known, the important developments of grammatical theory since the 1960s have given great impetus to an almost simultaneous burst of research on agrammatic behavior. Several redefinitions and reinterpretations have been proposed, but it must be noted that some of this literature has merely updated old questions and controversies raised around the turn of the century by shrewd pioneering aphasiologists. Nevertheless, the fast-changing tool of grammatical theory has contributed significantly to the creation of fine-grained tests and has consequently led to the gathering of much novel experimental data. Moreover, such theory has also guided principled examination of spontaneous agrammatic discourse, as reported, for example, by Menn, Obler, and Goodglass (in press), who examined pathology data derived from 14 languages. One more point must be made before we discuss the core problems. Strictly experimental materials are left aside in most of what follows because they necessarily tap metacognition, whereas in the present Chapter we wish to focus on natural, spontaneous discursive behavior. Thus "natural psycholinguistics" is the general theoretical framework at issue here. (Experimental psycholinguistics involves elicited responses, whereas natural psycholinguistics explores spontaneous behaviors.)

## Definitions

Because there is no consensus on exactly what agrammatism is in any investigation of the true psychological nature of the underlying disturbance that gives rise to agrammatic discourse, a number of preliminary assumptions are required. First, let us accept the impressionistic clinical labeling of discursive behavior as "agrammatic" when, on the surface, closed-class items do not seem to be used as often and as well as expected. We consider that this simplistic assertion is general enough and sufficiently all-embracing to avoid controversy at the outset. The possible inappropriateness of the label "agrammatic" as a clinical (sub)category need not concern us at this point, for all we seek at this juncture is some workable terminology for this avenue of investigation to be fruitful. One could have similar reservations with respect to the label "closed class" as a linguistic (sub)category, although nothing has yet been said here about the ins and outs of the involvement of closed-class items.

In our view, at least one more assumption has to be made with regard to the universality of the agrammatic phenomenon, notwithstanding that the determination of an adequate level of analysis for its theoretical apprehension may call for a great amount of further research. Following the first assumption, if indeed agrammatic behavior always does imply improper use of closed-class items, it should somehow refer to a universal entity. The reason is straightforward: In accordance with what is actually known about the natural languages of the world, and however great any structurally defined distance between particular grammars may be, no one has ever encountered a language that is devoid of closed-class items. Therefore until the eventual—and improbable—finding of a natural language that contains no closed-class vocabulary, agrammatism must be considered a universal phenomenon.

We trust that, to this point, the frame seems sound or at least viable, although it is certainly limited to purely observational considerations on what emerges at the surface. Because as soon as the "how" and "why" questions are asked, profound disagreements emerge, and the proffered tentative explanations diverge rather dramatically. The list below is meant to illustrate this situation quickly by indicating major proposals for the apprehension of agrammatism and by pointing out some of their representative proponents.

1. Perspective
   a. Positive: Kolk (in press)
   b. Negative: most American authors
2. Problem
   a. Secondary: Goodglass (1976)
   b. Primary: Berndt and Caramazza (1980)
3. Deficit
   a. Lexical: Bradley, Garrett and Zurif (1980)
   b. Phonological: Kean (1979)
   c. Morphological: Lapointe (1983)
   d. Syntactic: Grodzinsky (1984)

## Discussion

Some authors consider agrammatism the positive result of a recourse to an adaptive communication strategy, whereas others define it negatively as a patholinguistic residual that manifests after improvement in the clinical context of Broca's aphasia (see Perspective, item 1, above). When a negative point of view is adopted, as one finds in most American literature on the subject, agrammatism generally corresponds to one typical symptom of Broca's aphasia. This concept implies that the agrammatic deficit is present from the onset of the disease, at least in a latent state, and that its overt semiology is simply conditioned by a sufficient evolution of the syndrome, thereby allowing some discursive speech. From a positive point of view, on the other hand, the surfacing of agrammatism stems from an unimpaired psychological capacity of adaptation in a propitious context, notwithstanding that a patient's awareness of his/her patholinguistic problem may, in a sense, constitute the initial motivation for using an elliptical language strategy.

According to some studies, agrammatism is just an epiphenomenon of the motor deficit that generally accompanies Broca's aphasia, whereas others hold that it is a primary linguistic deficit (see Problem, item 2, above). Finally, several linguistic descriptions of agrammatism have been proposed where different claims are put forth. As noted above, the agrammatic deficit is described variously in lexical, phonological, morphological, or syntactic terms.

In fact, however, this remarkably confusing state of affairs should surprise no one. On the one hand, we must take into account the fast-changing character of grammatical theory; and on the other hand, we must reckon with omnipresence of variability in aphasia. In this study, we concentrate on a specific type of variability that has to do with observed differences in agrammatic discourse across languages. It must be mentioned immediately that our tentative suggestion in this regard does not claim to provide a general solution for all variabilities or even approach it (Nespoulous, 1987; Miceli, this volume, Chapter 1, 1–19). Much more limited in scope, our proposal seeks only a better understanding of cross-linguistic variability within agrammatic behavior. In our view, this single issue is of great importance because, as was previously stated, agrammatism must refer to some universal entity.

One of the main difficulties when trying to conceive of such a universal entity is that the manifest linguistic symptomatology of agrammatism seems neither unitary nor truly homogeneous across languages. In effect, some symptoms apparently differ so much from one language to another that we have not yet obtained a consensus on the kind of inferred grammatical impairment these somewhat heterogeneous signs hypothetically reflect. The global agrammatic symptoms noted below, as a broad observational basis of empirical facts, satisfies our present purpose, which is to discuss the possibility of viewing this semiological set as the reflection of a linguistic or grammatical disturbance per se.

1. Use of simplified sentence-level units
2. Omissions and/or substitution errors in the use of the free grammatical morphemes
3. Omissions and/or substitution errors in the use of bound grammatical morphemes

First, it has long been recognized that the semiology of agrammatism reveals difficulties of a greater or lesser importance in combining sentential elements. Even most simple Noun + Verb sequences are reported by many authors to be difficult to produce in severely affected patients. In mild to moderate cases, some true sentence-level units are indeed displayed, although rarely otherwise than as syntactically independent single-clause sequences in either isolated or coordinated juxtaposition. The scarceness of clause-level embedded constructions has always been noted in agrammatism and is evidenced across languages.

Second, agrammatic discourse exhibits smaller phrase-level disturbances, which is also an amply documented phenomenon across languages. Expected free morphemes such as determinants, auxiliaries, and prepositions are frequently lacking. Moreover, substitutions are well and widely attested to: They are present not only in experimentally constrained contexts, where they often make up the sole grammatical error type to be found, but also in unconstrained spontaneous discourse. Substitution errors are important to keep in mind, notably because they challenge the syntactic deficit hypothesis of agrammatism, at least insofar as they testify to the preservation of syntactic structure, as these errors are within-category substitutions.

Finally, word-level units are also affected because, on the surface, words frequently either appear stripped of expected bound morphemes or, alternatively, are interspersed with improper ones. This situation, once again, is seen across languages. Note that this word-level problem has been discussed mainly with respect to inflecting morphology, but similar word-level disturbances are also reported for compounding morphology in languages that have no inflectional systems whatsoever. (See Packard's chapter on Chinese agrammatism in Menn et al., in press.)

In fact, what is difficult to capture across languages is the precise nature of the alleged grammatical trouble. In essence, this trouble seems sometimes more related to syntax and at other times more related to morphology. In order to understand agrammatism as a universal entity, we suggest that the needed logical construct must include general principles through which the overall potential for agrammatic deviance is predetermined. In other words, one ought to seek theoretical notions that would range over both morphological and syntactic functions. Things being the way they are, it appears that current formal conceptions of grammatical theory cannot serve this purpose, and it remains true even though the specific properties of given particular grammars obviously constrain, and thus partially define, the agrammatic deviance potential for the pertaining languages. In our view, the major point is that actual theories of grammar, independent of their specific orientations toward phonology, morphology, or syntax, are meant to shed light on linguistic knowledge itself but not on why and how this knowledge is put to use in behavior.

Because agrammatism is a deviant or a special performance pattern rather than a type of knowledge, and because phonological, morphological, or syntacttic behaviors in themselves do not make much sense, one might then see all tentative descriptions and explanations of agrammatism, when presented in purely theoretical grammatical terms, as doomed to failure on strict logical grounds. Moreover, at least two sorts of evidence argue strongly in favor of this assertion: (1) the accurateness of grammaticality judgments elicited from so-called agrammatic subjects, as documented by Linebarger et al. (1983); and (2) the fact that agrammatic symptoms show up with considerable unpredictability, i.e., always intermittently. The rationale is as follows: Given that the closed system of rules that largely constitute current linguistic theory permits only all-or-nothing hypotheses with respect to knowledge of grammar, i.e., with respect to competence, and given that the speech production of so-called agrammatic subjects involves typical problems with grammatical elements, logically the only inferrable linguistic explanations are hypotheses of competence loss(es) (Zurif and Caramazza, 1976). Thus, there is an obvious double paradox in postulating some loss of grammatical competence that, on the one hand, does not significantly reduce capacities for grammaticality judgments and, on the other hand, is concomitant with intermittently agrammatic performance. In this sense, grammatical theory, as it stands, does not seem to be an appropriate logical construct either to explain or to describe agrammatism, as it would not even meet the requirements of observational adequacy.

However, we believe that a way out of this uncomfortable situation can be found within a psycholinguistic theory that would contain and define a common denominator of grammars whose specified methods of combining morphemes vary, although we agree that grammatical theory should continue to state that morpheme combination pertains to morphology for word-level representation and to syntax for phrase-level representation. Common conceptions of morphology and syntax, as separate structural components, may well be perfectly suitable for linguistic theory in itself, and issues of grammatical modularity are not called into question in this discussion. Nonetheless, the case could—and maybe should—be different with respect to psycholinguistic theory. Incidentally, we conceive of agrammatic discourse as an indication of the necessity for psycholinguistic theory to represent general formation processes in a unified fashion rather than through distinct types of morphological and syntactic rules.

Almost from the time linguistics came into existence, authors have noted, on the one hand, that open-class morphemes convey referential meaning, whereas closed-class morphemes, whether bound or free, express relational meaning. On the other hand, they have also noted that the way to express relational meaning varies within and across languages. For example, the bearing of the indirect object function by common noun phrases is indicated in English either by a syntactic preposition or by a particular word ordering, whereas it can be indicated only by such a preposition in French or by a similar postposed particle in Japanese. In Polish, moreover, it is marked by case inflection on the noun as well as on the adjective, if there is one; conversely, in German it is signaled altogether by the lexical form of the determinant, if there is one, by case inflection on the adjective, if there is one, and by suffixing −$n$ to the noun, if it is plural. Looking back at the list of agrammatic symptoms, it appears that any discursive sequence, characterized by the semantic merging of at least one referential meaning with at least one relational meaning, is likely to be deviant in agrammatism. Of course, we in no way wish to argue that agrammatism results from a semantic knowledge deficit because, as pointed out above, we think it has to do only with the dynamic use of knowledge.

What we do suggest, however, is that the functioning of the processes responsible for the formation of such semantically complex surface units may occasionally be altered in aphasia, and that agrammatic behavior is due to these alterations. We suggest further that such alterations fall within the domain of short-term memory and attention. Moreover, the general formation processes in question would have to constitute a unified class at some level in psycholinguistic theory—if we want this theory to help in the understanding of agrammatic behavior, e.g. as a universal phenomenon. As for the description of what is going on in agrammatism, we trust that such a psycholinguistic framework can provide more appropriate notional tools to deal with cross-language variability, even if, obviously, much of it remains sketchy.

Inasmuch as explanatory matters can be addressed here at all, it is clear that the theoretical position adopted in the foregoing implies that agrammatic behavior would not unveil a causative linguistic deficit per se but would, rather, result from special uses of grammatical knowledge in the psychological context of episodically limited short-term memory and attentional availability. The essential idea therefore is simply that agrammatism calls for a psycholinguistic model in which there would be at some point a single level for the processing of both word and phrase information, i.e., for the unified processing of what belongs to the distinct representational levels of morphology and syntax in grammatical theory.

*Acknowledgments.* Special thanks to A. Caramazza and J. Bayer for comments on critical points of the original presentation and to R. Whalen for help with the written form.

## References

Berndt, R.S., & Caramazza, A. (1980). A redefinition of the syndrome of Broca's aphasia: implications for a neuropsychological model of language. *Applied Linguistics, 1,* 225–278.

Bradley, D.C., Garrett, M.F., & Zurif, E.B. (1980). Syntactic deficits in Broca's aphasia. In D. Caplan (ed.), *Biological Studies of Mental Processes.* Cambridge: MIT Press, pp. 269–286.

Goodglass, H., (1976). Agrammatism. In H. Whitaker & H.A. Whitaker (eds.), *Studies in Neurolinguistics,* Vol. 1. New York: Academic Press, pp. 237–260.

Grodzinsky, Y. (1984). The syntactic characterization of agrammatism. *Cognition,* *16*, 99–120.

Kean, M.L. (1979). Agrammatism: a phonological deficit? *Cognition, 7*, 69–83.

Kolk, H.H.J. (in press). Intentions and language pathology in aphasia. In G. Kempen (ed.), *Natural Language in Generation. Recent Advances in Artificial Intelligence, Psychology and Linguistics*. Dordrecht: Kluwer Academic.

Lapointe, S. (1983). Some issues in the linguistic description of agrammatism. *Cognition, 14*, 1–39.

Linebarger, M.C., Schwartz, M.F., & Saffran, E.M. (1983). Sensitivity to grammatical structure in so-called agrammatic aphasics. *Cognition, 13*, 361–392.

Menn, L., Obler, L.K., & Goodglass, H. (eds.), (in press). *Agrammatic Aphasia: Cross-Language Narrative Sourcebook*. Amsterdam: John Benjamins.

Nespoulous, J.L. (1987). La variabilité dans les performances verbales des aphasiques. Presented at the Journal-Club du Laboratoire Théophile-Alajouanine, Montreal.

Zurif, E.B., & Caramazza, A. (1976). Psycholinguistic structures in aphasia: studies in syntax and semantics. In H. Whitaker, H.A. Whitaker (eds.), *Studies in Neurolinguistics*, Vol. 1. New York: Academic Press, pp. 261–291

# 11
# Principle of Sonority, Doublet Creation, and the Checkoff Monitor

Hugh W. Buckingham jr.

Syllable markedness as a means to characterize patterns observed in the production of phonological errors in aphasia is considered in this chapter. Specifically, the markedness theory incorporated here is the well known principle of sonority, and the error type in question is the often-observed "doublet creation." Consonantal doublet creation, where an exact replica of some target-word consonant is duplicated and is either added to the string (in the sense of epenthesis) or substitutes from some other already existing consonant in the target word, is discussed. A basic assumption here is that syllable markedness can form a knowledge base for language production mechanisms; or, put slightly differently, productive mechanisms derived from psycholinguistic model construction should embody principles arrived at through linguistic inquiry. It is a sine qua non that linguistic theory must have an impact on the psychological constructs derived from performance domains.

The productive mechanism at issue in this chapter is the "checkoff monitor," whose responsibility it is to mark as used (or delete—thus check off) phonological segments that have been taken from a short-term buffer and copied onto their respective productive syllable positions. As with many productive mechanisms for language, the checkoff monitor was proposed to account for certain types of slips-of-the-tongue observed in the misfiring of normal speakers. In typical fashion, the mechanism is subsequently considered as part of the computational machinery for normal language production and accordingly may be considered as a component that may or may not be disrupted as a consequence of brain damage. What is claimed in this chapter is that the checkoff monitor can be said to "know" or "be sensitive to" (pick your intentional predicate) the principles that deal with sonority and that the mechanism's operations are conditioned accordingly.

The line of reasoning is as follows. Doublet creating errors arise through serial ordering derailments, where a segment is misordered and appears either earlier or again later in productive order. For there to be a doublet, the moved segment must also remain in its originating slot, or at least it must not be checked off after being misordered. The next point is that not all serial ordering errors involve doublet creation, which is to say that often a moved segment is checked off from its site of origin. The question then becomes that of determining when we get doublets and when we do not. It is proposed here that the checkoff monitor is sensitive enough to sonority constraints to ensure that its operations fall in line accordingly, so that, if by checking off a moved segment a more marked sequence of segments would result, it refrains from its normal operation. It that case, the doublet has been created; in the other cases, there is no doublet.

## Sonority Principle (Hierarchy) of Syllable Structure

There are several sources, or levels, at which one may look for linguistic justification for the principle of sonority. Clements (1988) demonstrated that this principle can be characterized at a deep phonological level, but at the same time its properties and characteristics are reflected in one way or another at surface phonetic levels as well as at the acoustic/perceptual level. At an underlying/abstract level, syllable structure is characterized from the left periphery to the vowel segment in terms of an increase in syllabicity, which has an articulatory counterpart in terms of vocal tract openness and an acoustic counterpart in terms of perceptual salience. Underlyingly, the sonority hierarchy is ordered from least to most sonorant in the following fashion: O(bstruent)—N(asal)—L(iquid)—G(lide)—V(owel). The hierarchy is reversed from the vowel to the right periphery of the syllable. The unmarked syllable abides by this ordering.

Clements (1988) demonstrated how certain phonological processes may give rise to more marked syllable types or sequences that contradict sonority, but his claim was that in most cases the surface phonetic counter-examples reflect morphological or phonological processes rather than any necessary inconsistence in sonority in general, especially as characterized at the underlying level. Extrasyllabicity, late morphological affixation, glide formation, unitary treatment of geminates, and the like most often account for surface forms that might appear to contradict sonority.

A major portion of sonority theory deals with the scalar relations among the segments. Most phoneticians and phonologists have characterized syllables in terms of increases in sonority from the left periphery to the vowel and from there a decrease in sonority up to the right periphery of the syllable. The first point to note is that there does not appear to be any interaction between the nature of the sonority increase from C to V and that from V to C. That is, we must separately consider sonority slopes in the first part of the syllable (C...V) and in the second part of the syllable (V...C). In Clements' (1988) view, these two units are referred to as "demisyllables," a term he credited to previous phoneticians. "Preferred" slopes of sonority variation are different for the initial and final demisyllables. The unmarked slope of initial demisyllables is steep, which is to say that the maximally preferred initial CV is obstruent—vowel. The unmarked slope of the final demisyllable is more gradual, the final consonant being more sonorous than the leftmost consonant of the initial demisyllable. In general, it can be said that the preference of human languages for discontinuity between vowels and consonants arises from demands of sonority, as fluctuation in sonority among segments enhances perceptual processing. The same may be said for adjacent consonants. Preferred sequences consist of two consonants that do not share the same place on the hierarchy or that are not contiguous on the scale. A sort of "attraction of opposites" (Donegan and Stampe, 1978) is inherent in the principle of sonority. Again, note that there are no absolutes here. Some languages allow initial /pf-/ clusters composed of segments that share the same spot on the sonority hierarchy (both are obstruents).

Distance on this scale can easily be quantified, O to V having a distance of 4, O to N a distance of 1, N to V a distance of 3, and so on. Some languages reveal a strict constraint whereby no consonant cluster can consist of segments of a distance less than 3, for instance. Harris (1983) demonstrated that Spanish clusters require a minimum distance of 2. That is, in Spanish there are no initial clusters O-N or N-L; O-L clusters are acceptable. Obviously, then, a highly undesirable situation is one where two contiguous segments share the same location on the sonority scale, e.g., two nasals together, two liquids together, two vowels together. In fact, this constraint is part of the rationale underlying the treatment of geminates as *single* segments, sharing the root and supralaryngeal tiers as well as the place tier (Clements, 1988). Obviously, geminates are homorganic, but other nongeminate homorganic clusters do not share root and supralaryngeal nodes and thus are not considered single units. Vowels, for the same reason, are rarely if ever found tautosyllabically contiguous. In many cases, high vowels next to other vowels undergo glide formation, and the unwanted situation thereby is avoided, V-V changing to G-V, or V-G.

A "core" syllabification process according to Clements (1988) initially isolates the vocalic component and subsequently works to the left in order of decreasing sonority, assigning each consonant to the syllable of that vowel. The assignment stops once the next consonant in line is higher in sonority. This onset assignment process is computed simultaneously in polysyllabic words. In those cases where phonotactics outlaws a certain onset cluster that would otherwise be produced, the syllabification process is thereby altered. For example, the word *padlock* in English does not show an onset cluster of $dl- for the second syllable, although /d/ is less sonorous than /l/. After onsets are assigned, the remaining consonants are assigned to coda positions. The syllabification algorithm thus predicts a more gradual sonority decrescendo for final demisyllables only when they are word-or phrase-internal. In any event, one of the consequences of the "core" syllabification process is the "law of syllable contact." This law stipulates that a syllable contact sequence X$Y is more preferred where X is more sonorous than Y, which, as is stressed later, provides a reasonable explanation for the highly undesirable situation of adjacent rimes.

Finally, sonority is tightly involved with the so-called phonotactic patterns of language, as demonstrated above in terms of different sonority distances for contiguous consonants. Specific language surface phonotactic patterns must be considered as in some way overriding general sonority in two ways. First, as demonstrated by such studies as that of Bell and Saka (1983), reversed sonority may be seen in consonant clusters (Hankamer and Aissen, 1974). Also, although sonority admits of the possibility of O-N clusters (i.e., the order is not reversed), many languages simply do not allow them; some do, however. This point is important in the study of phonemic paraphasia, as addition paraphasias never introduce a nasal after an obstruent in initial demisyllables of English, but an /l/ may be introduced in this fashion. Sonority does not explain this fact; specific English phonotactics does. In addition, some sonority scales split oral stops from fricatives, claiming that oral stops are less sonorant, which always leaves the problem of the initial S + oral stop clusters, as that would be a reversal. Some have argued that in these cases the /s/ should be considered "extra-syllabic" and thus outside the syllable. Those who simply place O(bstruent) on the scale claim that it would represent a sonority "plateau," with a strictly horizontal slope line (i.e., no increase or decrease in sonority). In any event, the plateau as well as the reversed sonority order are unwanted situations, and we would expect that any segmental ordering computational mechanism would "know" enough to avoid the situation as much as possible.

## Scan Copier and the Checkoff Monitor

A brief description of the scan copier and the checkoff monitor is in order. Shattuck-Hufnagel (1979, 1983) proposed these mechanisms to account for various types of segmental slips-of-the-tongue; and Buckingham (1980, 1983, 1985, 1986, 1987) interrelated these mechanisms and adapted them to the positional level of computation in the overall production model of Garrett (1975, 1976, 1980, 1982, 1984, 1988). Essentially, the scan copier's responsibility is to scan the representative segmental structure of content words that have been placed in an operating buffer. The window size of the string of content words in the buffer is roughly the phrase, but because many sound errors span phrases (i.e., they cross the NP-VP boundary) it is not unreasonable to admit of a window size of up to a clause. The scan copier not only scans, it copies the segments onto separately formed productive order syllable templates. The scanner "knows" when it is copying onset consonants, vowels, and final consonants; and in fact the scanner appears to be able to look at syllable positions simultaneously. That is, the scanner can look at several onset positions simultaneously, copying in order of syllable position. This situation looks to be the case, as most all ordering errors abide by the constraint that stipulates that onset consonants move to other onset slots, vowels move to vowel slots, and final consonants move to other final consonant slots. The only time this constraint regularly breaks down is when the scanner is, for whatever reason, within a single syllable. Coda consonants often move to onset slots if those slots are tautosyllabic. After a segment is copied onto (or assigned to) its respective utterance order slot, the checkoff monitor deletes it from the buffer or somehow marks it as used and not to be copied again. The interactive activationists would claim that after the segment was activated and assigned its slot its activation level would return to zero. Garrett (1988) claimed that these accounts are compatible. In any event, the segment, once copied, must be eliminated from the buffer; otherwise some form of reiteration occurs.

In sum, the copier and checkoff mechanisms work in tandem and are conceived as computational devices that manipulate symbols. In this case the symbols are phonological units, and those units are in their abstract forms because at this point in the production scheme their phonetic shapes have not been determined. The manipulations are those of copying and deleting, and the level at which these operations occur is the positional level in the Garrett model (Buckingham, 1986; Garrett, 1988).

The doublet creating error arises when *both* mechanisms fail to operate normally. Shattuck-Hufnagel (1979) characterized slip-of-the-tongue constraint No. 6 as follows.

Anticipatory and perseveratory errors often involve the "double use" of a target segment, once in its appropriate location and once as an intrusion.

She subsequently offered an account of this situation in terms of her ordering mechanisms (1979).

. . .if both the scan copier and the checkoff device misfire on the same segment, so that a misselected segment also fails to be marked as used, then it is available to be copied again and can appear twice.

Here, then, is the essential description of the genesis of the doublet. Note, however, that no *explaination* is provided.

## Doublet Creating Errors (Pair Creation)

Doublets may be created by misscanning segments to either the left (anticipation) or the right (perseveration). The segment that is misordered may be added to an unfilled slot in the word, or it may actually substitute for some item. The addition type of doublet adds a segment to the original word, whereas the substitutive doublet creating error does not result in an increase in the number of segments in the word involved. Figure 3.3 in Nespoulous, Joanette, Ska, Caplan, and Lecours (1987) listed clear examples of prepositioning phonemic errors with and without substitution and with and without pair creation. There is a four-way distinction shown.

1. Scan error with doublet creation (additive)
       a v i k y l t œ R
       k a v i k y l t œ R
2. Scan error with doublet creation (substitutive)
       a v i k y l t œ R
       a k i k y l t œ R
3. Scan error without doublet creation (additive)
       a v i k y l t   œ R
       l a v i k y t œ R
4. Scan error without doublet creation (Substitutive)
       a v i k y l t   œ R
       a l i k y t œ R

For the doublet creating errors of (1) and (2) the consonants move from onset position to onset position. In each case they move from a phonetic environment of V$__V. The nondoublet creating errors involve the movement of coda consonants to onset positions (thus breaking the above-mentioned syllable position constraint). In each case the moved segments stem from a phonetic environment of V__$C. Note that the doublet error in both cases involves the misordering of an intervocalic consonant. This situation was not the case with the nondoublet creating error.

Recall the syllable contact law. A V$V is marked because vowels share equal status on the sonority scale. The V$C is preferred because the V is more sonorous than the consonant. Just *how* much sonority difference needs to obtain does not seem to matter much, so long as there is some. V$t is sharper in sonority difference, but l$t would abide by the constraint as well.

Buckingham (1987) presented a brief analysis of the doublet creations found in the phonemic paraphasias reported in Lecours and Lhermitte's (1969) influential paper on paraphasia. In that analysis it was noted that the significant majority of doublets involved the misordering of intervocalic consonants. Let us take an in-depth look at two of those errors.

5. a b ɔ m i n a b l   (target word)

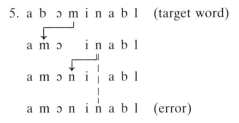

a m ɔ   i n a b l

a m ɔ n i | a b l

a m ɔ n i n a b l   (error)

In the descriptive analysis of Lecours and Lhermitte (1969), they represent complex transformations. However, the descriptive system used in their article is not followed here. The general analyses are equivalent in any event. In (5), /m/ is misscanned and substitutes for /b/, leaving the V__V position. The /n/, however, is misscanned and fills the V__V left by /m/. The /n/ leaves an intervocalic position as well; but, interestingly enough, it remains in its original slot, and so the doublet involves the /n/.

6.

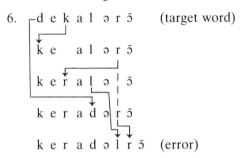

keradəlrɔ̃   (error)

Here /k/ is misscanned and substitutes for the initial /d/, leaving an inter-vocalic position. The /r/ is misscanned and comes to fill that intervocalic position, /r/ originating in an intervocalic slot itself. However, /r/ remains in its place of origin, and therefore the doublet in this error involves the /r/. Interestingly, the original /d/ of the target moves into the intervocalic slot of the /l/, and /l/ moves around the schwa. Admittedly, there is more complication with this error, as the misordering of the /l/ results in a sequence of two liquids (i.e., a sonority plateau). Let us now explore the important generalization that doublets involve intervocalic consonants in a significant number of cases.

It should be clear to the reader that two contiguous vowels represent a marked transsyllabic sonority plateau V$V—one where the segment to the left of the boundary is not of greater sonority than the segment to the right and is thus marked according to the syllable contact law. There seems to be something complex about the situation of adjacent rimes occurring in sequence with nothing to break the sequence. There would be little if any discontinuity on the acoustic spectrum. It is these cases where the checkoff monitor would fail to check off a moved segment. So, in a sense, the normal operation of this mechanism is blocked in those cases where, if it were to operate, a highly marked sequence would result.

Look back at examples (1) to (4). In both examples of pair creation, the segment involved was in the intervocalic position in the target word, i.e., in the /i$__y/ slot. In those errors where there were no doublets, the mis-ordered segment did not come from an intervocalic position, i.e., /y__$t/.

Supporting evidence comes from a study by Béland, Caplan, and Nespoulous (unpublished). In an analysis that did not include ordering errors, Béland et al. nevertheless found that interesting things happen to adjacent rimes. In the errors, one of the two rimes may drop, or a consonantal epenthetic error (addition paraphasia) may serve to break up the unwanted sequence of vowels. Even more importantly, Béland et al. stated that:

> Since vowel-vowel sequences are difficult for our subject, we would expect him not to create such sequences through deletion of intervocalic consonants. This is, in fact, confirmed in his performance since consonantal omissions are never observed when a consonantal segment stands between two vowels.

The absence of intervocalic consonantal deletion paraphasias serves to support my point about the necessary involvement of intervocalic consonants in doublet creation errors; consequently it is consistent with my claim that the checkoff monitor does not erase from the buffer a misordered copy if that copy is of an original intervocalic consonant. These observations are obviously two sides of the same coin. In doublet errors, intervocalic consonants remain (otherwise there would be no doublet); and in simple omission paraphasias, intervocalic consonants are rarely if ever deleted. The sonority principle is at work in both situations. Note further that Béland et al. went on to say that:

> For instance, a word such as /abit/ will never surface as */ait/ by consonantal omission of the /b/.

For the same reason, the form /abit/ would be a perfect candidate for a doublet creating error /babit/. Thus the interlocking constraints concerning omission paraphasias and doublet creating errors become crystal clear.

However, it is not known yet just what component serves as the source of pure omission errors in phonemic paraphasia. Scan copiers do only that: They scan and copy. It is the checkoff monitor that erases, or otherwise eliminates, segments from the buffer. Shattuck-Hufnagel postulated an additional mechanism that she called an "error monitor" to check for suspicious pairs or triples in the representative form. Sometimes, however, when an underlying word actually has two or three occurrences of some segment, the error monitor erroneously deletes one.

In slips-of-the-tongue [and in masking errors in spelling (Ellis, 1982)] omissions most often occur in words that have more than one occurrence of the omitted item. It is not clear if this is the case in omission errors in aphasia. From the Béland et al. study, it does not appear to be the case, which is why there is some question as to just which mechanism is doing the deleting in purely paradigmatic omission errors. Nevertheless, whatever it is, it is abiding by the principle of sonority.

There is another intriguing question that remains. Note in example (5) above, for instance, that the /m/ moved from its intervocalic position and was indeed checked off, as the doublet did not involve the /m/. That left the intervocalic position open, thus throwing together two vowels. In that case, however, the following intervocalic /n/ was misscanned and took over that slot, thereby avoiding the marked case for sonority. It was the /n/ in this case that was not checked off from its original site, and thus it was the doublet. Why in some cases the misscanned intervocalic consonant is checked off [another consonant most likely filling its place, such as the /r/ in example (6)] and in other cases it is not checked off remains a puzzle.

## Other Interlocking Principles and Operations

Although the mechanism treated in this chapter is the checkoff monitor as it relates to the principle of sonority, other mechanisms and principles interact as well. Examples, obviously, are the scan copier already mentioned as an integral component in doublet formation and the CV core syllable typology discussed at length by Clements and Keyser (1983) and Clements (1988). First, it was mentioned at the outset of the chapter that for initial demisyllables the preferred sonority rise is abrupt, and so the C would be an obstruent in the least marked case. We might, therefore, look to see if a misscanning error would improve the sonority situation. Where one obstruent moves to an onset position and substitutes for yet another obstruent, no change in markedness occurs. However, with the doublet error of *lelephone* for *telephone* (Buckingham, 1987), a more marked CV sequence in terms of sonority is set up.

When a target word has an initial vowel, e.g., the French word *avikyltoer*, any movement of an internal consonant to the unfilled onset C slot would lead to a less marked situation in terms of CV typology. Incidentally, this point ties in with sonority because an initial demisyllable of a V has no rise at all in sonority. Adding practically any consonant would improve the situation, especially an obstruent.

We noted above that intervocalic consonants rarely, if ever, undergo deletion in paraphasia. On the other hand, consonants are deleted from consonant clusters, but one interesting observation has been made (Garrett, 1988). In onset consonant clusters, it is the second of the consonants that is most often deleted. Given the fact that he second of two consonants in initial demisyllables is almost always more sonorous than the first, its deletion sets up a more preferred sequence, as the sonority rise is more abrupt. Unfortunately, it appears only to be a tendency, albeit an important one. For instance, Béland and Nespoulous (1985) observed cases where the reverse took place in initial demisyllables. In that study, they noted cluster simplification errors such as $bR \circ S \to R \circ S$. However, they also noted cluster simplification errors such as $g \circ lf \to g \circ l$, where a more gradual sonority decline in the final demisyllable is borne out. It would not have been the case had the /l/ been deleted. That is, sonority principles account for the error $g \circ l$, but they are contradicted with the omission of the obstruent in the initial demisyllable. Béland and Nespoulous's (1985) point was that deletion at syllable peripheries is conditioned by the fact that the peripheral slots are in "weak" positions and therefore tend to drop. This hypothesis interlocks with the sonority theory only with respect to final, word- or phrase-internal demisyllables. The principle of sonority would predict far more cluster simplification errors such as $g \mathfrak{d} lf \rightarrow g \mathfrak{d} l$ than $bR \mathfrak{d} S \rightarrow R \mathfrak{d} S$. As far as I know, however, this point has not been quantified.

Blumstein (1978) observed that many addition paraphasias follow the principle of sonority. In her corpus, 22% of addition errors involved the addition of a liquid or a semivowel to the right of an initial stop or continuant. Obviously, if one is to add some consonant to a singleton to form a cluster, it is expected that the dictates of sonority would be followed. In fact, it is precisely what Blumstein found. The epenthesized /l/'s and /r/'s were always to the right of the less sonorous consonants. To this point, however, must be added three comments.

First, is it the undesirability of reversed sonority order that is conditioning the addition errors, or is it the dictate that sonority slopes must rise in initial demisyllables? These points are perhaps two sides of the same coin, but some languages do in fact permit bizarre reversals, such as Pashto /lm-/, /wl-/, and /wr-/ (Bell and Saka, 1983). It would be interesting to look at paraphasias and slips-of-the-tongue in those kinds of language to verify this point.

Second, note that although initial demisyllable sequences of O(bstruent) —N(asal) are perfectly acceptable in sonority theory, no addition paraphasia of an English-speaking aphasic would involve a change in *box* to *bnox*. In this case, one would need to go slightly beyond the general guidelines of sonority and consider language-specific phonotactic patterns, which in English rule out initial obstruent/nasal clusters.

The third point is that in the analysis of addition paraphasias it is important to indicate whether the additional segment comes from the surrounding environment or has no source. We have seen above that many misordered segments are additive in their new positions not substitutive. The no-source addition is puzzling, as we do not know where it comes from or what kind of mechanism produces it. The same puzzle holds for the no-source substitution (Shattuck-Hufnagel, 1979). Lecours and Caplan (1975), in their review of Blumstein (1973), pointed out that although Blumstein had a category for environmental errors (ordering errors) she did not make the source/no source distinction when analyzing the addition errors. That is, some of the addition errors could have been contextual misorderings. When we can be sure that addition paraphasias come from misfires of the scan copier, we can attribute knowledge of the sonority to that mechanism. Suffice it to say that, when analyzing phonemic paraphasias in terms of the computational mechanisms that may be involved, one is puzzled over the no-source errors because they do not appear in the buffer to be manipulated. (See Béland et al., unpublished, and Chapter 14 in this volume for further comments on these issues.)

Finally, it is often the case that the vowel skeleton of a word remains intact, with the consonants apparently looser and moving around those vowels in various ways. Word-initial consonants are looser yet (Shattuck-Hufnagel, 1987). Note that the vowel array in the paraphasias (1) to (6) remain virtually undisrupted (Buckingham, 1987). This primacy (or fixedness) or the [+syllabic] segment of words may, at least theoretically, be in some way related to Clements' (1988) cyclically organized formulation of syllable sonority mentioned above. In his scheme, the ordered procedures are realized on segment strings to build syllables. Importantly, the *first* operation searches for [+syllabic] segments and introduces the syllable node over them. Subsequent operations depend on the setting of the vowels. Clements (1988) claimed that:

This step presupposes that syllabic segments are already present in the representation at this point, whether created by rule or underlying.

In this way the primacy of the vowel is established, with all other operations unfolding around them. As outlined above, the second operation in the cycle adds segments *to the left* that have successively lower sonorance. The third operation does the same for the final demisyllable on the right. The point here is that if productive ordering is at all related to this "core syllabification principle" vowels would ipso facto be more resistant to distortion or misordering. Perhaps there is some sort of harder cast to the vocalic slots in their utterance-order syllabic templates onto which underlying vowels are copied. In any event, there seems to be something in the nature of the vowel that renders it less liable to alteration in either slips-of-the-tongue or in paraphasia.

## Conclusion

Admittedly, emphasis in this chapter has been limited in most part to adjacent rimes, where the sonority plateau involves two vowels and the syllable contact law is thereby disobeyed. Needless to say, the principle of sonority involves far more than this environment; but where doublet creation is concerned, it certainly seems to be the case that intervocalic consonants at once shift position and remain in their original context. It is the job of the checkoff monitor to ensure that segments are eliminated from the buffer after they have been copied onto their respective utterance order slots. When this erasure would result in two vowels falling together, however, the mechanism refrains from its normal operation, and a doublet is accordingly created. Therefore in a real sense, the checkoff monitor can be said to operate, at least in part, under the principle of sonority.

## *References*

Béland, R, & Nespoulous, J-L. (1985). Recent phonological models and the study of aphasic errors. Presented at the 23rd Annual Meeting of the Academy of Aphasia, Pittsburgh.

Béland, R., Caplan, D., & Nespoulous, J-L. (unpublished). Phonological constraints on phonemic paraphasias in a reproduction conduction aphasic.

Bell, A., & Saka, M.M. (1983). Reversed sonority in Pashto initial clusters. *Journal of Phonetics*, *11*, 259–275.

Blumstein, S.E. (1973). *A Phonological Investigation of Aphasic Speech*. The Hague: Mouton.

Blumstein, S.E. (1978). Segment structure and the syllable in aphasia. In A. Bell & J.B. Hooper (eds.), *Syllables and Segments*. Amsterdam: North Holland.

Buckingham, H.W. (1980). On correlating aphasic errors with slips-of-the-tongue. *Applied Psycholinguistics*, *1*, 199–220.

Buckingham, H.W. (1983). Apraxia of language vs. apraxia of speech. In R.A. Magill (ed.), *Memory and Control of Action*. Amsterdam: North Holland.

Buckingham, H.W. (1985). Perseveration in aphasia. In S. Newman & R. Epstein (eds.), *Current Perspectives in Dysphasia*. Edinburgh: Churchill Livingstone.

Buckingham, H.W. (1986). The scan-copier mechanism and the positional level of language production: evidence from phonemic paraphasia. *Cognitive Science*, *10*, 195–217.

Buckingham, H.W. (1987). Review: phonemic paraphasias and psycholinguistic production models for neologistic jargon. *Aphasiology*, *1*, 381–400.

Clements, G.N. (1988). The role of the sonority cycle in core syllabification. *Working Papers of the Cornell Phonetics Laboratory*, No. 2, April.

Clements, G.N., & Keyser, S.J. (1983). *CV Phonology: A Generative Theory of the Syllable*. Linguistic Inquiry Monograph 9. Cambridge, MA: MIT Press.

Donegan, P.J., & Stampe, D. (1978). The syllable in phonological and prosodic structure. In A. Bell & J.B. Hooper (eds.), *Syllables and Segments*. Amsterdam: North Holland.

Ellis, A.W. (1982). Spelling and writing (and reading and speaking). In A.W. Ellis (ed.), *Normality and Pathology in Cognitive Functions*. London: Academic Press.

Garrett, M.F. (1975). The analysis of sentence production. In B. Gorden (ed.), *The Psychology of Learning and Motivation: Advances in Research and Theory*. New York: Academic Press.

Garrett, M.F. (1976). Syntactic processes in sentence production. In R.J. Wales & E. Walker (eds.), *New Approaches to Language Mechanisms*. Amsterdam: North Holland.

Garrett, M.F. (1980). Levels of processing in sentence production. In B. Butterworth (ed.), *Sentence Production. Vol. 1. Speech and Talk*. London: Academic Press.

Garrett, M.F. (1982). Production of speech: observations from normal and pathological language use. In A.W. Ellis (ed.), *Normality and Pathology in Cognitive Functions*. London: Academic Press.

Garrett, M.F. (1984). The organization of processing structure for language production: applications to aphasic speech. In D. Caplan, A.R. Lecours, & A. Smith (eds.), *Biological Perspectives on Language*. Cambridge, MA: MIT Press.

Garrett, M.F. (1988). Processes in language production. In F. J. Newmeyer (ed.), *Linguistics: The Cambridge Survey. Vol. 3. Language: Psychological and Biological Aspects*. Cambridge, England: Cambridge University Press.

Hankamer, J., & Aissen, J. (1974). The sonority hierarchy. In A. Bruck, R.A. Fox, & M.W. Le Galy (eds.), *Papers from the Parasession on Natural Phonology*. Chicago: Chicago Linguistic Society.

Harris, J.W. (1983). *Syllable Structure and Stress in Spanish*: *A Nonlinear Analysis*. Cambridge, MA: MIT Press.

Lecours, A.R., & Caplan, D. (1975). A review of Blumstein (1973). *Brain and Language*, *2*, 237–254.

Lecours, A.R., & Lhermitte, F. (1969). Phonemic paraphasias: linguistic structures and tentative hypotheses. *Cortex*, *5*, 193–228.

Nespoulous, J-L., Joanette, Y., Ska, B., Caplan D., & Lecours, A.R. (1987). Production deficits in Broca's and conduction aphasia: repetition versus reading. In E. Keller & M. Gopnik (eds.), *Motor and Sensory Processes of Language*. Hillsdale, NJ: Lawrence Erlbaum Associates.

Shattuck-Hufnagel, S. (1979). Speech errors as evidence for a serial ordering mechanism in speech production. In W.E. Cooper & E.C.T. Walker (eds.), *Sentence Processing*: *Psycholinguistic Studies Presented to Merrill Garrett*. Hillsdale, NJ: Lawrence Erlbaum Associates.

Shattuck-Hufnagel, S. (1983). Sublexical units and suprasegmental structure in speech production planning. In P.F. MacNeilage (ed.) *The Production of Speech*. New York: Springer-Verlag.

Shattuck-Hufnagel, S. (1987). The role of word-onset consonants in speech production planning: new evidence from speech error patterns. In E. Keller & M. Gopnik (eds.), *Motor and Sensory Processes of Language*. Hillsdale, NJ: Lawrence Erlbaum Associates.

# 12
# Phonological Paraphasias Versus Slips of the Tongue in German and Italian

WOLFGANG U. DRESSLER, LIVIA TONELLI, and EMANUELA MAGNO CALDOGNETTO

Whereas cross-linguistic work on aphasia has been well established, speech error research has been mostly carried out within single languages (except Berg, 1987, 1988). Following Dressler's (1982) first outline of similarities and differences between speech errors and phonological paraphasias in several languages, we started a respective Italian-Austrian project (Dressler, Magno Caldognetto, and Tonelli, 1986; Dressler, Tonelli, and Magno Caldognetto, 1987).

Our main aims have so far been as follows.

1. To improve on, and decide between, alternative classifications and classificatory subdivisions of phonological slips of the tongue
2. To establish quantitative and qualitative differences between slips and paraphasias in view of their importance for production models, phonological and neurolinguistic theory, and aphasia therapy (e.g., for differentiating mild aphasia and normal speech errors at the end of therapies)
3. To distinguish presumably universal versus system-specific disturbances in regard to the great differences between the phonological systems of Italian and German

The phonological model used is the framework of natural phonology as founded by Stampe (1969), elaborated by Dressler (1984, 1985), and applied to the phonological study of aphasia by Dressler (1974, 1982), Wurzel and Böttcher (1979), and Kilani-Schoch (1982).

The German speech error data are the Austrian ones of Meringer (1908) and Meringer and Mayer (1895); the more than 500 Italian lapsus have been collected in Padua since 1982. The German aphasia data were selected by chance from four Wernicke's, six Broca's, and seven global Viennese aphasics (investigated in a project studying 80 aphasics by Heinz and Jacqueline Stark, and Dressler; see Dressler and Stark, 1988). The Italian aphasic data are those of 10 Wernicke and 5 Broca patients studied at the Clinica Neurologica di Padova by F. Denes. In this study we are not concerned with differences between types of aphasia but with differences between phonological paraphasias and slips of the tongue.

## Simplifications Versus Complications

To compare phonological "simplifications" and "complications" in slips and paraphasias, we started with the assumption (as argued in our previous publications) that phonological paraphasias consist of two main types.

1. Processes that are also typical for slips of the tongue
   a. Anticipations, e.g., it andato (gone) → antato
   b. Perseverations, e.g., si gira (one turns) → si sira
   c. Metatheses, e.g., politici (politicians) → policiti
2. Phonological substitutions identifiable with universal natural phonological processes as postulated in natural phonology (see also "markedness effects" in Nespoulous, Joanette, Béland, Caplan, and Roch Lecours, 1984).
   a. Lenitions, e.g., chiuderlo (to close it) → chiuzerlo
   b. Simplifications of syllable structure via consonant cluster reductions (or syllable final consonant deletion) or vowel insertions into consonant clusters, e.g., G. Zebra ['tse:bra] → ['tse:bara] or ['tse:ba]

Wurzel and Böttcher (1979) argued that paraphasias tend to simplify syllable structure in the direction of the optimal syllable, which consists of one consonant and one vowel. Examples are the above-mentioned paraphasias of the German word for zebra. However, these investigators did not allow for complications such as in the following.

G. Geist ['gaest] (ghost) → [sgaest]
It. passava (passed by) → paspava

However, our material—like that of many others (Blumstein, 1973)—shows that both simplification and complication of syllable structure occurs in phonological paraphasias. They are not evenly distributed, however. First, as predicted by the model of natural phonology for languages at large, complications concentrate in strong prosodic positions, such as word-initially as in the above-mentioned paraphasia [sgaest]; and simplifications concentrate in weak prosodic positions, such as unstressed word-internal or word-final syllables. Second, and more important for our topic, there are interesting quantitative differences both within paraphasias and between paraphasias and slips, as shown in the following distributions, first within a balanced sample from our Viennese patients (Table 12.1).

Table 12.2 shows, in round figures, that the relations between simplifications and complications in slips and paraphasias strongly diverge. Although the differences are less marked in Italian than in German (maybe because syllable structure is simpler in Italian than in German) the preponderance

TABLE 12.1. Simplifications/complications in Viennese paraphasias.

| Parameter | Wernicke | Broca | Global |
|---|---|---|---|
| Simplifications | 9 | 56 | 19 |
| Complications | 7 | 26 | 9 |

TABLE 12.2. Simplifications versus complications in paraphasias/slips

| Study | Paraphasias | Slips |
|---|---|---|
| German (Vienna) | 2:1 | 1:5 |
| Italian (Padua) | 1:1 | 1:3 |

of complications in slips of the tongue is striking in both languages (similar results in Berg, 1988).

## Discussion

Most phonological slips can be seen as phonological blends (in a broad sense). In terms of Baars' (1980) "competing plans hypothesis" (Stemberger, 1985) two wordo shapes with similar degrees of activation may compete for being produced in the same slot, a hypothesis compatible with many models of parallel processing. If neither of the two competitors wins out completely, one probable outcome is a blend of the two competitors (or sources of the error) in the form of either a contamination (blend in its narrow sense) or an anticipation or perseveration.

Fare una frase (to make a sentence) [Italian]
    → frare una frase (additive anticipation) *or*
    → fare una fase (subtractive perseveration)

If we compare such additive and subtractive outputs, both sources/competitors (viz. "fare" and "frase") leave behind clear traces in the first, additive output, whereas the traces of the second source in the second, subtractive output are less clear. This tendency of two competitors to add rather than to subtract their traces in the erroneous output becomes most evident in contaminations where words such as 'smoke" and "fog" typically result in "smog" (four phonemes) rather than "foke" (three phonemes) (Dressler, 1976). The same argumentation can explain why additive errors outweigh subtractive ones in slips of the tongue in general.

It is generally acknowledged that slips involve consonants more often than vowels, and that vowels are rarely added or subtracted because it would change the rhythmical pattern of the target word. Therefore phoneme additions usually are consonant additions in the form of syllable structure complication, which explains the preponderance of complications over simplifications shown earlier in the chapter.

Because phonological paraphasias contain many errors that are explainable in terms of the same mechanisms as nonpathological slips of the tongue, there must be instances of complications in paraphasias as well. As we have claimed above, however, there are among paraphasias universal process type substitutions (Kilani-Schoch, 1982) where simplifications outweigh complications, as proposed by Stampe (1969), Dressler (1974), and Wurzel and Böttcher (1979).

## Phonological Repair

When normal speakers become aware of their own phonological slips, they correct them immediately, and these corrections are usually immediately successful. It is rather rare that a further correction becomes necessary (Fromkin, 1973; Levelt, 1983; Meringer and Mayer, 1985). Aphasic repair, however, often involves successive approximations. In our opinion, quantitative analyses of such repair sequences of phonological approximations (Joanette, Keller, and Roch Lecours, 1980) are adequate only if the paraphasia that initiates the sequence is adequately characterized. We therefore propose the following hypotheses, which so far have proved to be successful in our ongoing research.

1. Ceteris paribus, an aphasic is more likely to correct a phonological paraphasia the more severe and thus the more salient the paraphasia is, as the awareness of an error is likely to increase with its salience—and presumably the eagerness to correct it as well.
2. Paraphasias that resemble typical normal slips of the tongue are less salient than others that do not, i.e., that are clearly of a pathological type (see above).
3. The least salient among these paraphasias are those that consist of one substitution only. Such simple substitutions prevail in aphasia (Magno Caldognetto, Tonelli, and Luciani, 1986; Söderpalm, 1979).

      G. beruflich (professional) → berufloch

an error that the patient immediately and successfully corrected.
4. More salient are paraphasias that involve multiple substitutions independent of each other (Dressler, 1982), as in

      G. tropft (drops) → Topf

where the omissions (deletions) of the second phoneme /r/ and the final phoneme /t/ are independent of each other.

5. Most salient are phonological paraphasias that involve multiple interdependent substitutions, i.e., substitutions that cumulate in connection
with each other so that they are more likely to be noticed. An example
of the last type is as follows:

It. sigaretta (cigaret) → [risa 'get:a]

Here we can reconstruct the following two alternative error paths from
the intended word to the erroneous output via two metatheses:

/siga/ → [gisa] *or* /sigare/ → [rigase]
[gisare] → [risage]     [rigase] → [risage]

In both alternatives the two metatheses involved are interdependent,
i.e., the second metathesis presupposes the first one (or the first metathesis "feeds" the second one).

G. Mittwoch (wednesday) ['mItvOx] → ['fIdOx]

The simplest error path is made up by the two interdependent substitutions:

replacive anticipation /mItvOx/ → ['vItOx]
voicing metathesis [vItOx] → ['fIdOx]

An alternative but longer error path would be as follows:

assimilation /mItvOx/ → ['mItfOx]
replacive anticipation ['mItfOx] → ['fItOx]
intervocalic voicing ['fItOx] → ['fIdOx]

Of course, still more complicated error paths may be proposed, but in
any case the substitutions assumed cannot be enacted independently of
each other.

Our hypotheses predict that paraphasias that involve multiple interdependent substitutions are more often corrected than those that involve
multiple independent or simple substitutions only. This theory holds for
the data in Table 12.3, although the trends are not statistically significant.

TABLE 12.3. Repair of multiple substitution paraphasias.

| Condition | Independent (No.) | Interdependent (No.) |
|---|---|---|
| Viennese substitutions | | |
|   Corrected | 38 | 47 |
|   Not corrected | 23 | 15 |
| Paduan substitutions | | |
|   Corrected | 15 | 12 |
|   Not corrected | 71 | 31 |

# Discussion

Even when we are able to corroborate our predictions with statistically significant results, we must concede that our analysis of repairs presupposes the assumption of substitutions that correspond either to processes of slips (e.g., anticipations) or to universal natural phonological processes. There is independent evidence that the substitutions assumed by us are not mere artifacts of our analysis, as aphasics often seem to rely on such substitutions during repair. A successful strategy of successive phonological approximations (repair) consists in, for example, reenacting backward the phonological substitutions assumed by our reconstructive analysis of error paths from intended source to erroneous output.

We assumed (above) the two substitution processes of /r/ deletion and /t/ deletion in the error path:

$$\text{G. tropft (drops)} \rightarrow \text{Topf (pot)}$$

The Wernicke patient, in his successive approximations, exhibited the following:

$$\text{einen Topf}\ldots\text{einen Topft}\ldots\text{na, tropft (a (acc.) pot}\ldots\text{a)}$$
$$\text{(pot-t}\ldots\text{no, drops)}$$

He thus seemed to roll back or reenact backward the two deletion substitutions, one after the other.

# Summary

In this overview we briefly discussed two aspects of an ongoing project of contrasting (1) speech errors (lapsus, slips of the tongue) and phonological paraphasias in general and (2) in German versus Italian in particular. The first aspect was the different distribution of simplification and complication of syllable structure in slips and paraphasias. The second concerned phenomena of repair (successive approximations) and the likelihood of their occurrence.

# References

Baars, B.J. (1980). The competing plans hypothesis: a heuristic viewpoint on the causes of errors in speech. In H. Dechert & M. Raupach (eds.), *Temporal Variables in Speech: Studies in Honor of Frieda Goldman-Eisler*. The Hague: Mouton, pp. 39–40.

Berg, T. (1987). *A Cross-Linguistic Comparison of Slips of the Tongue*. Bloomington: Indiana University Linguistics Club.

Berg, T. (1988). *Die Abbildung des Sprachproduktionsprozesses in einem Aktivationsflußmodell: Untersuchungen an deutschen und englischen Versprechern*. Tübingen: Niemeyer.

Blumstein, S. (1973). *A Phonological Investigation of Aphasic Speech*. The Hague: Mouton.

Dressler, W. (1974). Aphasie und Theorie der Phonologie. *Incontri Linguistici, 1*, 9–20.

Dressler, W. (1976). Tendenzen in kontaminatorischen Fehlleistungen (und ihre Beziehung zur Sprachgeschichte). *Die Sprache, 22*, 1–10.

Dressler, W. (1982). A classification of phonological paraphasias. *Wiener Linguistische Gazette, 29*, 3–16. (Revised in Dressler & Stark, 1988.)

Dressler, W. (1984). Explaining natural phonology. *Phonology Yearbook, 1*, 29–53.

Dressler, W. (1985). *Morphonology*. Ann Arbor: Karoma Press.

Dressler, W., Magno Caldognetto, E., & Tonelli, L. (1986). Phonologische Fehlleistungen und Paraphasien im Deutschen und Italienischen. *Grazer Linguistische Studien, 26*, 43–57.

Dressler, W., Tonelli, L., & Magno Caldognetto, E. (1987). Analisi contrastiva dei lapsus e delle parafasie fonologiche rispetto alla sillaba. In W. Dressler, C. Grassi, R. Rindler Schjerve, & M. Stegu (eds.), *Parallela 3*. Tübingen: Narr, pp. 54–60.

Dressler, W., & Stark, J. (eds.) (1988). *Linguistic Studies in Aphasia*. New York: Springer.

Fromkin, V.A. (ed.) (1973). *Speech Errors as Linguistic Evidence*. The Hague: Mouton.

Joanette, Y., Keller, E., & Roch Lecours, A. (1980). Sequences of phonemic approximations in aphasia. *Brain and Language, 11*, 30–44.

Kilani-Schoch, M. (1982). *Processus Phonologiques, Processus Morphologiques et Lapsus dans un Corpus Aphasique*. Bern: Lang.

Levelt, W.J.M. (1983). Monitoring and self-repair in speech. *Cognition, 14*, 41–104.

Magno Caldognetto, E., Tonelli, L., & Luciani, N. (1986). Lapsus e parafasie a confronto: classificazione e distribuzione. *Acta Phoniatrica Latina, 9*, 51–59.

Meringer, R. (1908). *Aus dem Leben der Sprache: Versprechen, Kindersprache, Nachahmungstrieb*. Berlin: Behr.

Meringer, R., & Mayer, K. (1895). *Verprechen und Verlesen: Eine psychologisch-linguistische Studie*. Stuttgart: Göschen.

Nespoulous, J-L. Joanette, Y., Béland, R., Caplan, D., & Roch Lecours, A. (1984). Phonologic disturbances in aphasia: is there a "markedness effect" in aphasic phonetic errors? *Advances in Neurology, 42*, 203–214.

Söderpalm, E. (1979). *Speech Errors in Normal and Pathological Speech*. Malmö: Gleerup.

Stampe, D. (1969). The acquisition of phonetic representation. *Papers of the 5th Regional Meeting, Chicago Linguistic Society*, pp. 443–454.

Stemberger, J.P. (1985). *The Lexicon in a Model of Language Production*. New York: Garland.

Wurzel, W.U., & Böttcher, R. (1979). Konsonantencluster, phonologische Komplexität und aphasische Störungen. In M. Bierwisch (ed.), *Psychologische Effekte sprachlicher Strukturkomponenten*. Berlin, DDR: Akademie Verlag, pp. 401–445.

# 13
# Syllable Structure in Wernicke's Aphasia

Heinz Karl Stark and Jacqueline A. Stark

Analysis of speech production of Wernicke's aphasics confronts one, at first glance, with nearly unsolvable problems on all linguistic levels of analysis. Linguistic theory is thus greatly challenged when accounting for the symptomatology of Wernicke's aphasics. We believe that linguistic theory can help explain one of the most interesting and puzzling phenomena in aphasic symptomatology, i.e., neologistic jargon. In the present study we analyzed the performance of two aphasics who produce phonemic jargon on a repetition and a naming task. The aim of this investigation was to elucidate the interactions between prosodic and morphosyntactic structures of neologisms and paraphasias within the framework of metrical phonology. In particular, we addressed the following questions: (1) Is there a hierarchy of impairment for the various constituents of syllable structure? (2) In what ways do the various levels/components interact on the prosodic and morphosyntactic hierarchy?

In phonemic jargon, stress and intonation patterns are considered to be relatively unimpaired, as is the proper application of phonemic sequence structure rules or phonotactics (Dressler, 1985). Among stretches of speech composed of either semantic or phonemic jargon, i.e., neologisms, jargon aphasics produce comprehensible words. Most impaired in these aphasics is the selection of the proper target phonemes of major lexical items. Intonation contours and stress patterns are also relatively intact (Butterworth, 1985; but see Cooper and Zurif, 1983; Danly, Cooper, and Shapiro, 1983). Additionally, affixes or endings of words have been demonstrated to be better preserved (Blumstein, 1973; Buckingham and Kertesz, 1976). Thus even in passages of jargon, certain structures are relatively preserved, e.g., syllable structures, stress or rhythmic patterns or relative prominence relations (strong/weak) between the syllables in phonological neologisms, and the metrical foot structure of the target word. Several rules are also correctly applied, including language-specific sequence structure rules or phonotactic rules.

Consider the following neologism "Schnafenarber ['Snafən''arbɛɐ] for "Flasche+n+öffn+er" (bottle opener) taken from a repetition task (pa-

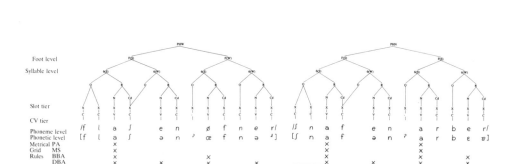

FIGURE 13.1. Example of a neologism produced by patient J.E.

tient J.E.). In this example (Fig. 13.1), the phonological neologism is not severely impaired on the underlying representational (UR) level, where segments are represented by categorical or underspecified feature matrices. However, it is severely impaired on the lexical representational (LR) level and on the superficial representational (SR) level, where the minimal feature specification of consonants and vowels takes place. The syllable structure of this neologism matches that of the target item. The foot structure is also intact, although the prominence relations on the foot level are impaired. The most impaired structure is the morphosyntactic structure: The root morphemes of the target item are neologistic, although the affixes can be reconstructed with caution. If we consider the preserved and impaired structures in the above neologism we can conclude that there are different cues available for the analyses of neologisms in reconstructing the target items in addition to the pragmatic context or grammatical category information (e.g., affixes).

## Nonlinear Aphasia Studies

In many of the studies on phonology in jargon aphasia, linear generative phonological theories based on sound patterns of English (Chomsky and Halle, 1968) or natural phonology (Dressler, 1985, 1988) have been applied. Although some investigations cover the prosodic dimensions (e.g., intonation, stress, duration, pitch) and the morphosyntactic structures, there is still a gap in integrating the different independent but interacting components in a representation model (van der Hulst and Smith, 1985).

We believe that this gap can be filled by applying nonlinear metrical phonology to the study of aphasia because this theory provides an elaborate system of representation of the levels and units that can be selectively/simultaneously impaired in aphasics. The nonlinear phonological studies on aphasia—although they are fairly rare to date—support this claim (Béland, Caplan, and Nespoulous, in press; Dogil, 1985; Stark, Deutsch, Stark, and Wytek, 1988).

## Basic Theoretical Concepts of Metrical Phonology

Because we analyze the data in terms of the syllable structure, we briefly describe how this structure is treated in metrical theory (Hayes, 1984; Selkirk, 1984).

### Prosodic Hierarchy

The prosodic hierarchy represents a modified tree structure of the phonological word as the highest node in the tree, which consists of metrical feet, syllables, or both. A metrical foot consists of at least two and at most three syllables. The metrical foot dominates the syllable. The syllable, as a basic language-processing unit for speech perception and production (Robinson, 1977; Treiman, 1983; Troyer-Spoehr and Smith, 1973), has a constituent structure that is considered to be hierarchical. It is composed of the onset and rhyme; the rhyme, in turn, is defined as the nucleus and coda of a syllable. If, for example, a phonological word has two feet (at least four syllables), the relative prominence of the syllables is labeled strong/weak (s/w) or weak/strong (w/s).

The nucleus is the only obligatory syllable constituent (Treiman, 1983). It always consists of at least one segment. The onset and the coda can have no segments or more than one segment. These syllable constituents are attached to the segment slots on the slot tier or skeleton tier. The slots are timing units in which the sound segments are to be inserted or, rather, connected because they are placed on the CV tier or melodic tier (Béland et al., in press; van der Hulst and Smith, 1985). As is the case with metrical feet, syllables also alternate in their stress relations or relative strength strong/weak or weak/strong. A tier for distinctive feature matrices can be attached to the CV tier, which in turn is associated with the skeleton tier (Hogg and McCully, 1987).

### Morphosyntactic Hierarchy

The morphosyntactic hierarchy, connected to the slot tier, is independently attached to the segment slots. (Aspects of the metrical grid and foot structure are referred to only in the examples. These data will be reported in a follow-up study.) Having laid out this background, we now turn to our repetition and naming experiment.

## Procedures

### Subjects

Data from two Wernicke's aphasics are analyzed in this study.[1] Both patients produced phonemic jargon in spontaneous speech, naming, and repetition; and auditory comprehension was moderately impaired as assessed by a standardized aphasia examination.

Patient 1 (J.E.) is a 70-year-old retired baker with 9 years of schooling. He suffered a cerebrovascular accident (CVA) 2 months prior to the testing reported here. Based on results from the Aachen Aphasia Test (AAT), his language impairment is best characterized as Wernicke's aphasia, with severe to moderate impairment.

Patient 2 (O.R.) is a 57-year-old high school graduate who was a tour guide prior to his CVA. He was tested 6 months after onset for the present analyses. O.R.'s language impairment is also best described as a severely to moderately impaired Wernicke's aphasic (determined by the AAT).

Extensive language testing was carried out on both patients, and the patients were found to be comparable in terms of their overall language impairment and lesion localization. Computed tomography revealed that both patients had a large lesion in the left temporal and parietal lobes.

### Methods

Each patient was tested twice with a 3-week interval between testing sessions. The responses were tape recorded on a Uher 4200 Report Stereo recorder and transcribed in a narrow phonetic transcription (according to the International Phonetic Alphabet). The test items are listed in Appendix 1. The naming and repetition tasks were carried out separately. The number of items included in the analysis differed minimally for each patient (J.E. 176 items, O.R. 169 items). The first response was scored. The control subject's pronunciation from the repetition task was used as a baseline for the analysis. The data were analyzed according to the structure of the target item: one- to five-syllable words consisting of one to five morphemes.

---

[1] The data reported on here stem from an ongoing aphasia project financed by the Austrian Research Foundation (Fonds zur Foerderung der wissenschaftlichen Forschung) (W. Dressler, J. Stark, H. Stark). A control subject was also tested (H.S.) to allow a comparison of specific variables including pitch accent, main stress, rhythmic alternation, and stress clash.

# Results

When interpreting the results on the syllable constituent structure level, we referred in a rather abstract manner to its preterminal interface, the slot or skeleton tier, with which the syllable constituents are connected. Impairment of, or changes in, the syllable constituents refer to changes on the slot tier with reference to the target item. A change in the syllable constituent means that the number of segments is increased (branching) or decreased (debranching, deletion). An example of branching from O.R.'s repetition data is the target item "buch" "book."

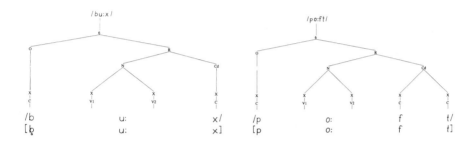

An example of debranching from J.E.'s repetition data is the target item "stift" "pencil" or "crayon."

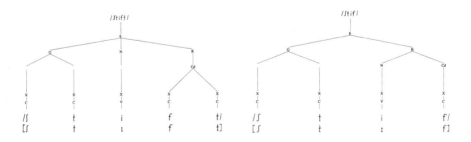

## *Overall Error Rate for Constituents of the Syllable Structure*

The two tests revealed no statistically significant results for the variables examined in this study. The data from the two sessions were pooled. In

254 of the 345 items tested (73.6%) a syllable showed impairment on the syllable structure level. It must be stressed that, although the syllable structure was intact—in particular the number of elements of the syllable constituents—on the syllable structure level in 24.6% of the cases, the aphasic's production was not necessarily correct in terms of the phonological level. In more than 50% of the cases in which a correct syllable structure was produced, the patients' response was a neologism. The example given in Figure 13.1 exemplifies this point. The syllable structure of the target word "flaschenoeffner" (bottle opener) was maintained; however, the response produced by J.E. was a neologism.

Regarding the question of whether any syllable constituent was impaired, a comparison of the items according to number of syllables revealed that in 67 items (56.2%) of the 117 one-syllable words a syllable was impaired in some way in the syllable structure constituents, 85 items (70.2%) of the 121 two-syllable words, 28 items (90.3%) of the 31 three-syllable words, and 54 items (96.4%) of the 56 four-syllable words; all of the 20 five-syllable words were impaired (Fig. 13.2). The rate of impairment is given in Table 13.1 for J.E. and O.R. according to the number of syllables of the target item (collapsed across syllable position). A syllable constituent was affected in 70.4% of the test items for J.E. (124 of 176) and in 76.9% (130 of 169) for O.R. The error rate is highly correlated with the number of syllables (chi-square after Pearson, DF 4, $p < .000$ for each patient). Overall, an increase in error rate is associated with an increase in number of syllables.

TABLE 13.1. Overall error rate of syllable structure constituents for each patient according to number of syllables of test items.

| No. of syllables | Error rate (%)[a] | | |
| --- | --- | --- | --- |
| | J.E. | O.R. | Mean |
| One | 54.2 | 60.3 | 56.2 |
| (n = 117) | (32/59) | (35/58) | (67/117) |
| Two | 63.5 | 77.6 | 70.2 |
| (n = 121) | (40/63) | (45/58) | (85/121) |
| Three | 100.0 | 81.3 | 90.3 |
| (n = 31) | (15/15) | (13/16) | (28/31) |
| Four | 93.0 | 100 | 96.4 |
| (n = 56) | (27/29) | (27/27) | (54/56) |
| Five | 100 | 100 | 100 |
| (n = 20) | (10/10) | (10/10) | (20/20) |
| Mean rate | 70.4 | 76.9 | 73.6 |
| | (124/176) | (130/169) | (254/345) |

[a] The error rates for J.E. and O.R. differ highly significantly for all numbers of syllables (Pearson chi-square, DF 4, $p < .000$).

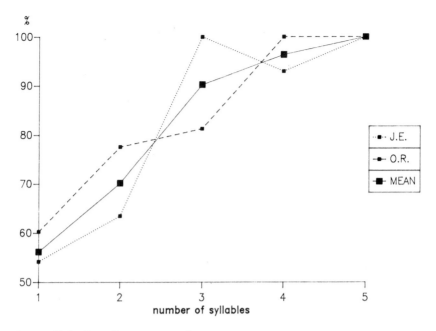

FIGURE 13.2. Overall mean rate of errors.

The syllable structure of one-syllable words was affected in 54.2% of the items in J.E.'s corpus and in 60.3% of the items in O.R.'s corpus. In contrast, not a single five-syllable item was correctly produced by either patient (10 of 10). Although O.R. made more errors than J.E., the increase in overall error rate as a function of syllable number was true of both patients. We therefore present pooled data, noting only exceptions.

## Total Error Rate for Onset, Nucleus, or Coda

The total number of errors for onset, nucleus, or coda are given in Table 13.2 and Figure 13.3 according to the number of syllables and the syllable position (collapsed for both patients and tasks). The one-syllable words show a mean error rate of 24.5%, two-syllable words 31.5%, three-syllable words 44.4%, four-syllable words 49.8%, and five-syllable words 58.7%. For the two-syllable words there is an 8% increase in the mean percentage of total errors from the first syllable to the second syllable of these items. The mean error rate for the first syllable is minimally increased in comparison with the one-syllable words (24.5% versus 27.6%).

The three-syllable items also show a minimal increase across the three syllables. The error rate for each syllable is still greater than that for the same position in the two-syllable items (27.6% versus 41.9% and 35.5% versus 44.0%). The mean error rate for the four-syllable words averaged

TABLE 13.2. Total number of errors (onset, nucleus, coda) on syllables according to number of syllables of test items and syllable position.

| No. of syllables | Errors by syllable position[a] | | | | | Mean rate | Significance |
|---|---|---|---|---|---|---|---|
| | 1 | 2 | 3 | 4 | 5 | | |
| One | 24.5 | | | | | 24.5 | |
| (n = 117) | (86) | | | | | | |
| | | | | | | | $p < .05$[b] |
| Two | 27.6 | 35.5 | | | | 31.5 | |
| (n = 121) | (100) | (129) | | | | | |
| | | | | | | | $p < .05$ |
| Three | 41.9 | 44.0 | 47.3 | | | 44.4 | |
| (n = 31) | (39) | (41) | (44) | | | | |
| | | | | | | | n.s. |
| Four | 50.6 | 44.7 | 57.7 | 46.3 | | 49.8 | |
| (n = 56) | (85) | (75) | (97) | (77) | | | |
| | | | | | | | n.s. |
| Five | 26.7 | 43.3 | 61.7 | 85.0 | 76.7 | 58.7 | |
| (n = 20) | (16) | (26) | (37) | (51) | (46) | | |
| Mean total | 34.3 | 41.9 | 55.6 | 65.6 | 76.7 | | |

[a] Statistically significant differences for syllable position for one- to five-syllable words for position 1 (K-W: $p < .000$) and for position 4 for four- and five-syllable words (K-W: $p < .000$).
[b] Two percentages were tested for significant differences. One-syllable words were compared with two-syllable words, etc.

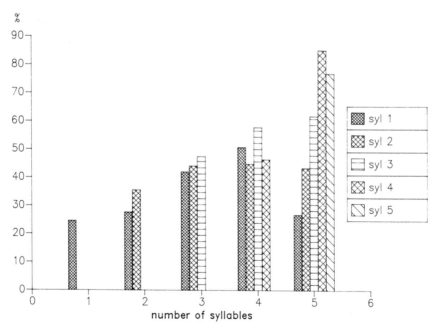

FIGURE 13.3. Total percent of errors.

across syllable positions shows a 5% increase over the three-syllable words and is double that of the one-syllable items. The error rate for the four-syllable positions reveals that the second and fourth syllables are less impaired than the first and third syllables. This pattern seems to correlate with the stress pattern of the items of this group, e.g., "tasch$e+n$+ lam$pe" (flashlight). The mean rate of total errors for onset, nucleus, or coda for the five-syllable words is 58.7%. There is a constant increase in number of errors from the first syllable to the fourth. The fifth syllable is less impaired than the fourth.

The mean total errors according to syllable position increases in pro-portion to the position of the syllable in the two- to five-syllable words. The first syllable is impaired in 34.3%, the second syllable in 41.9%, and the third in 55.6% of the items. Comparison of the first syllable position according to number of syllables of the items reveals an increase from one- to four-syllable words (24.5% → 27.6% → 41.9% → 50.6%). The first syllable position of the five-syllable words is an exception. We alluded to this situation previously. The differences between the first syllable position are statistically highly significant according to number of syllables of item (K-W, $p < .0006$). The second syllable position shows an increase from two- to three-syllable words but remains constant for the three- to five-syllable words. It is not statistically significant.

The error rate for the third syllable position reveals a steady increase from three- (47.3%) to four- (57.7%) to five-syllable (61.7%) items. This increase according to number of syllables, however, is not significant. The highest increase in error rate is for the four-syllable words with reference to syllable position four. This highly significant difference ($p < .0004$) amounts to almost 40%.

Summarizing Table 13.2 and Figure 13.3, the mean error rate for the one- to five-syllable items collapsed across syllable position and the mean total percentage of errors according to the first to fifth syllable position show a similar pattern: The greater the number of syllables of an item, the higher is the mean percentage of total errors. Moreover, the later a syllable is positioned in a two- to five-syllable word, the greater is the tendency for a syllable to be impaired. In both cases, the direction of the syllable struc-ture changes is the same. The longer the word, the higher is the percentage of total errors. Two exceptions have been noted. The first exception is the first syllable of the five-syllable items. Here we find an increase according to syllable position but not in terms of the first syllable position of five-syllable words in comparison to four-syllable words (four-syllable words 50.6% versus 26.7% of the five-syllable words). We can account for this pattern in terms of stress patterns, i.e., weak versus strong syllables.

The second exception noted is the alternation in the four-syllable words from more (50.6%) to less (44.7%) to more (57.7%) to less (46.3%) impaired. The example given in Figure 13.1 illustrates this point. This pattern goes in one direction, i.e., across the units of the four-syllable word. It does not affect the increase in error rate from three-syllable to four-syllable words according to syllable position. (The decrease for syllable position two from four- to five-syllable items (44.7% to 43.7%) is marginal.)

## Simultaneous Impairment of the Onset, Nucleus, and Coda

The error rates given in Table 13.2 and Figure 13.3 refer to all errors made on a particular syllable. In contrast, the simultaneous impairment of onset, nucleus, and coda represents a more severe error. Only three items of the 117 one-syllable words—onset, nucleus, and coda—were simultaneously impaired (2.6%). In words of two or more syllables the stability of these three components decreases according to the number of syllables of the item. The mean error rate for one-syllable words is 2.6%, for two-syllable words 9.0%, for three-syllable words 21.5%, for four-syllable words 31.3%, and for five-syllable words 43.0%. All three components are more impaired the later a syllable is positioned in a word: 12.2% rate of simultaneous impairment for syllable one, 15.8% for syllable two, 34.6% for syllable three, 40.8% for syllable four, and 60% for syllable five.

## Simultaneous Impairment of the Nucleus and Coda

The rhyme is considered to consist of the nucleus and coda of a syllable. The nucleus was shown to be the least impaired and the coda the most impaired syllable constituent. The error rate for simultaneous impairment of these constituents thus gives us the rate of impairment for the rhyme of a syllable. The mean error rate for simultaneous impairment of nucleus and coda collapsed across syllable position is 6.8% for one-syllable items (8 of 117), 20.2% for two-syllable words, 30.1% for three-syllable words, 37.5% for four-syllable words, and 51.0% for five-syllable words. With regard to syllable position: The later a syllable in an item is, the more the rhyme is impaired (18.8% for position one to 65% for syllable position five). The onset is more impaired than the rhyme (simultaneous impairment of nucleus and coda).

## Mean Error Rate for Patient J.E. versus Patient O.R.

In Table 13.2 and Figure 13.3 we collapsed the patient data for onset, nucleus, or coda because an increase in errors was observed for these syllable structures. Does the steady progression in error rate of the items of greater number of syllables hold up in comparisons of the two patients? In Table 13.1 and Figure 13.2, the results are given for each patient in terms of whether any syllable was affected. The types of errors made by the

TABLE 13.3. Mean error rate for onset, nucleus, and coda for
J.E. versus O.R. according to number of syllables of test items
(collapsed across syllable position).

| No. of syllables | Error rate (%) | | | | | |
|---|---|---|---|---|---|---|
| | Onset | | Nucleus | | Coda | |
| | J.E. | O.R. | J.E. | O.R. | J.E. | O.R. |
| One (n = 117) | 25.4 | 15.5 | 18.6 | 5.2 | 30.5 | 51.7 |
| Two (n = 121) | 30.2 | 28.5 | 27.0 | 25.9 | 31.8 | 46.6 |
| Three (N = 31) | 48.9 | 39.6 | 37.8 | 27.1 | 60.0 | 54.2 |
| Four (n = 56) | 42.3 | 63.9 | 31.0 | 51.7 | 44.8 | 66.7 |
| Five (n = 20) | 52.0 | 66.0 | 54.0 | 56.0 | 56.0 | 68.0 |

patients are not specified: Is it the case that the same error frequency holds
for both patients for the onset, nucleus, and coda; or do they have a different hierarchy of susceptibility with reference to the syllable structures?
We addressed this question in Table 13.3 and Figure 13.4. The mean error
rate for onset, nucleus, and coda errors are given (collapsed across syllable
position) for J.E. and O.R. separately.

The pattern of errors presented in Table 13.2 and Figure 13.3 also
mirrors the patients' mean error rate (except for three-syllable words for
J.E. and the coda for O.R. in two-syllable words). There is an increase in
error rate for all three-syllable constituents: onset, nucleus, and coda in
relation to the number of syllables of an item. This pattern is clearer in
O.R. His mean error rate for onset increased from 15.5% for one-syllable
words, to 28.5% for two-syllable words, to 39.6% for three-syllable words,
to 63.9% for four-syllable words, to 66.0% for five-syllable words. The
nucleus also shows this progression, although the nucleus of the one-
syllable words is much less impaired than the onset and coda. The nucleus
is impaired in only 5.2% of the one-syllable words, whereas it is impaired
in 25.9% of the two-syllable words, 27.1% of the three-syllable words,
51.7% of the four-syllable words, and 56.0% of the five-syllable words.
The coda is the most impaired syllable constituent structure for O.R. It is

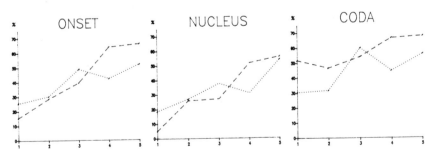

FIGURE 13.4. Mean error rate for onset, nucleus, and coda (patients J.E. and O.R.)

impaired in 51.7% of the one-syllable items, 46.6% of the two-syllable items, 54.2% of the three-syllable items, 66.7% of the four-syllable items, and 68.0% of the five-syllable items.

Patient J.E. displayed overall the same pattern of errors as O.R.; i.e., he showed an increase in error rate in relation to the number of syllables of the items. He also showed the same overall pattern, whereby the nucleus was least impaired followed by onset; the most impaired syllable structure is the coda. The error rates for J.E. for the syllable onset from one- to five-syllable words are 25.4% → 30.2% → 48.9% → 42.3% → 52.0%. J.E.'s mean error rate for the nucleus was initially higher than that of O.R. for the one-syllable words (18.6%), and it increased to 27.0% for the two-syllable words, to 37.8% for the three-syllable words, to 31.0% for the four-syllable words, to 54.0% for the five-syllable items. The coda was less impaired in J.E. than in O.R. except for the three-syllable words. It was impaired in 30.5% of the one-syllable words, 31.8% of the two-syllable words, 60.0% of the three-syllable words, 44.8% of the four-syllable words, and 56.0% of the five-syllable words. J.E.'s pattern of errors differed from the expected progression in that the three-syllable words were more impaired than the four- and sometimes the five-syllable words in terms of the syllable constituent structure. Words such as "schuhloeffel" (shoe horn) were more difficult for J.E. than four-syllable items such as "zwetschenknoedel" (plum dumplings). This finding is consistent for all syllable structure constituents.

## Syllable Deletion and Syllable Epenthesis

The most severe case of distortion of the syllable constituent structure in reference to the target item is syllable deletion and syllable epenthesis. These errors are devastating because they not only change the syllable structure, they also affect the metrical grid, i.e., the metrical foot and the rhythmic pattern. Syllables were deleted in 28.9% of the items (66 of 228), which means that more than one-fourth of the syllables were deleted. Syllable deletion was statistically significantly more in items consisting of three or more syllables. One or more syllables were deleted in 50.0% of the four- and five-syllable words. Syllable epenthesis is found in only a few instances (19 of 345, 5.5%). However, one-syllable items were even changed into two-syllable words.

## Influence of Morpheme Structure and Rhythmic Pattern on Syllable Constituent Structure Impairment

In the previous sections, the rate of impairment of the syllable constituent structures was analyzed in terms of the number of syllables and the position of a syllable in an item. The role of morphosemantic/morphosyntactic and rhythmical structure in the processing of syllable constituents was only indirectly alluded to at various points. However, when interpreting the data presented in Table 13.2, the influence of morpheme and rhythmical structure on the patients' performance becomes evident.

The two-syllable nouns, for example, consist of two types of morpheme structure: (1) two syllables equal one morpheme, as in the item "spra$che" (language) and (2) two syllables equal two morphemes, e.g., the item "hand+schuh" (glove). The second type is a compound noun with a greater degree of morphosemantic transparency. The difference in morpheme structure (and rhythmic pattern) between the two groups of two-syllable items is an important one with relation to whether any error is made on the different two-syllable words: In 57.5% of the items with the morpheme structure 1 some error was made. In contrast, in 91.5% of the morpheme structure 2 items some error affecting the syllable structure was made. Although the percentage for group 1 is already high, the two-syllable items of the morpheme structure 2 have almost the same error rate as the most difficult morpheme structures (90.5%, 97.6%, 94.4%, and 100.0% for the most complex morpheme structure). The cutoff point for correction production appears to be at the morpheme structure 2 level. Closer consideration of these examples reveals the following error pattern for the onset, nucleus, and coda of these two-syllable items.

|  | Morpheme structure 1 (%) | Morpheme structure 2 (%) |
|---|---|---|
| Onset 1 | 18.9 | 27.7 |
| Onset 2 | 25.7 | 53.2 |
| Nucleus 1 | 14.9 | 29.8 |
| Nucleus 2 | 25.7 | 42.6 |
| Coda 1 | 31.1 | 53.2 |
| Coda 2 | 36.5 | 40.4 |

Although both item types have two syllables, more errors are made on the morpheme structure 2 items. In these examples, the two consecutive syllables are isomorphic. As such, they are semantically heavy in terms of information load. In the morpheme structure type 1, the second syllable is a weak one. The influence of factors other than the number of syllables is thus demonstrated by the differential susceptibility of the syllable structure units.

In a further analysis we compared the same items with reference to impairment of metrical foot structure. In these terms the two-syllable groups differed highly significantly (chi-square, DF 2, $p < .000$; M-W $p < .000$): The first group (e.g., "sprache") showed impairment in 5.4% of the items (4 of 74) and the second group (e.g., "rindfleisch") in 37.1% of the compound words (13 of 35). Therefore the number of syllables is not the only factor determining the rate of impairment of the metrical foot. The difference in structure of the two syllables is also reflected in the syllable deletion rate. Syllables were deleted in 6.8% of the items in the first group and in 17.1% in the second group.

With reference to the three-syllable items, their structure varied. In some examples, the first and second syllables are semantically and prosodically heavy as in, for example, "spar$buech$se" (piggy bank) in contrast to the third syllable, which is unstressed. There are other three-syllable items with a semantically heavy third syllable, e.g., "re$gen$schirm" (umbrella) or "tasch$e+n$+tuch" (handkerchief). The difference in structure of the three-syllable items might be the reason for the evenly distributed error rate across the three syllables (41.9%, 44.0%, 47.3%, respectively). These three-syllable items were difficult for patient J.E.

As mentioned previously, the error rate for the four syllable positions reveals that the second and fourth syllables are less impaired than the first and third syllable (Table 13.2 and Fig. 13.1). This pattern seems to correlate with the stress pattern of the items of this group, e.g., "tasch$e+n$+lam$pe" (flashlight). In the examples of this morpheme structure the first and third syllables are strong ones and are semantically heavy, and the second and fourth syllables are the weak ones [affixes, or (C)V structure]. The strong syllables bearing main stress and secondary stress display greater impairment in the coda than in syllables 2 and 4, which are both weak.

With reference to the five-syllable words, the last syllable is an unstressed, or weak, one in terms of its morphosemantic structure and its prosodic structure: -el, -er, -ung. The last syllable of these items is often deleted. The five-syllable group of items consists of words with varying stress patterns and semantic weight. The first syllable is also an unstressed, or weak, one in several of the test items, e.g., the unseparable prefix "be," in "belichtungsmesser" (exposure meter). In the examples with an unstressed first syllable, the syllable structure of the first syllable is unimpaired, whereas in the five-syllable items in which the first syllable is stressed, e.g., "fleischpreissteigerung" (increase in meat price) or "sicherheitsnadel" (safety pin), the first syllable is impaired. In Figure 13.5 we present the patients' production of the item "belichtungsmesser." The first unstressed syllable is intact, although there are other errors in these responses.

In summary, particularly the two-, three-, and five-syllable word groups include items that show a confounding of the number of syllables, stress pattern, and morpheme structure. Comparison of the error rates shows that this confounding of various factors has an effect on the overall processing of a word item.

## Naming Versus Repetition

No statistically significant differences were found for either patient between the naming and repetition tasks. In general, more errors were made on the

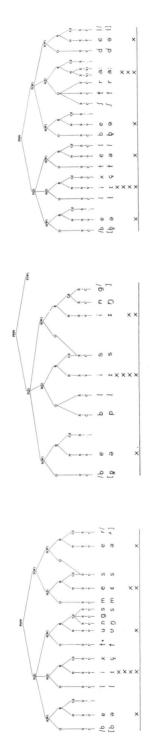

FIGURE 13.5. Comparison of a neologism produced by patient J.E. and patient O.R. in the repetition task for the target item "belichtungsmesser" (exposure meter).

naming task than on the repetition task. More examples are necessary for the naming task to address the issue of task-specific differences, as 25% of the items are from naming, in contrast to 75% from repetition.


## Discussion

With reference to the analysis of speech production of Wernicke's jargon aphasics within the framework of metrical phonology, we attempted to elucidate the following questions: In what way is the syllable constituent structure affected on the slot tier? Is it the case that (1) onset, nucleus, and coda are equally prone to impairment; or (2) onset and rhyme show the same error frequency?

The results from our study support the claim that difficulties in processing increase in relation to the structure and number of syllables and that the later a syllable occurs in a word the greater the probability of its impairment and deletion. The results also show that the various constituents of a syllable differ in their susceptibility to error. The patterns are pretty regular for both patients. The nucleus is the most stable, i.e., least impaired, syllable constituent structure followed by the onset. The coda is the most impaired structure. The rhyme is less impaired than the onset.

The distribution of errors illustrates that J.E. and O.R. were sensitive to structural variables even on the abstract level of syllable constituent structure: nucleus > onset > coda. Although their responses were often neologistic, their performance did not reflect "de novo organization" of unimpaired mechanisms with reference to the hierarchy of the syllable constituent structure. Thus our patients' performance confirms the assumption that the syllable is hierarchically organized. Moreover, the patients' data reflect the hierarchy postulated in phonological theory (Lass, 1985; Selkirk, 1984) and in the psycholinguistic literature (Treiman, 1983; Wijnen, 1988).

Exceptions to a steady increase in rate of impairment according to the number of syllables of an item were mentioned. These differences can be interpreted with reference to different "strategies" used by the patients and with regard to other confounding variables, such as morpheme structure and rhythmical pattern of the target items. These variables interact with the syllable constituent structure.

With reference to possible differences in "strategy," J.E. and O.R. revealed differences in processing three-syllable words. J.E. was less successful than O.R. in producing these items. He appeared to have relied on rhythmical factors: Either he deleted one of the syllables, e.g., in "sparbüchse", "piggy bank"

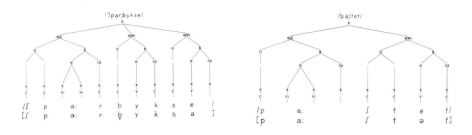

or he inserted a syllable, e.g., the item "schuhlöffel", "shoe horn."

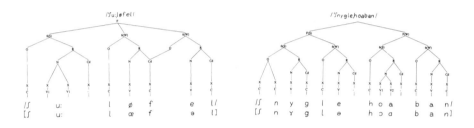

In both cases he produced a neologism. In both instances the patient's response was more rhythmical.

For the same item type, O.R. produced either three-syllable structures (mainly neologisms or phonological paraphasias), e.g., the item "schuhlöffel", "shoe horn."

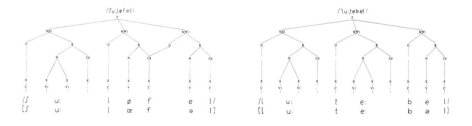

or he deleted a syllable, as in the item "shoe horn."

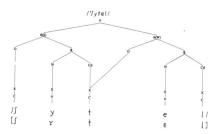

The patients were not substantially different in their overall performance. J.E. was more successful in the production of one- and two-syllable
words than O.R.; that is, he made fewer errors on the syllable structure
constituents (Tables 13.1 and 13.3; Figures 13.2 and 13.3). One- and
two-syllable words (nouns) consisting of one or two morphemes were
the easiest for both patients to produce. However, it made a difference
whether the target item was a two-syllable one-morpheme noun or a
two-syllable two-morpheme word. Not only did the complexity of the
syllable structures play a decisive role in whether an error was made on an
item, so did the higher degree of morphological and semantic information
to be processed (Dressler, 1988; Dressler, Mayerthaler, Panagl, and
Wurzel, 1987). Although the morphosemantic transparency of the two-
syllable two-morpheme items is greater than in the two-syllable one-
morpheme items, more errors were made on the former ones. From the
present results, a higher degree of morphosemantic transparency did not
make an item easier for J.E. and O.R. to process.

With reference to the two-morpheme items, i.e., compound nouns,
consisting of two syllables, the patients' difficulties in repetition are illustrated in the following examples. O.R. repeated the word "reisfleisch"
(rice and meat dish) as:

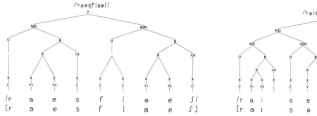

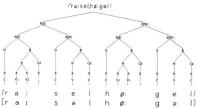

O.R. inserted two syllables and created a four-syllable neologism consisting of two trochaic feet (strong/weak). On the same item, J.E. also reduced the complexity of the syllable structures, but his neologism consisted of two syllables:

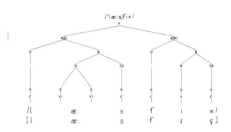

In other examples he inserted one or two syllables: "fleischpreis" (meat price) → ['Slaɛs,pœlsə].

The role of stress or rhythmic relative prominence must be taken into account when interpreting neologisms. They often display the same rhythmic pattern or parts of it as in the target. In repetition, it is important for items in which the first syllable bears main stress or in which the third syllable has main stress or second degree rhythmic prominence. In those cases rhythmic prominence does not result in fewer errors because these syllables are semantically heavy, i.e., content- or information-bearing units. In contrast, the weak syllables were retained in complex items, e.g., in the repetition of five-syllable items such as "belichtungsmesser" (Fig. 13.5).

In summary, although we focused our attention on the syllable constituent structure in this study, the concepts of nonlinear metrical phonology (Hayes, 1984; Selkirk, 1984; van der Hulst and Smith, 1985) were useful in providing a more adequate description of the jargon aphasic's performance and in particular the interaction among the prosodic and morphosyntactic hierarchies as postulated in metrical phonology.

*Acknowledgments.* We are greatly indebted to Ruth Kramer Ostrin for her constructive comments on the data, especially for helping us to see the forest *and* the trees among the syllable structure constituents. We also thank Rudolf Wytek for his statistical advice and Hans Fellbacher and Ilse Haaslinger for the computer program for representing the tree structure.

# References

Béland, R., Caplan, D., & Nespoulous, J-L. (in press). Phonological constraints on phonemic paraphasias in a case of reproduction conduction aphasia.

Blumstein, S. (1973). *A phonological Investigation of Aphasic Speech*. The Hague: Mouton.

Buckingham, H., & Kertesz, A. (1976). *Neologistic Jargon Aphasia*. Amsterdam: Swets & Zeitlinger.

Butterworth, B. (1985). Jargon aphasia: processes and strategies. In S. Newton & R. Epstein (eds.), *Current Perspectives in Dysphasia*. Edinburgh: Churchill Livingstone, pp. 61–96.

Chomsky, N., & Halle, M. (1968). *The Sound Pattern of English*. New York: Harper & Row.

Cooper, W.E., & Zurif, E. (1983). Aphasia information processing in language production and reception. In B. Butterworth (ed.), *Language Production*. Vol. 2. New York: Academic Press.

Danly, M., Cooper, W.E., & Shapiro, B. (1983). Fundamental frequency, language processing, and linguistic structure in Wernicke's aphasia. *Brain and Language*, *19*, 1–24.

Dogil, G. (1984). Nonlinear phonology in the area of speech and grammar pathology. In H. van der Hulst & N. Smith (eds.), *Advances in Nonlinear Phonology*. Dordrecht: Foris, pp. 161–178.

Dogil, G. (1985). Theory of markedness in nonlinear phonology. *Wiener Linguistische Gazette*, *24*, 3–21.

Dressler, W. (1985). Morphonology. Ann Arbor: Karoma Press.

Dressler, W. (1988). A linguistic classification of phonological paraphasias. In W.U. Dressler & J. Stark (eds.), *Linguistic Analyses of Aphasic Language*. New York: Springer Verlag, pp. 1–23.

Dressler, W., Mayerthaler, W., Panagl, O., & Wurzel, W. (1987). *Leitmotifs in Natural Morphology*. Amsterdam: John Benjamins.

Hayes, B. (1984). The phonology of rhythm. *Linguistic Inquiry*, *15*, 33–74.

Hogg, R., & McCulley, C.B. (1987). *Metrical Phonology: A Coursebook*. New York: Cambridge University Press.

Huber, W., Poeck, K., Weniger, D., & Willmes, K. (1983). *Aachener-Aphasie-Test (AAT)*. Goettingen: Hogrefe.

Lass, R. (1985). *Phonology: An Introduction into Basic Concepts*. London: Cambridge University Press.

Robinson, G.M. (1977). Rhythmic organization in speech processing. *Journal of Experimental Psychology: Human Perception and Performance*, *3*, 83–91.

Selkirk, E.D. (1984). *Phonology and Syntax: The Relation Between Sound and Structure*. Cambridge, MA: MIT Press.

Stark, H., Deutsch, W., Stark, J., & Wytek, R. (1988). Improvement of coarticulation in Broca's aphasia. In W.U. Dressler & J. Stark (eds.), *Linguistic Analyses of Aphasic Language*. New York: Springer Verlag, pp. 23–50.

Treiman, R. (1983). The structure of spoken syllables: evidence from novel word games. *Cognition*, *15*, 49–74.

Troyer-Spoehr, K., and Smith, E. (1973). The role of syllables in perceptual processing. *Cognitive Psychology*, *5*, 71–89.

Van der Hulst, H., & Smith, N. (eds.) (1985). *Advances in Nonlinear Phonology.* Dordrecht: Foris.

Wijnen, F. (1988). Spontaneous word fragmentation in children: evidence for the syllable as a unit in speech production. *Journal of Phonetics*, *16*, 187–202.

# Appendix 1: List of Test Items for the Repetition and Naming Task

| Test items | Repetition | Naming |
|---|---|---|
| One-syllable words (n = 27) | | |
| Buch (book) | + | |
| Bruch (breach, break) | + | |
| Dach (roof) | + | |
| Fass (barrel) | + | |
| Fest (festival, party) | + | |
| Fleisch (meat) | + | |
| Frass (feed, gluttony) | + | |
| Frist (deadline) | + | |
| Geld (money) | + | + |
| Ring (ring) | + | + |
| Rumpf (trunk, torso) | + | |
| Schach (chess) | + | |
| Schacht (shaft) | + | |
| Schlacht (battle) | + | |
| Schlich (by-way, secret way) | + | |
| Schloss (lock) | + | + |
| Schuh (shoe) | + | + |
| Schutt (rubble, refuse) | + | |
| Spruch (saying) | + | |
| Stadt (city) | + | |
| Stich (sting) | + | |
| Stift (pencil, convent) | + | |
| Strich (line) | + | |
| Strumpf (stocking) | + | |
| Taft (taffeta) | + | |
| Trumpf (trump card) | + | |
| Uhr (watch, clock) | + | + |
| Two-syllable words (n = 22) | | |
| Brille (eyeglasses) | + | + |
| Drache (kite, dragon) | + | |
| Fleischpreis (meat price) | + | |
| Gehstock (walking stick, cane) | + | + |
| Handschuh (glove) | + | + |
| Kalbfleisch (veal) | + | |
| Kluppe (clothes pin) | + | + |
| Knoedel (dumpling) | + | |
| Loeffel (spoon) | + | |
| Messer (knife) | + | |
| Muenzen (coins) | + | + |
| Patschen (slippers) | + | + |

| Test items | Repetition | Naming |
|---|---|---|
| Pfeife (smoking pipe) | + | + |
| Rache (revenge) | + | |
| Reisfleisch (meat and rice dish) | + | |
| Rindfleisch (beef) | + | |
| Schachtel (box) | + | + |
| Schluessel (key) | + | + |
| Schuerze (apron) | + | + |
| Sprache (language) | + | |
| Strohhalm (straw) | + | + |
| Strudel (pastry) | + | |
| Three-syllable words (n = 6) | | |
| Blechloeffel (brass spoon) | + | |
| Regenschirm (umbrella) | + | + |
| Schoepfloeffel (ladle) | + | |
| Schuhloeffel (shoe horn) | + | |
| Sparbuechse (piggy bank) | + | + |
| Taschentuch (handkerchief) | + | + |
| Four-syllable words (n = 10) | | |
| Aschenbecher (ashtray) | + | + |
| Dosenoeffner (can opener) | + | + |
| Fiebermesser (thermometer) | + | + |
| Flaschenoeffner (bottle opener) | + | + |
| Kirschenstrudel (cherry pastry) | + | |
| Rasiermesser (shaver's knife) | + | |
| Semmelknoedel (bread dumpling) | + | |
| Taschenlampe (flashlight) | + | + |
| Topfenstrudel (cream cheese pastry) | + | |
| Zwetschenknoedel (plum dumpling) | + | |
| Five-syllable words (n = 4) | | |
| Belichtungsmesser (light meter) | + | |
| Fleischpreissteigerung (meat price increase) | + | |
| Marillenknoedel (apricot dumpling) | + | |
| Sicherheitsnadel (safety pin) | + | + |

# Appendix 2: Abbreviations

phw = phonological word
F = metrical foot
σ = syllable
O = onset
N = nucleus
R = rhyme
Cd = coda
x = slot
x = grid
xx = grid

# 14
# Vowel Epenthesis in Aphasia

Renée Béland

Vowel epenthesis has been most adequately described using nonlinear phonology approaches. It has been shown that vowel insertion is predictable from the syllabic constraints imposed in a specific language. Halle and Vergnaud (1978) considered vowel epenthesis, as a rule, applied to fill empty nodes created in derivation. Piggot and Singh (1985) proposed that vowel epenthesis and consonant epenthesis are "repair strategies" that are used when assimilation, elision, and resyllabification have failed. Epenthesis can be universally characterized as the insertion of a segment into the appropriate slot that can be interpreted + or − syllabic depending on its position in the syllabic structure (Kaye and Lowenstamm, 1983). One of the most important observations from such analysis is that there is no need for an epenthesis rule. Epenthesis is applied to repair syllabifications that are disallowed in a specific language.

In this chapter we present aphasic and normal data collected during repetition and oral reading tasks of isolated word stimuli. Our purpose was to investigate two phonological analyses of the epenthesis phenomenon to: (1) provide a full description of epenthesis examples with respect to both the location and the quality of the epenthetic vocalic segments; and (2) see if the error examples produced by normal subjects differ from the examples produced by the aphasic subjects. Note that no distinction is made across the aphasic syndromes in our analyses because all syndromes have produced the same error types; that is, no distinction has been found with regard to the location and quality of the epenthetic vowels.

In the first section we present the subjects, methods, and data that were used. The second section is a review of proposals made for the representation of epenthesis and syncope in nonlinear phonology. We insist on the relation between these two operations of segmental insertion and deletion. The third section is a detailed investigation on the melodic representation of the intruding segments based on the Underspecification Theory as proposed by Archangeli (1984, 1985). In the fourth section, we investigate in analysis of vowel epenthesis based on the Theory of Charm and Government (Kaye, Lowenstamm, and Vergnaud, 1985). Finally, in the fifth

section we compare the two phonological analyses and conclude on the
phonological nature of the epenthesis phenomenon in aphasic speech.

## Methods and Data

Twenty-nine aphasic subjects (10 Wernicke, 7 Broca, 6 mixed, 6 conduction) with a left cerebral lesion were selected for this study. All subjects
(native French speakers) were paired with a normal control subject with
respect to age, sex, and educational level. The 58 subjects were submitted
to a repetition and a reading task of 321 words (stimuli). The stimuli were
selected on the basis of length (four phonemes) and syllabic structure. The
321-word list included examples of the 12 possible[1] string combinations of
consonant (C) and vowel (V) present in French (CVCV, VCVC, CCVC,
CVCC, CCCV, VCCC, VVCV, CVVC, VVCC, VCCV, CCVV). The
words were also selected for their segmental content. We tried to obtain
an even distribution of each consonantal segment. Subjects' responses
were tape recorded and transcribed in narrow IPA transcription (Béland,
1985). Here we present examples of vowel epenthesis collected in repetition and reading tasks of isolated word stimuli. The symbols N and A in
Tables 14.1 to 14.6 refer, respectively, to normal subject and aphasic
subject.

## Epenthesis and Syncope in Nonlinear Phonology

### Syncope of schwa in French

Selkirk (1978), Halle and Vergnaud (1978), and Bouchard (1981) have
proposed rules for the syncope of French schwa based on a metrical analysis. For this chapter I adopted the two rules formulated by Bouchard
(1981) to account for vowel syncope in French.

$$\phi$$
$$|$$
Rule A: V → θ/  W (obligatory)
$$|$$
$$-$$

Rule B: Reduce a vowel under W in a two-stress foot[2] (optional).

These rules can account for any schwa syncope in the word list repro-
duced in Appendix 1. For normal control subjects as well as for aphasic

---

[1] As for as noncompound words are concerned.
[2] Where a two-stress foot is a foot that does not have primary or secondary stress;
i.e., it is dominated by more than one node in a stress domain (Bouchard, 1981).

TABLE 14.1. Epenthetic vowel /œ/

| Repetition | Repetition |
|---|---|
| (3) /film/ (film) > /filmœ/ N,A | (21) /tyrk/ (turkish) > /tyrkœ/ N,A |
| (4) /mais/ (corn) > /maisœ/ A | (22) ./ivεr/ (winter) > /ivεrœ/ A |
| (5) /takt/ (tact) > /taktœ/ N,A | (23) ./dʒaz/ (jazz) > /dʒazœ/ A |
| (6) ./park/ (park) > /parkœ/ N,A | (24) ./tost/ (toast) > /tostœ/ N,A |
| (7) ./swar/ (evening) > /swarœ/ A | (25) /εsɔr/ (flight) > /εsɔrœ/ A |
| (8) ./swaf/ (thirst) > /swafœ/ N,A | (26) ./flœr/ (flower) > /flœrœ/ A |
| (9) ./egal/ (equal) > /egalœ/ A | (27) ./koɔp/ (coop) > /koɔpœ/ N,A |
| (10) /naif/ (naive) > /naifœ/ A | (28) ./otœr/ (height) > /otœrœ/ A |
| (11) ./odœr/ (smell) > /odœrœ/ A | (29) ./gɔlf/ (golf) > /gɔlfœ/ N,A |
| (12) ./otεl/ (hotel) > /otεlœ/ A | |
| (13) ./gril/ (grill) > /grilœ/ A | Reading |
| (14) ./kɥir/ (leather) > /kɥirœ/ N,A | (30) /tsar/ (tsar) > /tsarœ/ A |
| (15) ./tjεr/ (third) > /tjεrœ/ A | (31) /piʃε/ (pitcher) > /piʃεtœ/ A |
| (16) ./vwar/ (to see) > /vwarœ/ A | (32) /ʒɥif/ (Jewish) > /ʒɥifœ/ N,A |
| (17) ./apεl/ (call) < /apεlœ/ A | (33) /dyεl/ (duel) > /dyεlœ/ A |
| (18) ./talk/ (talc) > /talkœ/ N,A | (34) /laik/ (laique) > /laikœ/ A |
| (19) ./ymœr/ (humour) > /ymœrœ/ A | (35) /eʃεk/ (check) > /eʃεkœ/ A |
| (20) /mysk/ (musk) > /myskœ/ N,A | (36) noεl/ (Christmas) > /noεlœ/ A |

N = error produced by a normal subject; A = error produced by an aphasic subject; N, A = errors produced by both normal and aphasic subjects. The periods preceding some of the examples indicate that these examples are also found in the oral reading task.

subjects, schwa was in fact the only vowel syncopated between two consonants. In one case, we observed that the high vowel /i/ had been syncopated in the word *tissu* (fabric). The reduction of high vowels in Québec French, as mentioned by Bouchard (1981), may result from an application of rule B to all nonbranching vowels.[3] As pointed out by Bouchard (1981), rule A applies in an obligatory manner except with a reading intonation. In the reading task, we found a number of examples where schwa failed to undergo syncope even if it was falling under obigatory rule A.[4] In addition, aphasic subjects and normal control subjects pronounced some /œ/'s that do not come from a nonapplication of rule A. These /œ/'s (Table 14.1) must then be considered epenthetic.

## Vowel Epenthesis

In linear phonology, the process of vocalic insertion was formulated without reference to the syllabic structure. Schane (1973) gave the following

---

[3] Distinction between branching and nonbranching vowels was first made by Halle and Vergnaud (1978).
[4] Aphasic and normal subjects did pronounce these /œ/ in the reading task in the same proportion (33%).

rule for vowel insertion of /u/ in Hanunoo, a language that does not allow cluster word initially.

(37)
$$\emptyset \to \begin{bmatrix} V \\ + \text{ high} \\ + \text{ round} \end{bmatrix} \quad / \quad \# \, C \, \underline{\qquad} \, C$$

Halle and Vergnaud (1978) give a new formulation to epenthesis rule in Harari using a nonlinear model.

(38)
$$C \diagup \diagdown \emptyset \to C \diagup \diagdown i$$

Epenthesis applies to fill empty nodes created through morphological modifications. Halle and Vergnaud postulated "... a rule that assigns minimal syllabic structure to these stranded consonants and inserts a vowel under the empty node." For Kaye and Lowenstamm (1983), the epenthesis rule has the following form.

(39)
$$\emptyset \to \alpha$$

where $\alpha$ is + or − syllabic, depending on its position in the syllable structure. For these authors, the empty nodes are part of the underlying representations, and their distribution is predictable as a function of the markedness index associated with syllabic structure in that specific language.

In the analysis proposed by Piggot and Singh (1985), epenthesis is one of the four strategies available in a language to recuperate a form that violates the well-formedness conditions. They ranked the four strategies in this order: (1) resyllabification; (2) assimilation; (3) syncope, and (4) epenthesis, where epenthesis is used as a last attempt when none of the first three strategies has succeeded. The difference between the analysis proposed by Kaye and Lowenstamm and the present analysis is that empty nodes are part of the underlying representation (UR) for the former and must be created in derivation for the latter. In both analyses there is no need for an epenthesis rule.

## Epenthesis and Syncope

As pointed out by Halle and Vergnaud (1978), epenthesis and syncope of schwa are closely related, epenthesis being the symmetrical counterpart of a vowel elision rule. Examples in Table 14.1 show in fact that if subjects (aphasic as well as normal control) delete the schwa in a weak branch of a foot they also create a branching foot by intruding an /œ/ after the final consonant of a word. Thus we can formulate the symmetrical counterpart of rule (1) as rule (40):

(40)
$$\emptyset \to V \quad / \quad \begin{array}{c} W \\ | \\ V \end{array} \quad \begin{array}{c} \phi \\ \diagup \diagdown \\ S \quad W \\ | \\ V \ \underline{\quad} \end{array}$$

This rule says that it is possible to create a branching foot by adding a V to the right of a nonbranching foot.

We now turn to an analysis of vowel epenthesis examples based on the underspecification theory as proposed by Archangeli (1984).

## Underspecification and Vowel Epenthesis

In French the vowel /œ/ is syncopated in specific context, and it can also be used for epenthesis. According to Archangeli (1984), /œ/ can be considered as a default vowel in French, which means it has no melodic representation in the UR. In a three-dimensional representation (Archangeli, 1984; Grignon, 1984; Levin, 1984; Steriade, 1982), the melodic representation is one of the two planes—the syllabic and the melodic plane, which are joined together by the skeleton. We assume here, following Steriade (1982) and Grignon (1984), that URs are not syllabified. The vowel /œ/, subject to rule (1) in a nonlinear representation, is represented by a skeletal place with no melodic representation as indicated in rule (41) for the word "samedi' (saturday).

(41)                UR  X  X  X  X  X  X
                        |  |  |     |  |
                        s  a  m     d  i

In words containing /œ/ that are not subject to rules (1) or (2), the skeletal position is dominated by R (rime constituent) in the UR, as indicated in (42) for the word gueuler ("to yell").

                          R
                          |
(42)              UR  X  X  X  X
                      |     |  |
                      g     l  e

From now on, the phonetic symbol /ə/, or schwa, corresponds to a skeletal "x" position that is not dominated by a rime (R) constituent on the syllabic plane and that is linked to an empty feature matrix on the melodic plane. The phonetic sumbol /œ/ corresponds to any skeletal position dominated by a rime (R) constituent on the syllabic plane and linked to an empty feature matrix on the melodic plane.

Examples of vowel epenthesis in words containing branching onsets or codas, e.g., "trône" (throne) and "bruit" (noise), or words including two consonants that cannot form a branching constituent and must be split by the syllabification algorithm, e.g., "aspect" (aspect) and "objet" (object), are shown in Table 14.2.

In examples (43) to (83), subjects inserted the default vowel /œ/ to break up admissible clusters (pR, tR,...). In examples (84) to (91), subjects

TABLE 14.2. Epenthesis in words with branching or non-branching onset and coda

| Repetition | Reading |
|---|---|
| (43) /yblo/ (scuttle) > /ybœlo/ A | (70) /arbr/ (tree) > /arbœrœ/ A |
| (44) /mœbl/ (furniture) > /mœblœ/ A | (71) /sãtr/ (center) > /sãtrœ/ A |
| (45) ./aprã/ (I learn) > /apœrã/ A | (72) /gril/ (grill) > /gœril/ A |
| (46) ./tron/ (throne) > /tronœ/ A | (73) /plaʒ/ (beach) > /pœlaʒ/ A |
| (47) /ʒãdr/ (son-in-law) > /ʒãdrœ/ A | (74) /ekrã/ (screen) > /ekœrã/ A |
| (48) ./brɥi/ (noise) > /bœrɥi/ N,A | (75) /stri/ (stria) > /stœri/ N |
| (49) /frɛl/ (thin) > /frɛlœ/ A | (76) /klas/ (class) > /kœlas/ N |
| (50) /lɛvr/ (lip) > /lɛvrœ/ A | (77) /tras/ (trace) > /tœras/ A |
| (51) /katr/ (four) > /katrœ/ A | (78) /ʒ̃ɔgl/ (juggle) > /ʒ̃ɔgœlœ/ A |
| (52) /astr/ (star) > /astrœ/ A | (79) /ãtre/ (entry) > /ãtœre/ A |
| (53) /ekrã/ (screen) > /e$kœrã/ A | (80) /flyɛ/ (thin) > /fœlɥɛ/ A |
| (54) ./stri/ (stria) > /sœtri/ A | (81) /ãvwa/ (sending) > /ã$vœwa/ A |
| (55) ./brɔs/ (brush) > /bœrɔs/ A | (82) /trwa/ (three) > /tœrwa/ A |
| (56) /tãdr/ (tender) > /tãdrœ/ A | (83) /klue/ (nailed) > /kœluwe/ A |
| (57) /fabl/ (tale) > /fabœlœ/ A | |
| (58) ./ãgrɛ/ (fertilizer) > /ãgœrɛ/ A | Repetition |
| (59) /ẽfly/ (influx) > /ẽfœly/ A | (84) ./ɔbʒɛ/ (object) > /ɔbœʒɛ/ A |
| (60) ./abri/ (shelter) > /abœri/ A | (85) ./arpɔ̃/ (harpoon) > /arœpɔ̃/ A |
| (61) /ãglɛ/ (English) > /ãgœlɛ/ A | (86) ./aspɛ/ (aspect) > /asœpɛ/ A |
| (62) ./plɥi/ (rain) > /pœlɥi/ A | (87) ./apsã/ (absent) > /apœsã/ A |
| (63) ./frɥi/ (fruit) > /fœrɥi/ A | |
| (64) /frɥi/ (fruit) > /fœryɥi/ A | Reading |
| (65) ./skwa/ (squaw) > /sœkwa/ A | (88) /disk/ (record) > /di$sœ$kœ/ A |
| (66) ./frwa/ (cold) > /fœrwa/ A | (89) /bask/ (Basque) > /basœkœ/ A |
| (67) ./drwa/ (right) > /dœrwa/ A | (90) /admi/ (admitted) > /adœmi/ A |
| (68) ./grwe/ (snout) > /gœrwẽ/ A | (91) /arnɛ/ (harness) > /arœnɛ/ A |
| (69) ./prwa/ (prey) > /pœrwa/ A | |

The symbol "$" in the narrow IPA transcripton indicates a silent pause.

inserted the default vowel /œ/ in place of the syllabic boundary. These insertions correspond to the symmetrical counterpart of rule (2), as subjects created a branching foot by adding a weak branch to the right of a nonbranching foot. Using the Underspecification Theory within a three-dimensional representation, we can say that subjects insert an additional slot position in the skeleton that is automatically incorporated in the syllable by the syllabification algorithm and that is further interpreted as an /œ/ on the melodic plane by application of the redundancy rules set [see (103)].

In Table 14.3 the intruded slot is not automatically interpreted as an /œ/. The intruded vocalic segment is a copy of a vocalic segment in the string. The copied vocalic segment is usually the one that is closest to the intruded skeletal slot, e.g., "brûle" (burns) > [byryle]. Table 14.3 gives some examples of epenthesis in monosyllabic word stimuli. For monosyllabic words, there is only one vocalic segment available for copying. In fact, most of the time subjects used the default vowel interpretation instead

TABLE 14.3. Vowel Spreading.

| Repetition | Reading |
|---|---|
| (92) /gril/ (grill) > /gIril/ A | (96) /plaʒ/ (beach) > /pa$la$ʒœ/ A |
| (93) /ɔbʒɛ/ (object) > /ɔbɔʒɛ/ A | (97) /bryle/ (burned) >byryle/ N,A |
| (94) ./apsã/ (absent) > /apasã/ A | (98) /blɸi/ (blued) > /bɸlɸi/ A |
| (95) ./grwẽ/ (snout) > /gurwẽ/ N,A | (99) /ɔpte/ (opted) > /ɔpete/ A |
| | (100) /brɔs/ (brush) > /bɔ$rɔ$sœ/ A |
| | (101) /brɥi/ (noise) > /byryɥi/ A |

of copy. Given the limitations of the present corpus, i.e., that each word includes at most four phonemes, it is not possible to state the direction of the copying mechanism. So far, we have seen that the epenthetic vowel can be specified (1) as the default vowel /œ/ and (2) as a copy of a vocalic segment in the string. Table 14.3 gives examples of words including a glide, e.g., (95) and (101). Assuming that glides are underlyingly undifferentiated from corresponding high vowels (Kaye and Lowenstamm, 1983), we can posit that the same copy mechanism applies to specify the intruded vowel.

We now turn to examples in Tables 14.4, 14.5, and 14.6, for which mechanisms suggested so far cannot derive the nature of the epenthetic vowel. We are going to derive these epenthetic vowels within the context of Underspecification Theory as formulated by Archangeli (1984). According to this theory, we derived the following underspecified feature matrices for the French vocalic system.[5]

$$
(102) \quad
i \begin{bmatrix} +high \\ -round \end{bmatrix} \quad
e \begin{bmatrix} -low \\ -round \end{bmatrix} \quad
\varepsilon \begin{bmatrix} \quad \\ -round \end{bmatrix} \quad
a \begin{bmatrix} +back \\ -round \end{bmatrix} \quad
y \begin{bmatrix} +high \\ \quad \end{bmatrix}
$$

$$
\phi \begin{bmatrix} -low \\ \quad \end{bmatrix} \quad
\text{œ} \begin{bmatrix} \quad \\ \quad \end{bmatrix} \quad
u \begin{bmatrix} +high \\ +back \end{bmatrix} \quad
\tilde{\text{œ}} \begin{bmatrix} \quad \\ +nasal \end{bmatrix} \quad
o \begin{bmatrix} -low \\ +back \end{bmatrix}
$$

$$
\text{ɔ} \begin{bmatrix} +back \end{bmatrix} \quad\quad
\tilde{\varepsilon} \begin{bmatrix} -round \\ +nasal \end{bmatrix} \quad
\tilde{\text{ɔ}} \begin{bmatrix} +back \\ +nasal \end{bmatrix} \quad
\tilde{a} \begin{bmatrix} +back \\ -round \\ +nasal \end{bmatrix}
$$

As can be seen, some Québec French vowels do not appear in (102). we restricted the inventory to the vowels common to the 58 subjects. Application of the following set of redundancy rules fulfills all feature matrices.

---

[5] Note that special distinction is needed to differentiate the nasal vowel /œ/ from the nasal consonant /n/. There is no /œ/ in the word stimuli, so we are not going to distinguish them here. Essentially, we would propose to distinguish /œ/ from /n/ in their UR only when it is necessary, i.e., when they are both eligible to a rime identification. In these contexts, the vowel /œ/ must be dominated by R (rime) on the syllabic plane. This solution is parallel to the one we adopted to prevent syncope of nonsyncopable /œ/.

(103) Redundancy rules set:
  1. [          ] → [−high]
  2. [          ] → [−low] / [+high] DR
  3. [          ] → [+low] CR
  4. [          ] → [+round] CR
  5. [          ] → [−back] CR
  6. [          ] → [−nasal] DR

Following Pulleyblank (1983) Archangeli (1984), automatic spreading at the underspecified representational level within this vocalic system is available only for the features [+high], [−round], [−low], [+back], and [+nasal]. The derivation of epenthetic vowels by spreading, again at the underspecified representational level, is restricted to these features and to the values + or − associated with these features. In Table 14.4. the vowel /ɛ/ in examples (104) to (107) can be derived by spreading [−round], the rest of the specifications being fulfilled by the application of the redundancy rules set.

TABLE 14.4. Epenthetic vowel /ɛ/.

| Reading | Repetition |
|---|---|
| (104) /tsar/ (tsar) > /tɛs$ar/ N | (106) /stri/ (stria) > /Stɛri/ N |
| (105) /abri/ (shelter) > abɛri/ A | (107) /tsar/ (tsar) > /tɛzar/ N |

Derivation of /tsar/ > /tɛsar/:
a. Underlying representation of /tsar/

```
X  X     X      X
|  |     |      |
t  s  ⎡+back ⎤  r
      ⎣−round⎦
```

b. Insertion of a skeletal position:

```
X  X  X     X      X
|     |     |      |
t     s  ⎡+back ⎤  r
         ⎣−round⎦
```

c. Spreading [−round]:

```
X       X     X     X      X
|       |     |     |      |
t  [−round]   s  ⎡+back ⎤  r
                 ⎣−round⎦
```

d. Application of the redundancy rules set:

```
X        X     X      X       X    application of rule 1. ([    ] →
|        |     |      |       |       [−high])
t  ⎡−high ⎤    s  ⎡−high ⎤    r
   ⎣−round⎦       ⎢+back ⎥
                 ⎣−round⎦
```

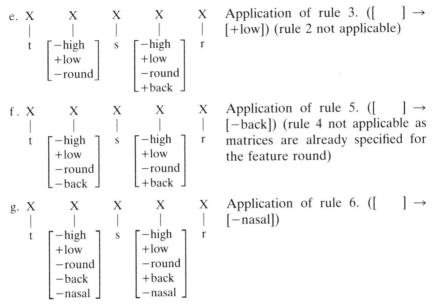

In Table 14.5 the vowel /ɔ/ in /apɔle/ (116) is derived by spreading [+back]. The two vowels /ɛ/ and /ɔ/ are thus derived by spreading one feature and its value to the inserted slot position. If we consider that an epenthetic process can arise as early as the underlying underspecified representational level, these epenthetic vowels are thus automatically derived by spreading, but there is no obvious reason why [+back], which spreads in example (116), does not spread in example (104). In other words, the problem is that the quality of the epenthetic vowel is not totally predictable on the sole basis of spreading. Sometimes only one feature spreads (example 104, where only [−round] spreads), and sometimes all features spread, i.e., a copy mechanism applies (Table 14.3, examples 92 to 101).

For the rest of the examples in Table 14.5 (108 to 115, 117 to 129) the epenthetic vowel /ɔ/ can be derived by spreading the labial feature: [+round]. In fact, the vowel /ɔ/ is always inserted in context of a labial consonant (/m/, /p/) and/or a labial glide. According to the Underspecification Theory, the nonlabial consonant /t/, being the default consonant in French,[6] labial consonants are underlyingly specified as [+round], thereby allowing the propagation of [+round] at the underlying representational level. As the propagation of [+round] is discussed is section on the

---

[6] In the absence of an epenthetic consonant in the phonological system of a language, Archangeli (1984) suggested that the default segment is the less marked segment of the consonantal system. There is, in fact, no epenthetic consonantal segment in French, and the universally unmarked segment /t/ corresponds to the less marked segment of the French consonantal system.

TABLE 14.5. Epenthetic vowel /ɔ/.

| Repetition | Repetition |
|---|---|
| (108) /frwa/ (cold) > /fɔrwɛ/ A | (120) /aswa/ (sit) > /asɔwa/ A |
| (109) /frwa/ (cold) > /fɔrwa/ A | (121) ./grwẽ/ (snout) > /gɔrwẽ/ A |
| (110) /āvwa/ (sending) > /āvɔ$wa/ A | (122) ./prwa/ (prey) > /pɔrwa/ N,A |
| (111) ./trwa/ (three) > /tɔrwa/ A | |
| (112) /emwa/ (emotion) > /e$mɔwa/ A | Reading |
| (113) /vwal/ (sail) > /vɔwa$lœ/ A | (123) /gwaʃ/ (gouache) > /gɔwaʃ/ A |
| (114) /frμi/ (fruit) > /fɔrwi/ A | (124) /trwa/ (three) > /tɔrwa/ A |
| (115) /pwal/ (stove) > /pɔwalœ/ A | (125) /drwa/ (right) > /dɔrwɛt/ A |
| (116) /aple/ (called) > /apɔle/ A | (127) /emwa/ (emotion) > /emɔwa/ A |
| (117) /amsɔ̃/ (hook) > /amɔsɔ̃/ A | (128) /amne/ (brought) > /amɔne/ N |
| (118) ./swar/ (evening) > /sɔwar/ A | (129) /kwɛt/ (bunches) > /kɔwɛt/ A |
| (119) ./krwa/ (cross) > /kɔrwa/ A | |

TABLE 14.6. Epenthetic vowel /i/ and /e/.

| Repetition | Reading |
|---|---|
| (131) /ɔpte/ (opted) > /ɔpite/ A | (134) /tsar/ (tsar) > /tisar/ A |
| (132) /apsā/ (absent) > /apisā/ A | (135) /aswa/ (sit) > /asiwa/ A |
| (133) /skwa/ (squaw)/ > /sikwa/ A | (136) /apsā/ (absent) > /apesā/ A |

Theory of Charm and Government, we do not discuss details here about the derivations within the Theory of Underspecification.

Another set of epenthetic vowels (Table 14.6) cannot be derived by automatic spreading of feature (or features) at the underlying representational level. In the examples in Table 14.6, epenthetic vowels cannot be derived by automatic spreading. Derivation of these vowels requires application of a dissimilation rule toward the vocalic segment on the left. According to the redundancy rule ordering constraint posited by Archangeli (1984), the redundancy rule supplying an alpha value for a feature F must be ordered before the first rule mentioning [F] in its structural description. The redundancy rule ordering constraint is as follows (Archangeli 1984, 1985).

(130)            Redundancy-Rule Ordering Constraint

A redundancy rule assigning α to F, where α is "+" or "−", is automatically ordered prior to the first rule referring to [F] in structural description.

Derivation of /i/ in example (132)—"absent" ("absent") > [apisā]— implies the following three steps:

(136)

1. spread [−round]
2. [      ] → [−high] CRule
3. $\emptyset$ → [−αhigh] / [αhigh]

Derivation of the epenthetic vowel /e/ in (135) [apesā] involves application of two redundancy rules prior to application of the dissimilation rule:

(137)

1. Spread [−round]
2. [          ] → [−high] CRule
3. [          ] → [+low] DRule
4. ∅ → [−αlow] / [αlow]

Derivation of the epenthetic vowel /i/ in (131) "opté" (opted) > [ɔpite] involves two dissimilation rules: one for the feature high and one for the feature round.

(138)

1. [          ] → [−high]
2. ∅ → [−αhigh] / [αhigh]
3. [          ] → [+low] DRule
4. [          ] → [+round] CRule
5. ∅ → [−αround] / [αround]

These sets of rules show that the dissimilation has its effect at different stages: (1) at the beginning of the specification (136); (2) slightly later (137); and (3) just before the feature specification (138). It thus appears that an algorithm could be postulated for this dissimilation effect. The utilization of these dissimilation rules is an ad hoc procedure, but if we consider that epenthesis can arise at different representational levels, we can suggest that derivations involving several dissimilation rules correspond to epenthetic processes that arise later in the feature specification processing.

To summarize our vowel epenthesis analysis, we can say there exists at least three ways in which an inserted vowel can receive a melodic interpretation: (1) by application of the redundancy rules set leading to /œ/; (2) by the spreading features of an adjacent vowel; and (3) by spreading followed by an application of one or several dissimilation rules. Both the spreading and default interpretations agree with the automatic character devoted to epenthesis in nonlinear phonology. In the third situation, phonological dissimilation rules are needed, but we have shown that an algorithm could be postulated to derive any of these vowels.

We now turn to a new interpretation of vowel epenthesis based on the new proposition made by Kaye et al. (1985) concerning the representation of segments.

# Epenthesis Within the Theory of Charm and Government

In the Theory of Charm and Government, distinctive features are no longer available to phonological processes. Distinctive features are used only for phonetic interpretation. Segments are represented by the elements (A,I,N,I,U,v) or by combinations of elements. For example, the French vowel /ɛ/ results from the following fusion: (A.I), where I is called the head and A the operator. Each element corresponds to a fully specified feature matrix. The result of the operation (A.I) is the complete set of features associated with the head I except for the hot feature of the operator A, which is [−high] (Kaye et al., 1985).

(139)

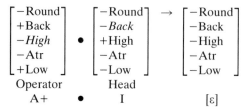

$$
\begin{bmatrix} -\text{Round} \\ +\text{Back} \\ -\textit{High} \\ -\text{Atr} \\ +\text{Low} \end{bmatrix} \bullet \begin{bmatrix} -\text{Round} \\ -\textit{Back} \\ +\text{High} \\ -\text{Atr} \\ -\text{Low} \end{bmatrix} \rightarrow \begin{bmatrix} -\text{Round} \\ -\text{Back} \\ -\text{High} \\ -\text{Atr} \\ -\text{Low} \end{bmatrix}
$$

Operator     Head

A+    •    I        [ɛ]

Hot features of elements, italicized in the matrices above, are the features associated with the line where the element stands. Three lines are needed to account for the French Québec vocalic system (Kaye, 1985).

(140)

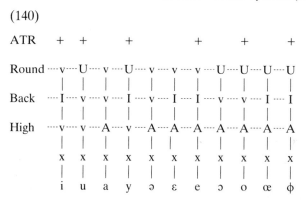

We do not go into further detail here about the theory itself, but we turn to an analysis of epenthetic vowels within this theoretical framework. Let us first consider the first group of examples involving the epenthetic vowel /œ/ (Table 14.1).

As stated earlier, epenthesis is the symmetrical counterpart of schwa omission. Adding a schwa in a word results in the creation of a branching foot, the added vowel being dominated by the weak branch of the foot. In the theory of elements, the phonological representation of schwa is as follows: (A.v), where v is the "cold" vowel, or the vowel with no hot feature. This cold vowel is found on each line not occupied by an element. This combination is allowed in the weak branch of a foot. The vowel /œ/ is the surface phonetic reflex of schwa in Québec French. As can be seen in (141a.), the first step is the creation of a point or a skeletal position, which is further interpreted as a schwa because this point is dominated by a weak branch of a foot. This phonological schwa is phonetically interpreted as /œ/ on the surface level. At this point, an equivalent interpretation could have been made with former theoretical approaches.

Let us now turn to a second group of examples (Table 14.5), including the epenthetic vowel /ɔ/. A close examination of the examples reveals that all epenthetic /ɔ/'s are produced in the context of a labial consonant. In the Theory of Charm and Government, the labial consonants have an element "U" in their combination. According to the above analysis of schwa epenthesis, the following steps are required for the derivation of epenthetic vowel /ɔ/: (1) the creation of a point that automatically is phonologically interpreted as a schwa; (2) the propagation of the element "U" on this position; and (3) the phonetic interpretation of the combination of schwa with the element "U" resulting in /ɔ/, as shown in (141).

(141)

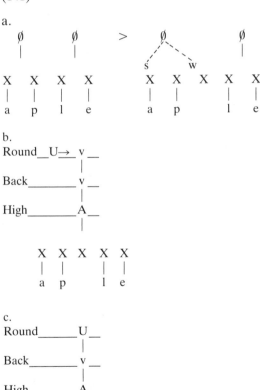

The exact representation of the labial stop /p/ needs to defined. At this point, the Theory of Charm and Government does not provide a full description of the consonantal system. Nevertheless, the representation of /p/ would incorporate the element "U" needed here in the present analysis.

Some examples with the epenthetic /ɔ/ also include a glide. In those examples we can state that it is the high vowel of the branching nucleus that is propagated. A similar process involving only the left branch of a light diphthong is found in Vata (Kaye, 1982).

Another group of examples are those including the epenthetic vowel /i/. In Québec French, the high vowels /i/ and /y/ are often syncopated when located between two voiceless consonants. Epenthesis being the symmetrical counterpart of syncopation, it is not surprising to find the high vowel /i/ reinserted in the same context. The high vowel /y/ could appear in the same context, but its presence would be more marked. In the last group of examples, the epenthetic vowel is a copy of vowel of the word stimulus. As can be seen in Table 14.3, most of the time, the vowel that is copied is the one closest to the intruded slot. It must be, stated that there is first insertion of a skeletal place. Second, there is a nucleus projection onto which feet are constructed. The intruded slot is further filled in with the closest nucleus projection. Here again, when projection is a branching nucleus, the high vowel is used for copying.

The quality of some epenthetic vowels can thus also be automatically derived by spreading within the Theory of Charm and Government. In addition, this theory makes strong predictions about the vowels that should not appear in specific contexts. For example, we should not find an epenthetic vowel /ɔ/ without the presence of an element "U" in the context. A form such as /akɔsã/ for "accent" ("accent") should not be attested to. We did not find any counter-example in our corpus which included 58 subjects (29 normal subjects and 29 aphasic subjects). The vowel /ɛ/ in example (104) (Table 14.4) appears in a closed syllable as indicated by the syllabic boundary "$." This vowel /ɛ/ is the phonological reflex of schwa in closed syllables, as attested to in morphological alternations such as *mener* (to lead) /mœne/ and "je mène" (I lead) /mɛn/. Kaye (1985) suggested that the vowel /ɛ/ results from an infrasegmental epenthesis of the element I. Because the vowel schwa is unable to govern, infrasegmental epenthesis gives rise to the vowel /ɛ/, which can govern the /n/ in the example of /mɛn/. The vowel /e/ in (137) cannot be derived within the context of the Theory of Charm and Government. In fact, all examples containing the epenthetic vowel /e/ come from the reading task. For this reason, it is not possible to ascertain the exact nature of these vowels. They can result from a literal reading of the letter "p" as /pe/ or "b" as /be/, and so on. In fact, the vowel /e/ never appeared with a consonant such as /ʃ/ for which the literal reading would be /ʃœ/ not */ʃe/. Thus we leave open the question of epenthetic vowel /e/ because of insufficient information.

# Conclusion

Epentheses examples have been produced by normal and aphasic subjects. Differences between examples produced by the two groups are quantitative, not qualitative. At the beginning of the chapter, following Piggot and Singh (1985), we identified epenthesis as a universal phonological process that can be used as a repair strategy. Epentheses examples collected from repetition and reading tasks revealed that normal subjects (but more often aphasic subjects) insert a vocalic segment between two consonantal segments that form a legal branching constituent in French. A repair strategy is applied in the absence of constraint violation. Description of the epenthesis phenomenon made by the two phonological theories investigated, the Underspecification Theory and the Theory of Charm and Government, have helped us to predict the place and the quality of the inserted vowels. The two theories agree on the fact that epenthesis is associated with the syllabification process. We have proposed that epenthesis can occur at different representational levels from the deep underlying levels to the surface levels. According to this viewpoint, epenthesis can be seen as an alternative route for the expected syllabification that is normally used for unsyllabifiable forms but that can be used—witness examples collected from normal and aphasic subjects—whenever the normal syllabification processing fails. The purpose of this chapter was to show not why but where and how this syllabification processing fails. The two phonological theories we have investigated have provided us with a full description of the epenthesis process without being able to take into account the variability observed in the quality of epenthetic vowels. For a same word (e.g., apsent /apsã/ *absent*) the vowels /a/, /i/, /e/, and /œ/ have been found inserted between the /p/ and the /s/ ([apasã], [apisã], [apesã], [apœsã]). If we consider that epenthesis can arise at different representational levels, the quality of the epenthetic vowel may depend on the degree of specification the feature matrices have undergone. The more specifications of the feature matrices are needed to derive the epenthetic vowel, the latest the epenthesis has occurred.

Phonological analyses of epenthesis proposed by the two phonological theories indicate that the form of epentheses produced by the normal and the aphasic subjects are predictable on a phonological basis. These errors are thus not randomly produced. Our claim is that these errors occur because the syllabification processing fails. The quality of the vowel depends on when the failure arose in the word processing, i.e., the representational level the speaking subject accessed. The application of a repair strategy such as epenthesis is an alternative route for normal syllabification. The application of a repair strategy is always simpler than use of the normal syllabification process because these repair strategies are normally used in the presence of a constraint violation, which, by definition, constitutes a more marked context than the context resulting from the application of the process.

## References

Archangeli, D.B. (1984). *Underspecification in Yawelmani Phonology and Morphology*, PhD dissertation, MIT.

Archangeli, D.B. (1985). Yokuts harmony: evidence for coplanar representation in nonlinear phonology. *Linguistic Inquiry, 16*, pp. 335–372.

Béland, R. (1985). *Contraintes Syllabiques sur les Erreurs Phonologiques dans l'Aphasie*. PhD thesis, Université de Montréal.

Bouchard, D. (1981). Avoice for 'e muet.'. *Journal of Linguistic Research, 1*, No. 4, pp. 17–47.

Grignon, A.M., (1984). *Phonologie Lexicale Tri-dimensionnelle du Japonais*. PhD thesis, Université de Montréal.

Halle, M., and Vergnaud, J.R. (1978). Metrical structure in phonology. Manuscript, MIT.

Kaye, J. (1982). Harmony process in Vata. *Structure of the Phonological Representations*. Part II. pp. 385–452. Harry van der Hulst, Novual Smith (eds.), Fonis Publications, Dordrecht, Holland.

Kaye, J. (1985). Sur les systèmes vocaliques. Presented at the 1985 CLA Annual Meeting, Université de Montréal.

Kaye, J. and Lowenstamm, J. (1983). De la syllabicité. *Forme Sonore du Language, Structure des Représentations en Phonologie*. Paris: Hermann.

Kaye, J., Lowenstamm, J. and Vergnaud, J.R. (1985). The internal structure of phonological elements: a theory of charm and government. *Phonology Yearbook 2*, 305–328.

Levin, J. (1984). Conditions on Syllable Structure and Categories in Klamath Phonology. Unpublished manuscript, MIT.

Piggot, G. and Singh, R. (1985). The phonology of epenthetic segments. *Canadian Journal of Linguistics 30*, 415–451.

Pulleyblank, D. (1983). *Tone in Lexical Phonology*, PhD dissertation, MIT.

Schane, S. (1973). *Generative Phonology*. Englewood Cliffs, NJ: Prentice-Hall.

Selkirk, E. (1978). The French foot: on the status of the mute 'e'. *Studies in French Linguistics, 1*, No. 2. pp. 141–150.

Steriade, D. (1982). *Greek Prosodies and the Nature of Syllabification*. PhD dissertation, MIT.

# Appendix 1: Word Stimuli Used in Repetition and Reading Tasks Including a Schwa

| CVCV | |
|---|---|
| *chemin* (road) /ʃœmē/ | *genou* (knee) /ʒœnu/ |
| *cheveu* (hair) /ʃœvø/ | *pesé* (weighed) /pœze/ |
| *dedans* (inside) /dœdā/ | *tenue* (outfit) /tœny/ |
| | *venin* (venom) /vœnē/ |

## VCVC

*abîme* (I damage) /abim/
*abuse* (I abuse) /abyz/
*achète* (I buy) /aʃɛt/
*affaire* (business) /afɛr/
*affiche* (poster) /afiʃ/
*affole* (I terrify) /afɔl/
*amuse* (I entertain) /amyz/
*arrête* (I stop) /arɛt/
*assise* (seated) /asiz/
*audace* (audacity) /odas/
*automne* (fall) /otɔn/
*échange* (exchange) /eʃɑ̃ʒ/
*échappe* (I escape) /eʃap/
*école* (school) /ekɔl/
*échelle* (ladder) /eʃɛl/
*Ecosse* (Scotia) /ekɔs/
*écoute* (I listen) /ekut/
*égal* (equal) /egal/
*élève* (student) /elɛv/
*empêche* (I prevent) /ɑ̃pɛʃ/
*encore* (again) /ɑ̃kɔr/
*engage* (he hires) /ɑ̃gaʒ/
*éponge* (sponge) /epɔ̃ʒ/
*époque* (time) /epɔk/
*épouse* (spouse) /epuz/
*équipe* (team) /ekip/
*essence* (gaz) /ɛsɑ̃s/
*étage* (floor) /etaʒ/
*étude* (study) /etyd/
*évêque* (bishop) /evɛk/
*habille* (I dress) /abij/
*habite* (I live) /abit/
*image* (picture) /imaʒ/
*immense* (huge) /imɑ̃s/
*infâme* (infamous) /ɛ̃fam/
*inonde* (I flood) /inɔ̃d/
*indigne* (unworthy) /ɛ̃diɲ/
*intense* (intense) /ɛ̃tɑ̃s/
*ovale* (oval) /oval/
*unique* (only) /ynik/

## CCVC

*biére* (beer) /bjɛr/
*blague* (joke) /blag/
*boîte* (box) /bwat/
*brosse* (brush) /brɔs/
*brûle* (burns) /bryl/
*chemise* (shirt) /ʃmiz/
*cheval* (horse) /ʃœval/
*chouette* (great) /ʃwɛt/
*classe* (class) /klas/
*cligne* (I blink) /kliɲ/
*couenne* (rind) /kwɛn/

*couette* (bunches) /kwɛt/
*cuivre* (copper) /kɥivr/
*diète* (diet) /djɛt/
*douane* (customs) /dwan/
*fièvre* (fever) /fjɛvr/
*frêle* (thin) /frɛl/
*glaise* (clay) /glɛz/
*gouache (gouache)* /gwaʃ/
*liane* (liana) /lijan/
*moelle* (marrow) /mwal/
*niaise* (silly) /njɛz/
*nièce* (niece) /njɛs/
*pierre* (stone) /pjɛr/
*plage* (beach) /plaʒ/
*poêle* (stove) /pwal/
*poigne* (grip) /pwaɲ/
*science* (science) /sjɑ̃s/
*souhaite* (he wishes) /swɛt/
*suave* (smooth) /sɥav/
*suite* (continuation) /sɥit/
*tiède* (luke warm) /tjɛd/
*toile* (cloth) /twal/
*trace* (trace) /tras/
*trône* (throne) /tron/
*viande* (meat) /vjɑ̃d/
*voile* (sail) /vwal/
*zouave* (zouave) /zwav/

## VCCV

*acheté* (bought) /aʃte/
*amené* (brought) /amne/
*appelé* (called) /aple/
*avenue* (avenus) /avny/
*échelon* (rung) /eʃlɔ̃/
*enlevé* (removed) /ɑ̃lve/
*ennemi* (enemy) /ɛnmi/
*hameçon* (hook) /amsɔ̃/

## VCCC

*arbre* (tree) /arbr/
*astre* (star) /astr/
*ordre* (order) /ɔrdr/

## CVVC

*béate* (blissful) /beat/
*bohéme* (bohemian) boɛm/
*chahute* (I rag) /ʃayt/
*déesse* (goddess) /dees/
*déhanche* (I sway) /deɑ̃ʃ/
*dehors* (outside) /dœɔr/
*géante* (giant) /ʒeɑ̃t/
*naïve* (naïve) /naiv/
*nuage* (cloud) /nyaʒ/
*nuance* (shade) /nyɑ̃s/

*poème* (poem) /poɛm/
*séance* (session) /seās/

CVCC

*barbe* (beard) /barb/
*basque* (Basque) /bask/
*battre* (beat) /batr/
*boxe* (boxing) /bɔks/
*buffle* (buffalo) /byfl/
*bulbe* (bulb) /bylb/
*caste* (caste) /kast/
*centre* (center) /sātr/
*cerne* (ring) /sɛrn/
*charge* (load) /ʃarʒ/
*chèvre* (goat) /ʃɛvr/
*chiffre* (number) /ʃifr/
*couple* (couple) /kupl/
*course* (run) /kurs/
*culte* (cult) /kylt/
*disque* (record) /disk/
*dorme* (sleep) /dɔrm/

*fable* (tale) /fabl/
*ferme* (farm) /fɛrm/
*fixe* (fixed) /fiks/
*gendre* (son-in-law) /ʒādr/
*gifle* (slap) /ʒifl/
*givre* (frost) /ʒivr/
*gorge* (throat) /gɔrʒ/
*jongle* (juggle) /ʒɔ̃gl/
*lèvre* (lip) /lɛvr/
*maigre* (slim) /mɛgr/
*marbre* (marble) /marbr/
*meuble* (furniture) /mœbl/
*mixe* (mix) /miks/
*palme* (palm) /palm/
*peuple* (nation) /pœpl/
*quatr* (four) /katr/
*rythme* (rythm) /ritm/
*tendre* (tender) /tādr/
*valse* (waltz) /vals/
*verve* (verve) /vɛrv/
*zèbre* (zebra) /zɛbr/

# 15
# Internal Structure of Two Consonant Clusters

Sylviane Valdois

Linguistic and behavioral data support the view that consonant clusters have a particular status. With respect to linguistic data, specific constraints apply to the distribution of phonemes within consonant clusters. Although virtually any consonant can occur in intervocalic position, there are severe restrictions on how consonants can be combined sequentially. For example, French allows word-initial clusters composed of three consonants. However, phonological sequential constraints limit the set of possible segments that can occur in each position: The first consonant must be /s/; the second is /p/, /k/, or /t/; and the third is a liquid or glide.

Evidence that specific constraints apply on consonant clusters also comes from the analysis of aphasic errors. Blumstein (1978) noted that 77.1% of aphasic substitution errors affect single consonants, whereas only 22.9% of such errors occur within consonant clusters. For example, the substitution of /m/ for /p/ can occur in intervocalic position, e.g., /epi/ "épi" (corn) → /emi/; but it is not expected in consonant clusters, e.g., /pRi/ "prix" (price). In the latter example, a production such as */mRi/ would violate a phonotactic constraint of French which reduces to stops and nonstrident fricatives the set of possible segments in the first position of clusters whose second member is a liquid. The distributional difference of substitution errors between singletons and clusters thus reveals specific constraints on the structure of consonant clusters. Aphasic errors therefore appear to reflect linguistic principles that govern the patterns of consonant clusters.

Few studies have investigated phonemic errors produced by aphasic subjects within this context (Blumstein 1973; Kilani-Schoch, 1982; Martory and Messerli, 1983; Nespoulous, Joanette, Béland, Caplan, and Lecours, 1984; Puel, Nespoulous, Bonafé, and Rascol, 1980). Typically, these studies provided only a global quantitative analysis of the transformations and focused exclusively on the nature of the omitted or added phonemes.

The purpose of the present study is to document the existence of some position effect within clusters. Addition and omission errors produced by aphasic subjects in the context of two-consonant clusters were analyzed.

The aim of this analysis was, first, to question whether the two consonantal segments that form clusters are equally prone to be omitted in clusters destruction. We also asked whether a consonant is as likely to be introduced in the first position of a cluster as in the second position in addition errors leading to the creation of clusters.

Specific predictions about the expected pattern of addition and omission errors were assessed. Some of them derive from a psycholinguistic investigation of slips-of-the-tongue data (Stemberger and Treiman, 1986) and are discussed below. Different predictions follow from the Theory of Phonological Government (Kaye, Lowenstamm, and Vergnaud, 1985), whose basic theoretical concepts about syllable structure are outlined below. Results from the analysis of addition and omission errors produced by aphasic subject in the context of two-consonant cluster are presented as well. They provide new insights about the internal representation of clusters and their psycholinguistic processing.


## Evidence from Slips-of-the Tongue

Since the investigation of slips-of-the-tongue conducted by Fromkin (1971), increased attention has been paid to the linguistic analysis of errors produced by non-brain-damaged subjects (Cutler, 1981; Fay and Cutler, 1977; Fromkin, 1973; Laubstein, 1985; Shattuck-Hufnagel and Klatt, 1979; Stemberger 1984). Results of speech error analysis are considered to shed light on processes involved in language production. Performance models of speech production have therefore been advanced to provide a comprehensive framework for studying the various types of error (Garrett 1975, 1982, 1984; Shattuck-Hufnagel 1979, 1983, 1987).

Nevertheless, few studies examined phonemic errors produced within the context of consonant clusters (Kupin, 1982; Stemberger and Treiman, 1986). The latter study investigated speech errors produced by normal English speakers in spontaneous speech as well as under experimental conditions. They extensively examined addition, omission, and substitution errors that occurred in word-initial clusters composed of two consonants, e.g. /pr/ of "pray" or /st/ of "state." In their study, clusters were symbolized as C1C2 sequences. The main purpose was to inquire into the relative accessibility of the two consonants in initial clusters. The hypothesis of a more accurate access of C1 was assessed by examining the error rates on consonants in either the C1 or C2 position. With respect to the analysis of addition, omission, and substitution errors produced in spontaneous speech, Stemberger and Treiman's results may be summarized as follows.[1]

---

[1] Note that experimentally induced speech errors yielded similar results.

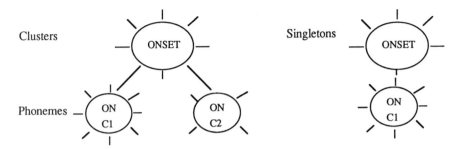

FIGURE 15.1. The internal structure of word-initial two-consonant clusters and singletons according to Stemberger and Treiman (1986). The design is inspired from Dell (1986).

1. The creation of word-initial clusters results more frequently from an addition in C2 than in C1 position, regardless of the type of cluster thus created (obstruent-liquid clusters or clusters beginning with /s/).[2]

2. C2 is the locus of omissions significantly more often than C1 in OL clusters (e.g., /R/ from "pray").

3. Omissions are also more frequent in the C2 position within word-initial /s/ clusters (e.g., /t/ from "state"), but this trend does not reach significance. Furthermore, /s/ clusters show significantly more omissions of C1 than other initial clusters.

4. Finally, noncontextual substitution errors show a greater error rate in the C2 position of OL clusters.

Stemberger and Treiman concluded from their analysis that the absolute serial position of a consonant in a word-initial cluster strongly influences the error rate, as a segment is less likely to be omitted, added, or substituted in C1 than in C2 position. They claimed that C1 and C2 must be represented differently in the language production system. They notably suggested that clusters must contain two distinct types of syllable position: a C1 position used for both singletons and clusters, and a C2 position exclusive to clusters. By reference to an activation theory, they hypothesized that C1 is more activated than C2 and added that activation of C1 is even greater in OL clusters than in /s/ clusters.

Figure 15.1 represents the internal structure of word-initial two-consonant clusters that may be inferred from their claim. The design is inspired from Dell's phonological network (Dell, 1986).

Aphasic data might support this representation in the same way as do normal data. Indeed, aphasic transformations have been demonstrated to

---

[2] In the remainder, an OL cluster stands for any obstruent-liquid cluster and an /s/ cluster for any cluster in which C1 is /s/.

be similarly characterized as slips-of-the tongue (Buckingham, 1980), and they are stated as reflecting structural properties of linguistic units as well (Béland 1985; Béland, Nespoulous, and Caplan, 1988; Blumstein, 1973, 1978). Predictions about the expected pattern of aphasic errors derive from Stemberger and Treiman's claims:

1. With respect to omission errors, a greater activation level on C1 notably predicts that C2 should be omitted more often than C1 in OL clusters as well as in /s/ clusters. However, this trend should be stronger in OL clusters, as C1 is more activated in these clusters than in /s/ clusters.

2. When a cluster is created, the added segment should be more frequently introduced in C2 than in C1 position, as a C1 position is already present in singletons. This trend should be observed in both OL clusters and /s/ clusters.

These predictions about word-initial two-consonant clusters are applied to the results of the analysis of aphasic errors. Our analysis of aphasic errors extends to word-medial and word-final clusters. The results lead to the determination of whether the internal representation of clusters proposed by Stemberger and Treiman is specific to word-initial clusters.

## Evidence from Phonological Theory

Within the framework of linear phonological theories, consonant clusters are analyzed as strings of sequentially ordered segments (Chomsky and Halle, 1968). However, other phonological theories have developed a nonlinear conception of the phonological representation of words (Halle and Vergnaud, 1980). Within this theoretical framework, consonant clusters are described in terms of syllabic constituents. They are therefore analyzed by reference to the notion of syllable. The existence of the syllable as a linguistic unit is now well established. However, different conceptions of the syllable have emerged that did not always agree about the internal structure of the syllable (Kahn, 1976; Kaye, Lowenstamm and Vergnaud, 1987; Kiparsky, 1979; Selkirk, 1982).

Kaye and colleagues (1985, 1987) developed the Theory and Phonological Government, which plays a determining role in the organization of the syllable structure. Because we refer to this theory for the analysis of aphasic data, its basic concepts about syllable must be briefly sketched. The theory, coming within the framework of three-dimensional phonology (Halle and Vergnaud, 1980), postulates that phonological representations lie on two planes, the melodic and the syllabic, linked by the skeleton (Fig. 15.2). The melodic plane consists of segmental representations, and the syllabic plane is concerned with syllabic structure. The skeleton specifies the number of slots or timing units that are present in the word (Kaye & Lowenstamm, 1984). The Theory of Phonological Government defines

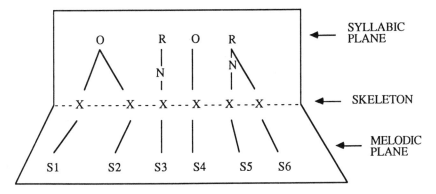

FIGURE15.2. An example of the three-dimensional phonological representation of the French word "travail" (work) [tRavaj]. This word is made of two syllables. The onset of the first syllable is branching: it is linked to two skeletal positions and corresponds to two segments, [t] and [R], in the melodic plane. In contrast, the onset of the second syllable is not branching and corresponds to only one segment, [v]. The rime of the first syllable does not branch while the rime of the second syllable is branching and dominates both the nucleus, linked to [a], and a rimal position corresponding to the final segment [j] in the melodic plane.

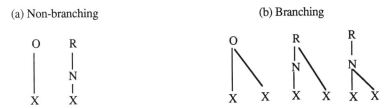

FIGURE 15.3. Possible configurations of syllabic constituents as postulated in the theory of phonological government (Kaye, Lowenstamm & Vergnaud, 1987).

syllables as onset-rime sequences. Onset, rime, and nucleus are obligatory constituents of the syllable. They are maximally binary; i.e., they can be linked to two slots at most.

Possible configurations of syllable constituents are shown on Figure 15.3. Each constituent appears in branching and non branching forms. A non branching onset is linked to a single slot (symbolized by "x"), itself corresponding to a single segment (symbolized by "s"). The structure of branching onsets differs from that of singletons, as the onset in linked to two adjacent skeletal positions and corresponds to two segments in the melodic plane.

A well formed branching onset is defined as a governing domain, where constituent government is strictly local and strictly directional (Fig. 15.4a). Government is defined as a binary asymmetrical relational holding be-

(a) Constituent government

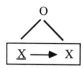

(b) Interconstituent government

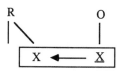

FIGURE 15.4. Two government domains. Government holds between two adjacent skeletal positions. Constituent government in (a) holds between the two positions corresponding to a branching onset. Interconstituent Government in (b) holds between an onset and a preceding rimal position.

tween two skeletal positions (Kaye, 1987; Kaye et al., 1987). The condition of strict locality requires that government applies to adjacent positions. Constituent government is strictly directional in that it is invariably left to right, the left-most positions being governing positions. Segments are associated with these left and right positions according to their governing properties. Segments have a governing property called "charm." Consonantal segments may be negatively charmed (S-), or they may be neutral (S°). Furthermore, charmed segments are governors, i.e., they may be associated with governing positions, whereas neutral segments are potential governees that may be associated with governed positions.

Concretely, obstruents and non strident fricatives are negatively charmed; other consonants are neutral. Thus a typical branching onset consists of a stop, or non strident fricative, followed by a liquid or glide.

Within this theoretically framework, OL clusters correspond to well formed branching onsets. Obstruents are charmed and liquids charmless, so that government relation is left to right, as expected in branching onsets. The situation is different for the other types of clusters, such as /st/ (e.g., "statue"), /Rt/ (e.g., "carton"), or /R1/ (e.g., "perle"). In these clusters the first member corresponds to a charmless segment, whereas the second member is charmed.[4] The governing relation is thus right to left and does not respect the condition of directionality appropriate for branching onsets. Such a relation, where the governor follows the governee, is specific to another form of government, the interconstituent government (Fig. 15.4b).

Thus, the theory distinguishes two types of cluster that correspond to different governing domains and have different syllabic representations. OL clusters form branching onsets. The obstruent is charmed and stands in the left-most governing position (C1). The liquid is neutral and is in the

---

[4] Some non-OL clusters involve two neutral segments, such as /R1/ or /lm/. Indeed, in all of them, the complexity of the consonant in the C2 position is greater than that in the C1 position. A government relation then applies from right to left between these neutral segments: "A neutral segment may govern if it has a complexity greater than its governee" (Kaye et al., 1987).

governed position (C2). All other clusters do not form branching onsets. The consonant that occurs in left-most position (C1) is neutral and stands in the governed position whereas the right-most consonant is charmed and occurs in the governing position (C2). It follows from the theory that word-initial clusters do not always form branching onsets. In word-initial /s/ clusters, the obstruent stands in the governing position and forms a non-branching onset at the syllabic level, whereas the left-most position, which is associated with /s/, is governed. Thus OL clusters and other cluster types have different syllabic structures whatever their location in the word.

If we assume that aphasic errors reflect structural properties of linguistic units, we can hypothesize that different error patterns will be observed in OL clusters and in other cluster types. Furthermore, we hypothesize that segments in governing positions are less likely to be omitted or added than segments in governed positions.

The latter hypothesis contrasts with previous predictions that follow from Stemberger and Treiman's work. In regard to the error rate on consonants in either the C1 or C2 position, we expect that (1) a consonant is more frequently omitted and added in the C2 than in the C1 position in OL clusters; whereas (2) in contrast, an error more often concerns a consonant in the C1 than the C2 position in other cluster types. The present hypotheses are evaluated below according to the results of the analysis of aphasic errors.

## Evidence from Aphasia

The addition and omission errors produced by aphasic subjects in the context of two-consonant clusters were analyzed.

### Subjects

The productions of nine prototypical aphasic subjects (Table 15.1) were analyzed. All subjects had suffered a single cerebrovascular accident

TABLE 15.1. Patient summary.

| Subjects | Type | Time P/O | Age | Sex | Education |
|---|---|---|---|---|---|
| 1 | Broca | 0;1 | 62 | M | 16 |
| 2 | Broca | 8;0 | 62 | M | 12 |
| 3 | Broca | 0;4 | 69 | F | 5 |
| 4 | Conduction | 0;1 | 60 | M | 8 |
| 5 | Conduction | 0;3 | 56 | M | 8 |
| 6 | Conduction | 0;1 | 58 | M | 20 |
| 7 | Wernicke | 0;2 | 68 | F | 4 |
| 8 | Wernicke | 1;0 | 62 | M | 4 |
| 9 | Anarthric | 0;2 | 41 | M | 18 |

Time post-onset (P/O) is indicated in years and months (y;m). Age and education are given in years.

(CVA) of the left hemisphere confirmed by computed tomography. All were native speakers of French and were right-handed. The productions were recorded in a single-word repetition task consisting of 481 French content words representing all French syllabic structures and a variety of segmental contents.

## Results

Only errors leading to the creation and destruction of clusters made up of two consonants were taken into account for the present analysis. Globally, 243 omission and 130 addition errors were collected.

Table 15.2 gives the number of addition and omission errors involving one segment in word-initial, word-medial, and word-final clusters. OL clusters were tabulated and analyzed separately from other cluster types. Note that only two types of cluster were considered word-initially: /s/ clusters and OL clusters. Other word-initial clusters, e.g. /pn/ (from "pneu," tire) /mn/ (from "mnésique," mnesic), or /ts/ (from "tsar," tzar), which occur in a small set of French words, were not represented in the repetition task. In contrast, various types of phoneme constitute word-medial and word-final clusters, (e.g., /kt/ from "docteur" (doctor); /Rt/ from "carton" (cardboard); /Rm/ from "permis" (license). They are referred to as "other cluster types." Results are presented separately for omission and addition errors.

TABLE 15.2. Addition and omission errors leading to the creation or destruction of word-initial, word-medial, or word-final clusters.

| Position | Omissions | Additions |
|----------|-----------|-----------|
| Initial | 51 | 25 |
| Medial | 143 | 62 |
| Final | 49 | 43 |
| *Total* | 243 | 130 |

### OMISSION ERRORS

#### Omission Errors in Word-Initial Clusters

Below are examples of omission errors within word-initial OL and /s/ clusters. Examples 1 and 2 show omission of C2, and examples 3 and 4 that of C1, in OL clusters. Examples 5 and 6 show omission of C2, and examples 7 and 8 that of C1 in /s/ clusters.

1. /plastik/ (plastic) → /pastik/
2. /tRibynal/ (court) → /tibynal/
3. /glas/ (ice) → /la:s/
4. /vRɛ/ (true) → /Rɛ/

TABLE 15.3. Omission errors involving C1 and C2 in word-initial OL clusters and /s/ clusters.

| Cluster types | C1 omissions | C2 omissions |
|---|---|---|
| OL | 3 (1%) | 38 (5.9%) |
| /S/ | 6 (5.5%) | 4 (3.7%) |

Percentages give the proportion of word-initial clusters which are concerned by an omission error.

5. /stasjɔ̃/ (station) → /sasjɔ̃/
6. /staty/ (statue) → /sǝty:/
7. /staty/ (statue) → /taty:/
8. /spesjal/ (special) → /pesjal/

Table 15.3 gives the number of omission errors involving a consonant in either the C1 or C2 position in word-initial OL and /s/ clusters. Data show that C2 is omitted significantly more often ($p < .05$) than C1 in Ol clusters. A reverse tendency is seen for /s/ clusters, with more omissions involving C1 than C2, but this trend does not reach significance.

Regarding the nature of the omitted segments, there is a trend for more errors involving liquids in the C2 positions, whereas obstruents that precede liquids in OL clusters and follow /s/ in /s/ clusters are typically preserved. Moreover, when a consonant is omitted in C2 position in /s/ clusters, it is always /t/. In all other /s/ clusters (other than /st/ clusters), the omitted segment in always /s/.

*Omission Errors in Word-Medial Clusters*

Examples of omission errors involving either C1 or C2 in word-medial consonant clusters are presented below. With respect to OL clusters the omission of C2 is exemplified in examples 9 and 10, whereas that of C1 is shown in examples 11 and 12. In regard to other cluster types, omissions are also observed in both C2 and C1 positions, as illustrated, respectively, by examples 13 and 14, and by 15 and 16.

9. /pRɔblɛm/ (problem) → /pRɔbɛ:m/
10. /pyblik/ (public) → /pyblk/
11. /ekRivɛ̃/ (writer) → /eRi-vɛ̃/
12. /telegRam/ (cable) → /teneRamœ/
13. /ɛstɔma/ (stomach) → /ɛsɔmɔ̃/
14. /elastik/ (elastic) → /elaslk/
15. /dɔktœR/ (doctor) → /dɔ:tœR/
16. /fuRmi/ (ant) → /fu:mi/

Table 15.4 gives the number of omission errors involving C1 and C2 in OL clusters and in other types of word-medial clusters. Results show a

TABLE 15.4. Omission errors involving C1 and C2 in word-medial OL clusters and other cluster types.

| Cluster types | C1 omissions | C2 omissions |
|---|---|---|
| OL | 4 (1%) | 29 (5.6%) |
| Other | 106 (15%) | 4 (0.6%) |

Percentages give the proportion of word-medial clusters that are affected by an omission error.

significant tendency ($p < .05$) for more C2 omissions in OL clusters, whereas C1 is significantly ($p < .01$) more often omitted in other clusters whose second member is not a liquid.

In regard to the nature of the omitted consonants, liquids are more frequently omitted within clusters whether they occur in the C1 or the C2 positions. Nevertheless, the number of omissions of C1 and C2 does not seem to reflect entirely the loss of some particular phonemes regardless of their position in clusters. If liquids were more prone to be modified, they might be lost in the C1 position (e.g., /l/ from /bɔlkɔ̃/) more often than the other phonemes to be found in this position, i.e., /s/ or stops in non-OL word-medial clusters (e.g., /s/ of /kaskɛt/ or /k/ of /dɔktœR/). This situation is not the case. Liquids, /s/, and stops are omitted in the same proportion in these clusters when they occur in the C1 position. This result suggests that omission errors are not strongly determined by the nature of the phonemes but, rather, are conditioned by their position within clusters. However, omission errors do not appear to be totally phoneme-type-independent.

*Omission Errors in Word-Final Clusters*

Examples of omission errors in word-final two-consonant clusters are given below. With respect to OL clusters, examples of C2 omissions are shown in example 17 and 18; no example of C1 omission was found in this context. In regard to other cluster types, omission errors may involve either C2, as in examples 19 and 20, or C1, as in examples 21 and 22.

17. /vinɛgR/ (vinegar) → /vinɛgœ/
18. /katR/ (four) → /kat/
19. /eʒipt/ (Egypt) → /eʒipœ/
20. /aRtist/ (artist) → /a:ti:sœ/
21. /alg/ (seaweed) → /a:gœ/
22. /sjɛst/ (nap) → /sjɛ:tœ/

Table 15.5 gives the number of omission errors involving C1 and C2 in OL clusters as well as in other cluster types. Data show that C2 is more frequently omitted than C1 in OL clusters, whereas C1 is omitted more

TABLE 15.5. Omission errors involving C1
and C2 in word-final OL clusters and other
cluster types.

| Cluster types | C1 omissions | C2 omissions |
|---|---|---|
| OL | 0 (0%) | 9 (12%) |
| Other | 34 (23%) | 6 (4.2%) |

Percentages give the proportion of word-final clusters which are affected by an omission error.

often than C2 in other cluster types. This difference is significant in both subtypes ($p > .05$ and $p > .001$, respectively).

When considering the nature of omitted phonemes, it appears that liquids are more frequently omitted in both subtypes of clusters. All omissions are that of liquids in OL clusters; 75% of the omissions that occurred in other cluster types concern also liquids.

ADDITION ERRORS

The analysis performed in this section is limited to the addition errors that lead to the creation of a two-consonant cluster. The cluster thus created results from the addition of a single consonant to a singleton in either C1 position (e.g., /Rɛgl/ → /gRɛgl/) or C2 position (e.g., /pyblik/ → /plyblik/). Clusters created in this fashion are classified as either belonging to the OL type or not.

*Addition Errors in Word-Initial Clusters*

Addition of a consonant in the C1 position is illustrated in examples 23 and 24, and examples 25 and 26 show the addition of a consonant in the C2 position to create an OL cluster. Example 27 exemplifies the addition of /s/ in the C1 position to create an /s/ cluster. No /s/ cluster was created by addition of a segment in the C2 position.

23. /Rɔbinɛ/ (tap) → /pRɔbinɛ/
24. /lɑ̃g/ (tongue) → /glɑ̃g/
25. /fabRik/ (factory) → /fRabRIk/
26. /tabuRɛ/ (stool) → /kRabuRɛ/
27. /kulwaR/ (corridor) → /skulwaR/

Table 15.6 (part A) gives the number of OL and /s/ clusters that were created by addition of a single consonant in either the C1 or C2 position. Data show that consonants are more often added in the C2 position than in the C1 position with respect to OL cluster creation ($p < .05$). In contrast, a consonant was added in the C1 position in the two examples of /s/ cluster creation.

TABLE 15.6. OL and other cluster types created by addition of a single consonant in either C1 or C2 position.

| Position | (A) Word-initial | | (B) Word-medial | | (C) Word-final | |
|---|---|---|---|---|---|---|
| | C1 | C2 | C1 | C2 | C1 | C2 |
| OL clusters | 5 | 18 | 10 | 26 | 0 | 27 |
| Other clusters | 2 | 0 | 26 | 0 | 8 | 8 |

*Addition Errors in Word-Medial Clusters*

In regard to the creation of OL clusters, examples 28 and 29 exemplify the addition of a consonant in the C1 position, and examples 30 and 31 that of a consonant in the C2 position. Examples 32 and 33 illustrate the addition of a consonant in the C1 position in cases where the created cluster did not belong to the OL type. No example of addition in the C2 position occurred in the latter context.

28. /elastik/ (elastic) → /eglastik/
29. /maRekaʒ/ (bog) → /makRakaʒœ/
30. /tRiko/ (sweater) → /tRiklo/
31. /flakɔ̃/ (bottle) → /flaklɔ̃/
32. /klinik/ (clinic) → /kliknik/
33. /fatig/ (tiredness) → faktigœ/

Table 15.6 (part B) gives the numbers of OL clusters and other cluster types that were created, in the word-medial position by addition of a single consonant in either the C1 or C2 position.

Consonants are added more frequently ($p > .05$) in the C2 position of created OL clusters. In contrast, all created clusters that are not of the OL type result from the addition of a consonant in the C1 position.

*Addition Errors in Word-Final Clusters*

Addition of a consonant in the C2 position is illustrated in examples 34 and 35 with respect to OL cluster creation. No consonant was added in the C1 position. In regard to the creation of other cluster types, examples 36 and 37 and examples 38 and 39 show addition of a consonant in the C1 and C2 positions, respectively.

34. /lãg/ (tongue) → /lãglœ/
35. /pRɛ̃sip/ (principle) → /pRɛ̃sipRœ/
36. /aRʒãtin/ (Argentina) → /aRʒãtilnœ/
37. /ɛskal/ (stop) → /ɛskaRlœ/
38. /mais/ (corn) → /maist/
39. /vag/ (wave) → /vagz/

Table 15.6 (part C) gives the numbers of OL clusters and clusters of other types that were created by addition of a consonant in either the C1 or C2 position.

All word-final OL clusters were created by addition of a consonant in the C2 position. A different pattern of errors emerges from the analysis of those created clusters that were not of the OL type. A similar number of additions in the C1 and C2 positions is found in the latter case.

SUMMARY AND DISCUSSION

Results from the analysis of addition and omission errors produced by aphasic subjects in two-consonant clusters are summarized on Table 15.7. With respect to OL clusters, a consonant is more often omitted or added in the C2 position, whatever the location of the cluster in the word. Results from the analysis of the other cluster types reveal a trend for the reverse pattern, C1 being more frequently omitted and added in most locations. However, there is no significant tendency for more omissions in the C1 position word-initially, and a consonant is added in the C1 position as often as in the C2 position word-finally.

The internal representation of word-initial clusters proposed by Stemberger and Treiman (1986) predicted that C2 is more prone to be omitted or added than C1 in OL clusters as well as in /s/ clusters. The present findings about word-initial clusters are not entirely compatible with this prediction. As expected, a consonant is more likely to be omitted or added in the C2 position to the destruction or creation of word-initial OL clusters. However, a similar pattern of errors does not emerge from the analysis of word-initial /s/ clusters. Although there is no significant tendency for more omission errors in either the C1 or C2 position, all created /s/ clusters result from the addition of a consonant in the C1 position.

The internal representation of word-initial clusters that Stemberger and Treiman put forth within an interactive activation framework cannot account for the error pattern observed in word-initial /s/ clusters. Indeed, their model cannot predict the more frequent addition of a consonant

TABLE 15.7. Summary of results.

| Position | Word-initial | Word-medial | Word-final |
|---|---|---|---|
| OL cluster | | | |
| Omission | C1–**C2** | C1–**C2** | C1–**C2** |
| Addition | C1–**C2** | C1–**C2** | C1–**C2** |
| Other clusters | | | |
| Omission | C1–C2 | **C1**–C2 | **C1**–C2 |
| Addition | **C1**–C2 | **C1**–C2 | C1–C2 |

The table shows the pattern of omission and addition errors in OL clusters and other cluster types. The most frequently affected positions within the cluster are in boldface.

in C1 position to the creation of /s/ clusters, as it assumes that a consonant is already present in the C1 position in singletons.

By reference to the Theory of Phonological Government (Kaye et al., 1985), we expected that two distinct patterns would emerged from the analysis, C2 being more often omitted or added in OL clusters and C1 in other cluster types. Although the pattern of addition and omission errors within OL clusters does conform to this prediction, no significant tendency for more errors in the C1 position emerges from the analysis of omissions and additions leading to word-initial clusters destruction and word-final clusters creation. The pattern of addition and omission errors that results from the analysis of OL clusters is therefore more stable than that from other cluster types. Data suggest that the latter clusters are less homogeneous than the former, thus leading to a less systematic pattern of errors. In fact, subtypes can be identified among non-OL clusters. The /st/ clusters show a pattern of addition and omission errors that differs notably from that of other non-OL clusters, including /s/ clusters. Indeed, all omission errors that involve a consonant in C2 position word-initially occur within /st/ clusters. Similarly, most of the non-OL clusters that are created word-finally by addition of a segment in C2 position are /st/ clusters. Consequently, with respect to /s/ clusters, a trend for more omission errors in the C1 position becomes apparent word-initially when /st/ clusters are excluded from the analysis. Similarly, although there is no tendency for a consonant to be added in either the C1 or C2 position when non-OL clusters are created word-finally, a trend for more additions in C1 position emerges when errors leading to the creation of /st/ clusters are not taken into account.

Results thus suggest the existence of two distinct patterns of error in the production of two-consonant clusters. A consonant is more likely to the omitted or added in the C2 position to the destruction or creation of OL clusters. In contrast, the destruction or creation of non-OL clusters typically results from the omission or addition of a consonant in the C1 position, at least when /st/ clusters are excluded. Therefore data show a trend for governed positions, C2 in OL clusters and C1 in other cluster types, to be more frequently omitted or added, whatever the type and location of the cluster in the word. The present results support the claim that OL clusters and other cluster types have different syllabic representations. They also suggest that segments in the governed position are more likely to be involved in the destruction or creation of clusters than segments in the governing position.

## Conclusion

Results from the analysis of addition and omission errors within two-consonant clusters support the claim that clusters must contain two distinct types of syllable position that are differently processed within the language production system. Indeed, the two distinct patterns of error that emerge from the analysis of OL clusters and other cluster types reflect the syllabic structure of these clusters. A unitary account of these error patterns may be provided within the Theory of Phonological Government, as errors typically involve consonants in the governed position in OL clusters as well as in other cluster types. The present findings suggest that errors occur at a level of representation that is phonological. Furthermore, syllables appear as units of the phonological representation that play a role in the language production system. An interpretation of the data in processing terms may be developed by reference to a spreading-activation theory of sentence production.

Dell (1986) proposed a network for phonological encoding that consists of nodes for different linguistic units, including syllables and syllabic constituents. He exposed a model of spreading-activation in which decisions about what unit to choose are based on the activation levels of the nodes representing these units. To account for our data within this theoretical framework, we must assume that governing positions have a greater activation level than governed positions. This assumption predicts more omissions on the governed position and accounts for the pattern of omission errors that emerges from our analysis of clusters destruction. In regard to the pattern of addition errors, we must argue that singletons form onsets and stand in governing position. Results from cluster creation support this claim, as the added consonant typically occurs in the governed position. Results from the analysis of addition and omission errors cannot be accounted for within a linear model of production where clusters are analyzed as C1C2 sequences, as the error pattern cannot be predicted by the absolute serial position of the segment in the string. In agreement with other studies in perception and production (Caramazza and Miceli, in press; Mehler, Dommergues, Frauenfelder, and Segui, 1981; Segui, 1984; Treiman and Danis, 1988) that demonstrated the role of the syllable at different levels of processing, this study further supports the idea that the syllable plays an important role in the processing of spoken language.

## Summary

Addition and omission errors were extensively examined within two-consonant clusters. Two distinct patterns of error emerged from the analysis: Consonants are more likely to be omittted or added in the second position of OL clusters, and more addition and omission errors involve segments in the first position within other cluster types. We propose that clusters must contain two distinct types of syllable position differently processed within the language production system.

*Acknowledgments.* The author gratefully thanks Professor Jonathan Kaye for his constructive discussions of the data and his helpful suggestions. We also thank Professors Yves Joanette and Jean-Luc Nespoulous for their comments.

## References

Béland, R. (1985). Contraintes syllabiques sur les erreurs phonologiques dans l'aphasie. Doctoral Dissertation. University of Montréal.

Béland, R., Nespoulous, J.L., & Caplan, D. (1988). *Phonological Constraints on Phonemic Paraphasias in a Reproduction Conduction Aphasic.* MS, Manuscript, University of Montréal.

Blumstein, S. (1973). *A Phonological Investigation of Aphasic Speech.* (*Janua linguarum 153*). The Hague: Mouton.

Blumstein, S. (1978). Segment structure and the syllable in aphasia. In A. Bell & J.B. Hooper (eds.), *Syllables and Segments.* Amsterdam: North Holland.

Buckingham, H. (1980). On correlating aphasic errors with slips of the tongue. *Applied Psycholinguistics, 1,* 199–220.

Caramazza, A., & Miceli, G. (in press). Orthographic structure, the graphemic buffer and the spelling process. In C. von Euler (ed.), *Brain and Reading.*

Chomsky, N., & Halle, M. (1968). *The Sound Pattern of English.* New York: Harper & Row.

Cutler, A. (1981). The reliability of speech error data. *Linguistics, 19,* 561–582.

Dell, G.S. (1986). A spreading-activation theory of retrieval in sentence production. *Psychological Review, 92,* 283–321.

Fay, D., & Cutler, A. (1977). Malapropisms and the structure of mental lexicon. *Linguistic Inquiry, 8,* 505–520.

Fromkin, V. (1971). The nonanomalous nature of anomalous utterances. *Language, 47,* 27–52.

Fromkin, V. (1973). *Speech Errors as Linguistic Evidence.* The Hague: Mouton.

Garrett, M. (1975). The analysis of sentence production. In G.H. Bower (ed.), *The Psychology of Learning and Motivation,* New York: Academic Press, pp. 133–177.

Garrett, M. (1982). Production of speech: observations from normal and pathological language use. In A. Ellis (ed.), *Normality and Pathology in Cognitive Functions,* London: Academic Press.

Garrett, M. (1984). The organization of processing structure of language production: application to aphasic speech. In D. Caplan, A. Smith, & A.R. Lecours, (eds.), *Biological Perspectives on Language.* Cambridge, MA: MIT Press.

Halle, M., & Vergnaud, J.R. (1980). Three dimensional phonology. *Journal of Linguistic Research, 1.*

Kahn, D. (1976). *Syllable-Based Generalizations in English Phonology.* Doctoral dissertation, MIT.

Kaye, J. (1987). *Government in Phonology: The Case of Moroccan Arabic.* MS, University of Montréal.

Kaye, J., & Lowenstamm, J. (1984). De la syllabicité. In F. Dell, D. Hirst, & J.R. Vergnaud (eds.), *Forme Sonore du Language.* Paris: Hermann.

Kaye, J., Lowenstamm, J., & Vergnaud, J.R. (1985). The internal structure of phonological elements: a theory of charm and government. *Phonology Year-book, 2*, 305–328.

Kaye, J., Lowenstamm, J., & Vergnaud, J.R. (1987). Constituent structure and government in phonology. Université du Québec à Montréal, Montréal.

Kilani-Schoch, M. (1982). *Processus Phonologigues, Processus Morphologiques et Lapsus dans un Corpus Aphasique*. Doctoral dissertation. Berne: Publications Universitaires Européennes.

Kiparsky, P. (1979). Metrical structure assignment. *Linguistic Inquiry, 10*.

Kupin, J.J. (1982). *Tongue Twisters as a Source of Information About Speech Production*. Bloomington: Indiana University Linguistic Club.

Laubstein, A.S. (1985). *The Nature of the Production Grammar Syllable*. PhD dissertation, University of Toronto.

Martory, M., & Messerli, P. (1983). Analyse comparée des troubles de l'expression orale. In P. Messerli, P.M. Lavorel, & J.L. Nespoulous (eds.), *Neuropsychologie de l'Expression Orale*. Paris: Editions du C.N.R.S., pp. 71–91.

Mehler, J., Dommergues, J.Y., Frauenfelder, U., & Segui, J. (1981). The syllable's role in speech segmentation. *Journal of Verbal Hearing and Verbal Behavior, 20*, 298–305.

Nespoulous, J.L., Joanette, Y., Béland, R., Caplan, D., Lecours, A.R. (1984). Phonological disturbances in aphasia: is there a markedness effect in aphasic phonemic errors? *Advances in Neurology, 42*, 203–213.

Puel, M., Nespoulous, J.L., Bonafé, A. & Rascol, A. (1980). Etude neurolinguistique d'un cas d'anarthrie pure. *Grammatica, 7*, 239–292.

Segui, J. (1984). The syllable: a basic perceptual unit in speech processing? *Attention and Performance, 12*, 165–181.

Selkirk, E.D. (1982). The syllable. *In The Structure of Phonological Representations*, Part II, Foris publications.

Shattuck-Hufnagel, S. (1979). Speech errors as evidence for a serial ordering mechanism in sentence production. In W.E. Cooper & E.C.T. Walker (eds.), *Sentence Processing*. Hillsdale, NJ: Lawrence Erlbaum Associates.

Shattuck-Hufnagel, S. (1983). Sublexical units and suprasegmental structure in speech production planning. In P.F. McNeilage (ed.), *The Production of Speech*. New York: Springer Verlag, pp. 109–136.

Shattuck-Hufnagel, S. (1987). The role of word-onset consonants in speech production planning: new evidence from speech error patterns. In E. Keller & M. Gopnik (eds.), *Motor and Sensory Processes of Language*. Hillsdale, NJ: Lawrence Erlbaum Associates.

Shattuck-Hufnagel, S., & Klatt, D.H. (1979). The limited use of distinctive features and markedness in speech production: evidence from speech error data. *Journal of Verbal Learning and Verbal Behavior, 18*, 41–55.

Stemberger, J.P. (1984). Structural errors in normal and agrammatic speech. *Cognitive Neuropsychology, 1*, 281–313.

Stemberger, J.P., & Treiman, R. (1986). The internal structure of consonantal cluster. *Journal of Memory and Language, 25*, 163–180.

Treiman, R., & Danis, C. (1988). Syllabification of intervocalic consonants. *Journal of Memory and Language, 27*, 87–104.

Valdois, S. (1987). *Les Erreurs d'Addition et d'Omission dans l'Aphasie: Rôle du Gouvernement Phonologique*. PhD dissertation, Université de Montréal.

Valdois, S. (1987). The internal structure of consonantal clusters: evidence from aphasia. Presented at the 25th Meeting of the Academy of Aphasia, Phoenix.

# 16
# Agrammatism: A Disruption of the Phonological Processing of Grammatical Morphemes?

JEAN-LUC NESPOULOUS and MONIQUE DORDAIN

From the pioneering work of Jakobson (1968), the main goal of neuro-linguistic research has always been to discover, in aphasic patients' symptomatology, stable although deviant effects of cerebral lesions on verbal behavior. Relying on a more and more sophisticated characterization of the intrinsic structure of natural languages provided by modern linguistics, scholars have thus attempted to account for the frequent behavioral dissociations evidenced in aphasia in terms of (1) linguistic "modules" (e.g., phonology, morphology, syntax) impaired or spared in a patient or a group of patients or (2) complexity scales, e.g., "markedness theory," (Trubetskoy, 1939), complex linguistic units and structures being expected to be more frequently "impaired" (or even "lost" in Jakobson's terms) than simple ones. Their ultimate goal, without any doubt, has always been to correlate clear-cut, coherent deviant linguistic behavior with (1) the clear-cut dysfunction of specific psycholinguistic processing devices and (2) clear-cut anatomophysiological modules.

For anyone in close contact with any aphasic patient, it is more than obvious that the above idealistic statement does not correspond to everyday clinical observation as often as one might wish.

1. Rarely does aphasia manifest as an all-or-none phenomenon.
2. More complex units and structures are far from being always and systematically disturbed in a single patient—hence the inadequacy of such a term as "loss," used by many (Jakobson first), to characterize aphasic impairments.
3. Simple units and structures can also be disturbed.
4. Finally, in terms of anatomoclinical correlations, it is far from being exceptional to observe symptomatological features in relation with "unexpected" lesion sites (Basso, Lecours, Moraschini, and Vanier, 1985).

One thus cannot but take performance variability into consideration when interpreting an aphasic patient's symptomatology—and the results of any neurolinguistic study, for that matter. Without doing so, and even (more than ever, one might want to say) when data analysis yields a statistically significant contrast between two subsets of structurally different phenomena, one would indeed oversimplify the underlying determinism of deviant surface manifestations in aphasia by overemphasizing their pathogenetic coherence. Surface manifestations, on more than one occasion, certainly have more than one causal factor. Thus even though the characterization of those factors responsible for such a variability in performance may tell us more about the patient's strategic adaptation to his deficit (or to the task at hand) than about the underlying causal deficit, they cannot be ignored by the neurolinguists mainly interested in brain-mind-behavior relations or the clinicians—neurologists or speech pathologists—whose principal aim is to help the patient to adapt to what is usually an irreversible impairment.

The present chapter illustrates the necessity, when observing verbal pathology data, to take the following factors into account (whenever possible): the nature of the causal deficit yielding deviant language behavior and surface manifestations, its locus in the functional architecture underlying language processing, and the plausible coming two play, in some patients at least, of adaptative strategies by which the nonanaosognosic aphasic patient tries to overcome his or her deficit whenever and as often as possible.

For this purpose, we present important additional data on the case of Mr. Clermont, a French-speaking agrammatic patient (Nespoulous, Dordain, Perron, Bub, Caplan, Mehler, and lecours, 1988), who was shown (1) to produce agrammatic verbal output in *all* sentence production tasks (from spontaneous speech to repetition and oral reading) whereas production of individual words, open or closed class, was intact and (2) to have no comprehension deficit whatsoever.

On the basis of such observations, we initially claimed (1) that the basic underlying deficit leading to the production of agrammatic sentences in this patient was not central, in Caramazza and Zurif's terms (1976); and (2) that such a deficit disrupted syntactic sentence processes on the production side only, thus preventing the patient from constructing complex (and even fairly simple) syntactic frames, which include, in Garrett's terms, grammatical morphemes.

The revision of such an initial interpretation offered here is based on the observation of three types of phenomenon.

## Phenomenon 1

The first phenomenon of interest has to do with the presence, together with the "classical" omission of function words, of *within-category substitu-*

*tions* of all types of free-standing grammatical morphemes (GMs) (Tables 16.1, 16.2, and 16.3).

To be sure, the (frequent) presence of such a phenomenon allows us to believe that, at least in those cases, the patient is able to compute adequate syntactic frames. If we thus set aside the "syntactic hypothesis" and tend to interpret the deficit as being *at the word level*, we are left with several plausible interpretations of the underlying deficit, particularly the following:

1. Is the apparently (?) "lexical" deficit observed in this patient to be interpreted as the consequence of a *lexical retrieval* difficulty specific to closed items whenever they have to be inserted into sentences (as our patient produced them adequately when they were presented in isolation)?
2. Is it to be interpreted as the consequence of a phonological deficit, in keeping with Kean's hypothesis (Kean, 1979) regarding the phonological status of GMs?

TABLE 16.1. Morpheme errors and distribution in narrative speech.

| Morpheme | Expected morphemes (No.) | Correctly supplied | | Substitutions | | Omissions | |
|---|---|---|---|---|---|---|---|
| | | No. | % | No. | % | No. | % |
| Articles | 156 | 113 | 72 | 23 | 15 | 20 | 13 |
| Other det. | 33 | 27 | 82 | 2 | 6 | 4 | 12 |
| Adjectives | 23 | 18 | 78 | 4 | 17 | 1 | 5 |
| Pro. | 59 | 49 | 83 | 1 | 2 | 9 | 15 |
| Cli. | 36 | 12 | 33 | 5 | 14 | 19 | 53 |
| Auxiliaries | 20 | 10 | 50 | 1 | 5 | 9 | 45 |
| Have-be verbs | 14 | 7 | 50 | 0 | 0 | 7 | 50 |
| Verbs | 131 | 120 | 92 | 4 | 3 | 7 | 5 |
| Relative pron. | 2 | 2 | 100 | 0 | 0 | 0 | 0 |
| Subord. conj. | 3 | 0 | 0 | 0 | 0 | 3 | 100 |
| Coord. conj. | 27 | 26 | 96 | 1 | 4 | 0 | 0 |
| Lexical prep. | 55 | 44 | 80 | 5 | 9 | 6 | 11 |
| Nonlexical prep. | 45 | 28 | 62 | 2 | 4 | 15 | 34 |

TABLE 16.2. Morpheme errors and distribution in sentence repetition.

| Morpheme | Expected morphemes (No.) | Correctly supplied | | Substitutions | | Omissions | |
|---|---|---|---|---|---|---|---|
| | | No. | % | No. | % | No. | % |
| Articles | 82 | 63 | 78 | 9 | 10 | 10 | 12 |
| Pro. | 16 | 11 | 69 | 4 | 25 | 1 | 6 |
| Cli. | 11 | 7 | 64 | 1 | 9 | 3 | 27 |
| Lexical prep. | 39 | 30 | 68 | 3 | 7 | 6 | 15 |
| Nonlexical prep. | 15 | 6 | 41 | 5 | 33 | 4 | 26 |

TABLE 16.3. Morpheme errors and distribution in sentence oral reading.

| Morpheme | Expected morphemes (No.) | Correctly supplied No. | Correctly supplied % | Substitutions No. | Substitutions % | Omissions No. | Omissions % |
|---|---|---|---|---|---|---|---|
| Articles | 105 | 82 | 79 | 18 | 17 | 5 | 4 |
| Pro. | 24 | 18 | 76 | 5 | 20 | 1 | 4 |
| Cli. | 15 | 11 | 74 | 2 | 13 | 2 | 13 |
| Lexical prep. | 48 | 43 | 92 | 4 | 6 | 1 | 2 |
| Nonlexical prep. | 38 | 29 | 78 | 3 | 7 | 6 | 15 |

## Phenomenon 2

The second phenomenon of interest—and relative to the first one—has to do with the *incomplete production* now and again in connected discourse of *prepositional locutions* (or "polymorphemic prepositions") of the following type: "à cause de" (on account of) → "cause de" (account of) or "à cause" (on account). Such a "truncated production" of prepositional locutions is of great explanatory value because, if confirmed, it would indicate that the preposition has indeed been adequately computed at the syntactic level, whereas it cannot be "exhaustively" processed at "lower" levels of processing (further downstream).

We decided to assess the processing of this specific type of polymorphemic function words in three distinct repetition and oral reading tasks comprising (all stimuli randomized) the following.

*Test A*: 20 isolated locutions ("à cause de")
*Test B*: 20 prepositional phrases including the same locutions ("à cause de Mitterand"...)
*Test C*: 20 full sentences, each including a prepositional phrase with the same locutions ("Les enfants sont punis à cause de Pierre")

The results[1] (Table 16.4) indicated the following.

1. In such tasks as well as in spontaneous speech, the patient had problems processing polymorphemic prepositions (in about 25% of the cases).
2. Errors *never* involved the "open class" lexical item belonging to such polymorphemic prepositions (e.g., "cause").
3. Errors on closed class items belonging to the polymorphemic grammatical morphemes (i.e., "à" and "de" in "à" cause de") are omissions

---

[1] These results were presented at the Annual Meeting the Academy of Aphasia, Montreal, October 1988.

TABLE 16.4. Morpheme errors on prepositional locutions (repetition vs. oral reading).

| Morpheme | In isolation (n = 20) | In prepositional phrases (n = 20) | In sentences (n = 20) |
|---|---|---|---|
| O REP (n = 10) | 1 | 3 | 6 |
| M | | | |
| I | | | |
| S O.R (n = 11) | 3 | 4 | 4 |
| S REP (n = 4) | 1 | 2 | 1 |
| U | | | |
| B | | | |
| S O.R (n = 3) | 3 | 0 | 0 |
| Total | 8 | 9 | 11 |

(21 of 28) and substitutions (7 of 28), present in equal proportion in both tasks (14 of 60 in both repetition and oral reading).

On the basis of the data summarized above and considering that our patient did not evidence any comprehension deficit (Nespoulous et al., 1988), we thus submit the following hypotheses.

1. The underlying deficit yielding agrammatic verbal output on the production side only was indeed *not syntactic*. Both the presence of within-category substitutions and the "truncated" production of polymorphemic prepositions seems to argue in favor of the retained capacity, in this patient at least, to compute adequately syntactic frames.
2. Such an underlying deficit has to be looked for further downstream (from the syntactic level) in a model of sentence production such as that of Garrett (1980).
3. The locus for such a deficit might well be at the level of the *implementation of the phonological form of closed class items*, which have phonological properties of their own, (Kean, 1979), when linear "positional" phonological representations are computed (Garrett, 1980).

The observation of production errors on polymorphemic prepositions—which, in contrast to monomorphemic GMs (which can only be omitted or substituted), allow the patient to produce only part of their phonological form—might well be crucial to substantiate the latter hypothesis (no. 3). Thus the apparent "class effect" observed in this patient would be phonologically based, as "phonological words" present in polymorphemic GMs are preserved whereas "phonological clitics" present in the same "complex" prepositions are often disturbed.

Before moving to the third phenomenon of direct interest, we must insist on the fact that it was also shown that this patient's difficulty to process adequately free-standing grammatical morphemes in all sentence production tasks could be, so to speak, manipulated and reduced in some tasks devised to force him to pay attention to those grammatical morphemes with which he was having difficulty.[2] The fact that Mr. Clermont's oral performance was definitely better when he was asked to pay particular attention to those grammatical morphemes that had been highlighted in pink in an oral reading task[3] seems to us of paramount importance on both theoretical and therapeutic grounds. It tends to document the possibility, for this patient at least, of bypassing a deficit up to a point by resorting to specific attentional strategies.

## Phenomenon 3

We thus decided to further assess the plausible interaction of linguistic, structural parameters and of such above-mentioned attentional strategies in Mr. Clermont's verbal production by devising a new test. Taking advantage of one of the structural properties of French, we asked Mr. Clermont to repeat and read aloud 115 noun phrases (NPs) of the /N of N/ type. Sixty-four NPs corresponded to "set phrases"—of the "oeil de boeuf" or "chemin de fer" type—and were thus "polymorphemic lexical items" rather than clear-cut NPs (despite identity in surface structure), whereas the remaining 51 NPs were newly coined (clear-cut) phrases. All stimuli were borrowed from a previous study with normals (Nespoulous, 1970) who had been asked to categorize /N of N/ phrases into three classes: set phrases versus newly coined phrases versus phrases for which they could not make up their mind about the degree of "lexical fossilization"; only the former two classes were retained to test the agrammatic patient's performance.

Our hypotheses were the following.

1. If the deficit is located at the phonological level, one should observe errors on prepositions present in both set and newly coined phrases.
2. If structural (and computational?) complexity alone plays a role, there should be more errors on prepositions present in newly coined phrases (which require additional syntactic processing) than in those present in set phrases, which, being unitary lexical entries, require no such syntactic processing.
3. If "controlled" selective attentional processes are indeed called for by the patient (see above), they might improve the patient's performance more on newly coined phrases than on set phrases because the subject would have to pay more attention to newly coined than to set phrases, the former being supposed to come out of the lexicon in one "chunk."

---

[2] As was made obvious by "letter cancellation tasks" in normals (Healy, 1976) as well as in aphasic subjects (Rosenberg, Zurif, Brownell, Garrett, and Bradley, 1985), free-standing grammatical morphemes tend to require less attention than open class lexical items.
[3] Results presented at the Annual Meeting of the European I.N.S., Lahti, 1988.

TABLE 16.5. Morpheme errors on set vs. newly coined phrases.

| Phrases | No. | Reading errors | | Repetition errors | |
|---|---|---|---|---|---|
| | | No. | % | No. | % |
| Set | 64 | 37 | 57 | 23 | 35 |
| Newly coined | 51 | 14 | 27 | 7 | 13 |

Results[4] (Table 16.5) indeed indicated that our patient produced (at least) twice as many errors (omissions) on set phrases than on newly coined phrases—57% versus 27% in oral reading and 35% versus 13% in repetition—even though in both tasks he was (obviously) given the full target phrase by the examiner.'

## Conclusion

The explanation that such results suggest is thus as follows. (1) The patient's underlying deficit is indeed basically "phonological" in nature, as the only common denominator between GMs ("de") present in set phrases and those (the same) present in newly coined phrases has to do with their phonological status ("phonological clitics") (Kean, 1979). (2) The across-task variability of his performances seems indeed to be dependent, at least partly, on the coming into play of attentional factors and processes (hence, probably, our former results on the Pink Element Test (Lahti, 1988). In other words, the patient having problems with his "rapid, unconscious, automatic processing" of some linguistic elements would then have to process such elements, much like a young child or a second language learner, in a more "controlled" way. (The more controlled, the better. The more automatic, the worse.)

Such a single case study thus emphasizes (1) the importance of "strategic" (?) attentional factors (Posner and Snyder, 1975) in language performance and (2) the potential role that such strategies—whether developed by the patient himself or induced by a speech therapy program—might play in language (re?)adaptive behaviors following brain damage.

## References

Basso, A., Lecours, A.R., Moraschini, S., & Vanier, M. (1985). Anatomoclinical correlations of the aphasias as defined through computerized tomography: exceptions. *Brain and Language, 26*, 201–229.

---

[4] Results were presented at the Annual Meeting of the European I.N.S., Antwerp, 1989.

Garrett, M. (1980). Levels of processing in sentence production. In B. Butterworth (ed.), *Language Production*. New York: Academic Press.

Healy, A. (1976). Detection errors on the word "the": evidence for reading units larger than letters. *Journal of Experimental Psychology: Human Perception and Performance*, 2, 235–242.

Jakobson, R. (1968). *Child Language, Aphasia and Phonological Universals*. The Hague: Mouton.

Kean, M-L. (1979). Agrammatism: a phonological deficit? *Cognition*, 7, 69–83.

Nespoulous, J-L., Dordain, M., Perron, C., Bub, D., Caplan, D., Mehler, J., & Lecours, A.R. "Agrammatism in sentence production without comprehension deficits: reduced availability of syntactic structures and/or of grammatical morphemes. *Brain and Language* (in press).

posner, M.I., & Snyder, R.R. (1975). Attention and cognitive control. In R. Solso (ed.), *Information Processing and Cognition. The Loyola Symposium*. Hillsdale, (NJ): Lawrence Erlbaum Associates.

Rosenberg, B., Zurif, E., Brownell, H., Garrett, M., & Bradley, D. (1985). Grammatical effects in relation to normal and aphasic sentence processing. *Brain and Language*, 26, 287–303.

# Author Index

# Subject Index